Atlas of —————————
Regional and Free Flaps for
Head and Neck Reconstruction

Atlas of
Regional and Free Flaps for
Head and Neck Reconstruction

Mark L. Urken, M.D., F.A.C.S.
Professor
Department of Otolaryngology
Mount Sinai School of Medicine
New York, New York

Mack L. Cheney, M.D., F.A.C.S.
Assistant Professor
Department of Otolaryngology
Harvard Medical School
Massachusetts Eye and Ear Infirmary
Boston, Massachusetts

Michael J. Sullivan, M.D., F.A.C.S.
Associate Professor
Department of Otolaryngology
The Ohio State University School of Medicine
Columbus, Ohio

Hugh F. Biller, M.D., F.A.C.S.
Professor and Chairman
Department of Otolaryngology
Mount Sinai School of Medicine
New York, New York

Illustrator
Sharon Ellis
New York, New York

Foreword by John J. Conley, M.D.

Raven Press New York

Raven Press, Ltd., 1185 Avenue of the Americas, New York, New York 10036

Made in the United States of America

Library of Congress Cataloging-in-Publication Data

Atlas of regional and free flaps for head and neck reconstruction/
  Mark L. Urken . . . [et al.]; illustrator, Sharon Ellis.
     p.   cm.
    Includes bibliographical references and index.
    ISBN 0-7817-0197-X
    1. Head—Surgery—Atlases. 2. Neck—Surgery—Atlases. 3. Flaps
(Surgery)—Atlases. 4. Surgery, Plastic—Atlases. I. Urken, Mark
L., 1954–
    [DNLM: 1. Head—surgery—atlases. 2. Neck—surgery—atlases.
  3. Surgical Flaps—atlases. 4. Surgery, Plastic—atlases. WE 17
  A8806334 1995]
  RD521.A846 1995
  617.5′10592—dc20
  DNLM/DLC
  for Library of Congress   94-15911

9 8 7 6 5 4 3 2 1

To
my parents,
for providing me with every opportunity
to pursue my education and my career
as well as instilling in me the pursuit of excellence,

my patients and their families,
for putting their faith in me,

Laura,
for providing her unwavering support and love
while enduring the hardships of completing this work.
M.L.U.

To my family,
Wendy, Luke, Jenna, and Sam,
with love.

And to Papa,
a wonderful grandfather.
M.L.C.

To
my nurturing parents,
Robert and Marilyn Sullivan
who gave me the opportunity and drive to learn,

my loving wife, Christine,
who gives me the support and encouragement to pursue my dreams,

my beautiful children,
Kyle, Eric, and Kathryn,
who give my life purpose and perspective.
M.J.S.

To Diane
for her love, support, and understanding.
H.F.B.

Contents

PART I. REGIONAL FLAPS

Muscle and Musculocutaneous Flaps

PART III. NERVE GRAFT DONOR SITES

Foreword

I was honored to be asked to write the foreword to this surgical atlas on head and neck reconstruction. Rehabilitative surgery of the head and neck involves the most sensitive areas of the body, embracing a high aesthetic value combined with special sense organs that have many highly organized physiological functions. The combination of emotional factors and essential functional performance add a special poignancy to performing crippling surgery in this area. This topic has been a passion of mine throughout my career in head and neck surgery and it is reassuring to me to see our specialty continue to have such a fervent interest and enthusiasm for the rehabilitation of head and neck cancer patients.

No single person or group has dominated the advancements that have been made in the field of head and neck reconstruction. Remarkable efforts of investigation, discovery, and ultimate application to the patient have stimulated new concepts of management. General surgeons, plastic surgeons, and otolaryngologists have all made significant contributions in this arena. Each of these surgical groups has contributed a unique expertise and perspective, all of which translate into improved care and quality of life for these patients.

We may be surprised to learn that the trapezius flap was reported 150 years ago and that the temporalis, sternocleidomastoid, and masseter flaps have been known, respectively, for 96, 86, and 83 years. The principle of exploiting regional tissue for reconstructive purposes had intrinsic restrictions due to the state of the art of surgery during that particular time frame. A period of building, expanding, and discovery was necessary to provide the possibility of more accurately reconstructing major ablative wounds in the area of the head and neck. By the 1960s and 1970s, understanding of the appropriate regional donor areas and regional vascular anatomy permitted the surgeon to utilize a greater variety of regional tissues for immediate and safe rehabilitation.

With the crescendo in expertise using regional flaps came the phenomenon of the development of free microvascular transplantation of tissue that occurred almost simultaneously. These are extremely important and sophisticated techniques in transplanting tissue that consists of skin, muscle, bone, mucous membrane, and nerves from a variety of donor areas throughout the body. The success of these transfers requires a greater attention to vascular anatomy and a more careful and meticulous surgical technique, both of which are so wonderfully presented in this book. Specific anatomic structures located in the extremities have been used with success, and the possibilities of other unique donor areas are still being discovered. The restoration of defects of the mandible is perhaps the clearest example of the impact that microvascular surgery has had in the head and neck region. I can clearly recall my own frustrations in trying to restore the bony architecture of the face with nonvascularized bone. Some two decades ago I began to transfer vascularized bone using regional flaps as the nutrient supply. However, these regional composite flaps were still fraught with complications when used in the primary setting and never provided the maximum degree of rehabilitation that has been achieved with micro-vascular bone flaps. I have marveled at the achievements in aesthetics and function with the application of dental implants that have permitted meaningful dental resto-ration. This sophisticated advance in reparative management has not eliminated the use of regional flaps but has added a new dimension in rehabilitative activity in this area.

The substance of this book handles in a clear and accurate style the use of regional skin, muscle, and musculocutaneous flaps as well as donor sites from distant regions of the body where vascularized skin, muscle, bone and nerves can be harvested and transferred to the head and neck. This book introduces these advances to the novice surgeon as well as delving into the subject matter in such detail as to provide a valu-able resource for the experienced head and neck reconstructive surgeon. The atten-tion to detail in the fresh cadaver dissections as well as the beautiful anatomic il-lustrations make this book a timely and a timeless addition to the medical literature.

There are many options that are now available to deal with the reconstruction of complex head and neck wounds. It is essential that the reader comprehend the sub-stance in this book and use its practical value to enhance the management of these very difficult problems. One must expect change in all areas of surgery and that is, of course, happening in head and neck surgery as well. It is imperative that all surgeons involved in the care of patients with head and neck cancer indulge in self critique and experience a sense of personal frustration with the plight of their patients following ablative surgery. This criticism is essential for new advances to be made and to pre-vent each and every one of us from lapsing into a state of complacency with our surgical successes. Such complacency and failure to embrace new ideas force us to practice surgery in the past and prevents us from finding new solutions. The future lies in our willingness to reach beyond the boundaries of our present understanding and work toward the ultimate reconstructive result.

John J. Conley, M.D.

Preface

The most attractive and challenging feature of head and neck reconstruction is the complexity of the anatomy and function of this region. The range of tissue types that must be duplicated is arguably greater than any other site in the body. Therefore, it is no surprise that a growing desire to achieve a higher level of rehabilitation has caused dissatisfaction with conventional regional cutaneous and musculocutaneous flaps. The ability to transfer flaps that are thinner, more pliable, contain vascularized bone, and have both motor and sensory potential, has driven the era of free flap surgery. However, the availability of free tissue transfer must not mean the abandonment of conventional techniques. Regional donor sites provide a valuable source of tissues that were ideal for many types of reconstruction. There are many different factors which enter into the decision regarding the optimum reconstruction for a particular patient and a particular defect. The adage, simpler is better, certainly applies to the selection of a donor site. However, the desire for simplicity by using a regional flap must be weighed against the quality of the end result that can be achieved when free tissue from a distant site is utilized.

Contemporary head and neck reconstruction involves a thorough appreciation of both regional and free flaps. This book covers a spectrum of donor sites and spans the innovations in technique from the 1960s through the early 1990s. The art of head and neck surgery with the diversity in reconstructive options has become a true creative endeavor. A mastery of different donor site options provides the surgeon with the confidence to find a solution for virtually every reconstructive problem, regardless of the complexity of the defect or the techniques that had been previously utilized in a particular patient.

In addition, there is a growing appreciation that one donor site may not suffice in the most complicated defects. We have often resorted to the use of multiple free flaps or the combination of a free flap and a regional flap to achieve the final result. Once again, expertise with many different flaps allows the surgeon to combine flaps as the situation dictates.

This book was conceived in large part, out of the requests of participants at an annual reconstructive course that my colleagues and I have given at Mount Sinai Medical Center over the past several years. The course has in many ways mirrored the evolution of head and neck reconstruction with an ever-increasing curriculum that reflects the expansion of available reconstructive options and an ever-increasing enrollment that reflects the growing interest and enthusiasm for this discipline. We realized that there was no single book that provided the head and neck surgeon with a detailed description of the anatomy and harvesting techniques for the major regional and free flap donor sites currently employed in head and neck reconstruction. We chose the medium of fresh cadaver dissections to provide the most realistic portrayal of the step-by-step details that would give the resident and attending surgeon a thorough understanding of each donor site. Since attention to detail is so vital to successful surgery, the descriptions in this book reflect that detail as closely as possible.

A thorough understanding of anatomy is the cornerstone of all surgery, and reconstructive surgery is certainly no exception. With an understanding of the intricate details of a donor site, the surgeon can creatively mold the tissue to fit the needs of the patient and the particular defect. Each chapter includes details of normal donor site anatomy as well as anatomic variations. In every section of the book the most important designs of each flap are presented as are the major applications to which that flap has been applied. With the tools of anatomy and surgical technique, the surgeon's imagination is the only limitation to solving a particular problem.

Chapters 23 and 24 detail the anatomy and harvest of nerve grafts from the sural and medial antebrachial nerves. With an emphasis on restoring function to the head and neck, sensory and motor reinnervation are key components and the head and neck surgeon will find it valuable to be well versed with these two donor sites.

By providing a discussion of anatomy, flap design and utilization, anatomic variations, preoperative and postoperative care, potential pitfalls, and harvesting techniques for each donor site, this book is oriented toward the resident as well as the practicing head and neck surgeon. However, it is not meant as a substitute for the essential painstaking learning processes of working in a microsurgical laboratory and in a cadaver dissection laboratory to master the techniques before applying them in clinical practice.

Just as the oncologic management of head and neck neoplasms will continue to evolve, so too will the reconstruction and rehabilitation of these patients. New donor sites will undoubtedly be introduced that further expand the range of tissue that is available. There will certainly be new techniques that may totally revolutionize this discipline. It is imperative that the surgeon approach these innovations with an open mind. Flexibility will permit change to occur and offer new hope to our patients.

Acknowledgments

We would like to pay tribute to the numerous contributions of the many pioneers in our specialty who paved the way for the current era of head and neck surgery and reconstructive surgery. The contributions of John Conley, Shan Baker, William Panje, and Sebastian Arena, to name a few, must be highlighted. We would like to pay particular tribute to the ingenuity and foresight of Max Som who issued in the era of clinical free tissue transfer with his work on the first free jejunal autograft performed in a human in 1958.

We would also like to acknowledge the outstanding photographic work of Lester Bergman and the tireless work of our superb illustrator, Sharon Ellis. The preparation and endless revisions of the manuscript could not have been possible without the help of Sylvia Giamarino, Carmen Hepfl, and Bessie Moss.

The quality of the production of this book is a direct result of the enthusiastic, caring and persistent professional staff at Raven Press, in particular Kathy Cianci and Joyce-Rachel John. Finally, this project would never have made it out of the conceptual stage and seen through to its fruition were it not for the unending support of Kathey Alexander. She put her unwavering faith in our ideas and never failed to find solutions to the many problems that we encountered along the way. We are indebted to her for her professionalism and friendship.

Atlas of Regional and Free Flaps for Head and Neck Reconstruction

I
PART

Regional Flaps

Pectoralis
Major

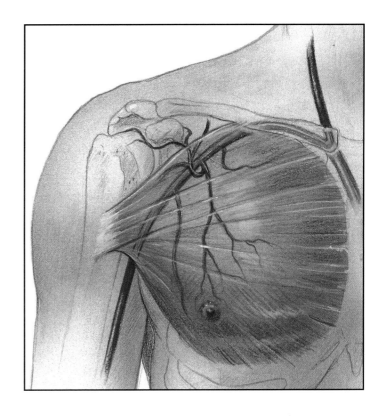

Mark L. Urken, M.D., and
Hugh F. Biller, M.D.

The pectoralis major muscle has been applied to the reconstruction of a variety of chest wall defects since 1947 when Pickerel et al. (42) reported its use as a turnover flap. Sisson et al. (52) used the pectoralis major as a medially based flap to provide great vessel protection and obliteration of dead space following mediastinal dissection for recurrent cancer of the laryngostoma after total laryngectomy. In 1977, Brown et al. (13) described the technique of bilateral island pectoralis major flaps for the reconstruction of a midline upper chest and lower neck defect. The muscle was completely isolated on its neurovascular pedicle following transsection of its origins and insertions. A skin graft was used for epithelial coverage after bilateral muscle advancement. In 1968, Hueston and McConchie (26) reported a case in which the pectoralis major was used as a carrier for the overlying skin in reconstruction of an upper sternal defect. The authors designed this flap with a broad base at the shoulder, which limited its arc of rotation. In addition, they performed a delay procedure to ensure the vascularity of the skin.

It was not until the latter part of the 1970s that Ariyan and Cuono (2) and Ariyan (1) recognized the tremendous potential of the musculocutaneous unit based on the pectoralis major for the reconstruction of a large number of head and neck defects. This discovery was of paramount importance because it enabled the single stage transfer of large amounts of well-vascularized skin for almost all ablative or traumatic defects of the upper aerodigestive tract, face, and skull base. In addition, the hardiness of the vascular supply permitted the creation of two skin paddles by de-epithelialization of an intermediate segment of skin so that the inner and outer lining could be transferred with a single flap for reconstruction of complex, composite defects.

The impact of this new reconstructive technique on head and neck surgery was recognized almost immediately. It rapidly replaced many of the existing reconstructive methods, and large series of cases from a variety of different medical centers were reported as testimony to the reliability, versatility, and ease of harvesting this flap. Although various modifications of the original description of this flap have been reported, along with a recognition of its shortcomings, it is still the mainstay of head and neck reconstruction (11,48).

The pectoralis major is a large fan-shaped muscle that covers much of the anterior thoracic wall. To a variable extent, it overlies the pectoralis minor, subclavius, serratus anterior, and intercostal muscles. The origins of the pectoralis major are divided into two or, sometimes, three portions. The cephalad segment arises from the medial third of the clavicle. The central, or sternocostal, portion has a broad origin from the sternum and the cartilages of the first six ribs. The third origin of this muscle, from the aponeurosis of the external oblique, is variable in size. The muscle fibers of this broad muscle converge to form a tendon that passes deep to the deltoid and inserts into the crest of the greater tubercle of the humerus. As it narrows in its course toward the humerus, it forms the anterior axillary fold (Figure 1-1). The medial aspect of the deltoid muscle is almost inseparable from the muscle fibers of the pectoralis major. The cleavage between these two muscles is referred to as the deltopectoral groove, through which runs the cephalic vein, which is a constant anatomic landmark.

The pectoralis major is surrounded by a layer of deep fascia. However, this is separate from the clavipectoral fascia that surrounds the pectoralis minor and extends cephalad from that muscle to the clavicle. Prior to attaching to the undersurface of the clavicle, this fascia splits to envelop the subclavius muscle. Both the vascular and nerve supply to the pectoralis major pass through the clavipectoral fascia en route to the deep surface of the muscle (Fig. 1-12).

The action of the pectoralis major is to adduct and medially rotate the arm. It becomes active in internal rotation of the arm only when working against resistance. The upper muscle fibers help to flex the arm to the horizontal level; the lower fibers assist in arm extension. Contraction of the pectoralis major helps to extend the arm to the individual's side, but it plays no role in hyperextension beyond that point.

The loss of the dynamic activity of the pectoralis major appears to be well tolerated, although the true impact on brachial function has not been studied extensively in any of the large series of pectoralis major musculocutaneous flap transfers. The additional morbidity of combining the loss of pectoralis major function and a radical neck dissection has also not been investigated in a systematic fashion. Much of the adductor activity is compensated for by the powerful, latissimus dorsi muscle, which makes up the posterior axillary fold.

FLAP DESIGN AND UTILIZATION

The major advantages of the pectoralis major musculocutaneous flap that distinguished it from the three major cutaneous flaps (deltopectoral, nape of neck, and forehead) that were in use at the time are the following:

1. Rich vascularity.
2. Large skin territory.
3. Ability to transfer without prior delay.
4. Improved arc of rotation.
5. Increased bulk.
6. Primary donor site closure.
7. Well-vascularized tissue coverage of the carotid artery in the event of a salivary fistula or cervical skin necrosis.
8. Ease of harvest in the supine position.
9. Ability to transfer two epithelial surfaces for inner and outer lining.

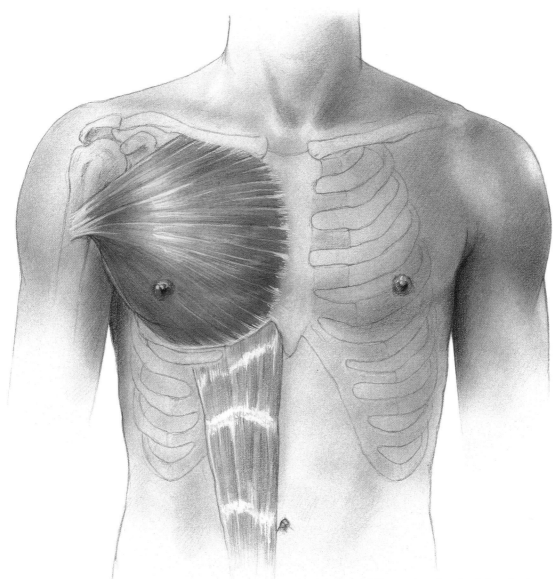

Figure 1-1. The pectoralis major is described as having three different heads of origin: clavicular, sternal-manubrial, and external oblique. The clavicular portion is distinct from the central and inferior portions of the muscle, both in function and in its neurovascular supply. The central portion of the muscle originates from the manubrium, the sternum, and the cartilages of the first six ribs. The pectoralis major both adducts and medially rotates the arm. The relationship of the cephalad portion of the rectus abdominis muscle to the caudal part of the pectoralis major should be noted.

The total skin territory of the pectoralis major is often greater than 400 cm². However, it is rare for the entire skin territory to be required to satisfy the demands of the ablative defect. With extensive use of this flap, its limitations have been identified, and modifications have been described to help overcome them. The major modifications are discussed according to these problem categories.

Methods to Improve the Arc of Rotation

Early in the history of this flap, it was recognized that a distal skin paddle placed over the caudal extent of the muscle was not only well vascularized but it also permitted a greater arc of rotation (4). Ariyan's (1) original description of this flap in-

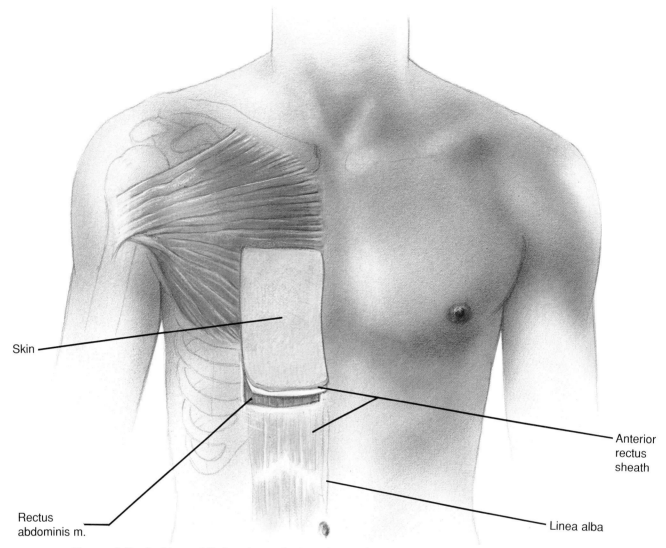

Skin

Anterior
rectus
sheath

Rectus
abdominis m.

Linea alba

Figure 1-2. A skin paddle has been designed over the caudal aspect of the pectoralis major and the cephalad portion of the rectus abdominis. A portion of the anterior rectus sheath that is beneath the skin flap is incorporated to enhance the skin's vascularity. A sufficient portion of the skin flap should overlie the pectoralis to ensure capture of the musculocutaneous perforators.

corporated a long segment of skin that extended from the clavicle to the caudal extent of the muscle. The skin component was oriented over the course of the pectoral branch of the thoracoacromial artery. The excess skin resulting from this flap design often required secondary trimming. An additional benefit to placing the skin paddle over the lower portion of the muscle was that it permitted the deltopectoral flap to be preserved for simultaneous or later use (55). Magee et al. (32) described the placement of the skin paddle over the lower portion of the pectoralis major, with an extension overlying the rectus abdominis muscle. Not only did this skin placement lead to less disfigurement of the breast in female patients, but as noted earlier, it also provided a mechanism to achieve a greater arc of rotation of this flap to more cephalad defects. Magee et al. described an array of vessels on the surface of the rectus sheath that necessitated the incorporation of this fascia to ensure the blood supply to the overlying skin. Although it is widely recognized that a portion of "random skin" can be harvested, it is also recognized that it may be unreliable. The foundation for the claim of Magee et al., that a segment of skin could be harvested entirely distal to the pectoralis, is tenuous. The general belief is that a significant portion of the skin paddle

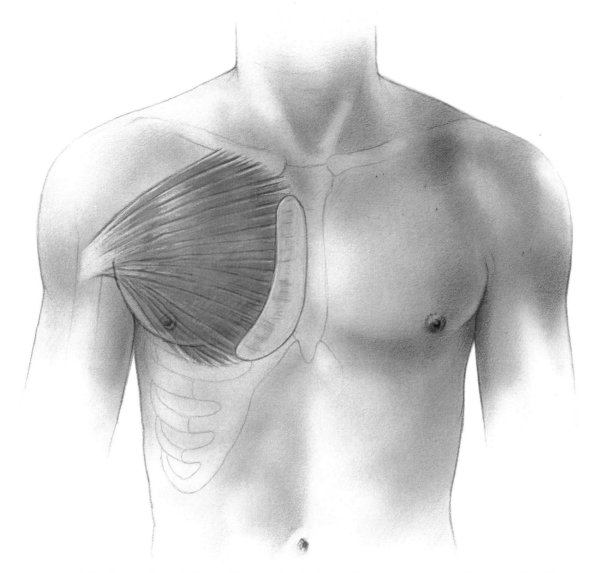

Figure 1-3. A parasternal skin paddle may be designed that crosses over to the opposite side of the sternum. The skin overlying the sternum markedly reduces the bulk of this flap.

must overlie the pectoralis major to capture a sufficient number of musculocutaneous perforators (Figure 1-2). The blood supply to the skin is discussed later in detail.

Additional measures that have been used to enhance the arc of rotation are related to the method of transfer of the muscular component of the flap. In the vast majority of cases, muscle is transposed over the clavicle and tunneled deep to the cervical skin. This is helpful to provide coverage of the carotid artery and to augment the soft tissue deficit following radical neck dissection. When a radical neck dissection is not performed, the bulk of the muscle may be problematic, requiring the use of a skin graft to achieve coverage. In Ariyan's (1) early description, the muscle was completely exteriorized and later removed after neovascularization had occurred. Fabian (21,22) and later Lee and Lore (31) proposed the removal of a segment of the clavicle to gain up to 3 cm of length. As a further modification of this approach, Wilson et al. (62) reported tunneling the muscle pedicle deep to the clavicle in a subperiosteal plane. They warned of the potential risk related to vascular compression. De Azevedo (19) described a similar modification by passing the flap through a subclavicular tunnel. In addition, he reported the preservation of the clavicular portion of the muscle by harvesting only a distal island of muscle beneath the desired skin paddle. The neurovascular supply to the proximal muscle was preserved with this technique, which

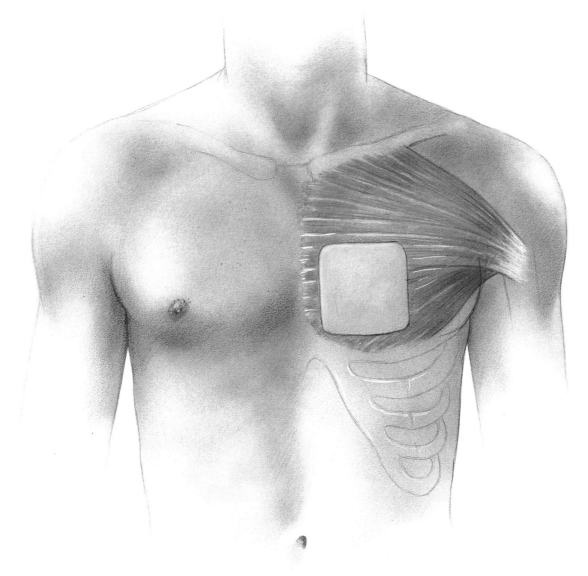

Figure 1-4. A two-stage procedure may be performed in which a skin graft is initially placed over the muscle. This composite flap is then transferred after a 2-week period, allowing the skin graft to heal to the muscle.

reportedly led to improved brachial function. In particular, he noted that patients were able to move their arms forward and downward against resistance.

Methods to Deal with Excessive Bulk

The body habitus of most patients with head and neck cancer rarely leads to concern about excessive bulk in a flap. However, this may be a problem in certain patients, especially when tubing of the skin is required to reconstruct the pharyngoesophagus, or the introduction of excess tissue in the oral cavity results in interference with normal lingual function (22). To reduce the bulk of the skin and subcutaneous tissue, Sharzer et al. (47) described harvesting a vertically oriented "parasternal" skin paddle that extended across the sternum to the opposite internal mammary perforators. Although the skin paddle had a substantial portion overlying the muscle, the component overlying the sternum achieved a considerable reduction in bulk (Figure 1-3).

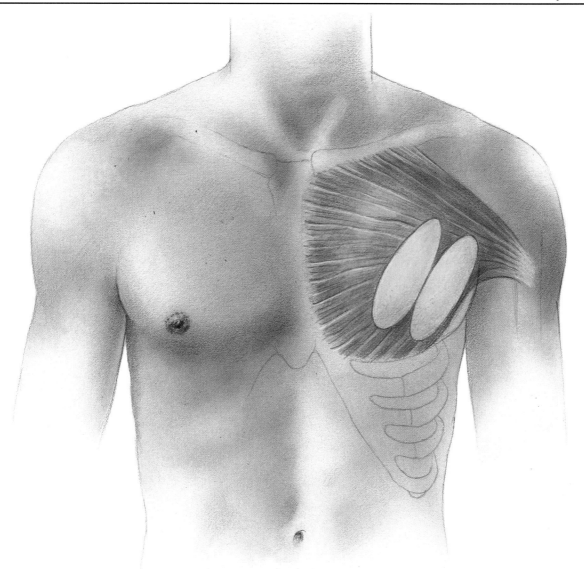

Figure 1-5. Two separate musculocutaneous units may be harvested with one based on the pectoral branch of the acromiothoracic artery and the other supplied by the lateral thoracic artery.

Alternative solutions to the problem of excessive flap bulk were achieved by eliminating the skin paddle entirely. Murakami et al. (39) described a two-stage procedure in which a split-thickness skin graft was placed over the muscle and then followed 3 to 4 weeks later by the harvest of the muscle–skin graft unit (Figure 1-4). They used this thinner flap for the reconstruction of the hypopharynx in four women in whom flap thickness was particularly problematic. This concept was extended by Robertson and Robinson (46) who reported the use of a quilted skin graft over the pectoralis major in a one-stage reconstruction of the pharyngoesophagus.

Small mucosal defects pose the additional problem of requiring only small segments of skin for reconstruction. By reducing the size of the skin paddle, there is a greater risk of missing a sufficient number of musculocutaneous perforators to achieve adequate flap vascularity. To prevent the necessity of including a larger skin paddle than needed, Johnson and Langdon (28) reported their experience with seven patients whose oral defects were reconstructed with the pectoralis major alone. Reepithelialization of the muscle was found to be rapid and produced a satisfactory long-term result.

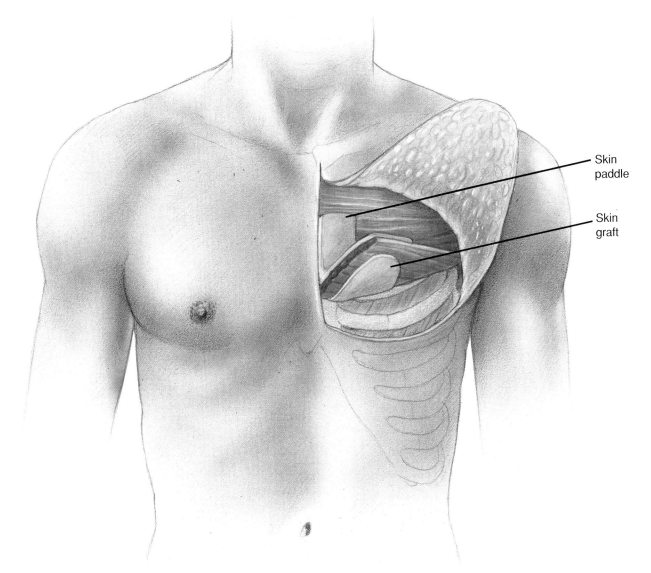

Skin paddle

Skin graft

Figure 1-6. The transfer of a Janus flap is achieved through a two-stage procedure in which a skin graft is initially placed on the deep surface of the muscle. After a 2-week delay, the musculocutaneous flap is harvested with a skin paddle on one side and a skin graft on the other side of the muscle.

Methods to Achieve Two Epithelial Surfaces for Reconstruction of Compound Defects

The reconstruction of compound defects involving the mucosa and overlying skin can be challenging. Early in the development of the pectoralis major flap, it was recognized that the rich vascularity of the skin permitted the design of two epithelial surfaces by removing the intervening bridge of skin (11). This design placed an added requirement that the flap be of sufficient length to allow it to be folded upon itself. This also produced additional bulk, which was either advantageous or disadvantageous, depending on the location of the defect. Weaver et al. (60) described a bilobular "Gemini" flap in which two separate skin paddles were harvested side by side to achieve opposing epithelial surfaces. These authors split the intervening skin and underlying muscle to achieve more complete separation between the two skin paddles. Tobin et al. (58) extended this concept one step further by raising two separate musculocutaneous units from the same pectoralis major, *i.e.*, one based on the lateral thoracic artery and the second based on the pectoral branch of the acromiothoracic artery (Figure 1-5).

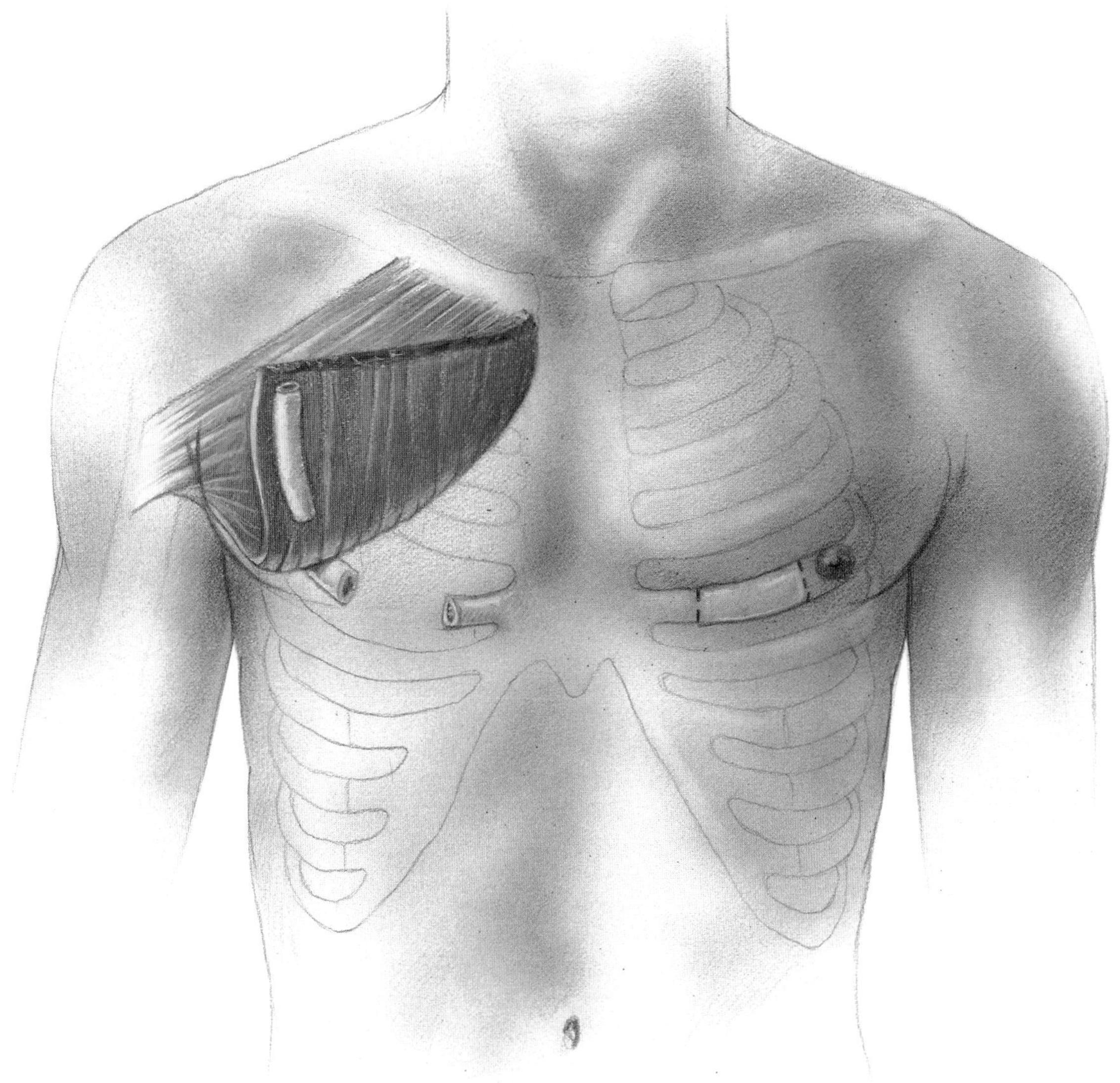

Figure 1-7. A segment of the fifth rib can be transferred as a vascularized bone composite flap. The blood supply to the rib is derived from the periosteal feeders coming from the muscle.

Preservation of the ipsilateral deltopectoral flap allows the transfer of a musculo-cutaneous and a cutaneous flap from the same side of the chest to achieve inner and outer lining (33). The benefit of the added vascularity of the deltopectoral flap creates the necessity of placing a skin graft on the chest wall donor site. Bunkis et al. (14) reported the combination of these two flaps to reconstruct full-thickness defects of the cheek. In those situations in which the deltopectoral flap is preserved but not primarily transferred, a delay procedure can be performed by making parallel inci-sions along the upper and lower limbs of the deltopectoral flap and raising the in-tervening skin to allow transfer of the pectoralis flap (18). Either simultaneous transfer or delay of the deltopectoral flap requires the preservation of the internal mammary perforators while harvesting the pectoralis major flap.

Dennis and Kashima (20) introduced the "Janus" flap as a solution to the problem of reconstructing a defect that requires both inner and outer lining. These authors reported a two-stage procedure in which a skin graft was placed on the deep surface of the pectoralis and allowed to heal. After 1 to 2 weeks, the musculocutaneous flap was harvested with the muscle sandwiched between the skin graft and the skin paddle (Figure 1-6).

Methods to Include Vascularized Bone in the Musculocutaneous Flap

The incorporation of vascularized bone with the pectoralis major musculocutaneous flap expanded the use of this technique to the reconstruction of composite defects of the head and neck. Experimental work in the early 1970s demonstrated the advantage of using vascularized bone in a contaminated and irradiated field (36,41). Cuono and Ariyan (17) were the first to report the use of the pectoralis osteomusculocutaneous flap for oromandibular reconstruction. They demonstrated the viability of the transferred fifth rib through fluorescence microscopy (Figure 1-7). Pulse labeling with different color markers showed the deposition of new osteoid and, hence, indicated active metabolism. However, the tenuous nature of the blood supply was reflected by additional investigators who used this composite flap and reported failure rates of 21% (30), 28% (9), and 75% (11). Additional complications associated with rib harvest included pneumothorax and pleural effusion.

An alternative source of vascularized bone for transfer with the pectoralis major is the sternum. Green et al. (25) described the transfer of the outer cortex of the sternum with a parasternal skin paddle. The harvest of this composite flap was associated with fewer pulmonary complications than was the rib, but this technique has not been embraced with much enthusiasm (Figure 1-8).

Additional Flap Modifications to Manage the Muscular Pedicle in the Neck

In most cases, the pectoralis major muscle provides coverage to the carotid artery and augments the radical neck dissection contour deformity. Depending on the muscular development of the individual patient, there may be a significant bulge as the muscle passes over the clavicle. Transection of the medial and lateral pectoral nerves helps to promote muscle atrophy. In patients who have not undergone prior radical neck dissection or in those patients with heavily irradiated cervical skin, it may be difficult to achieve primary closure of the skin of the neck over the muscle. In these cases, the cervical skin may be split and a skin graft placed over the exposed muscle. Alternatively, the muscle can be completely exteriorized and then resected after a 2- to 3-week period to allow neovascularization of the skin paddle. As noted previously, exteriorization of the muscle can provide additional length to the vascular pedicle.

Wei et al. (61) described an alternative solution by harvesting a skin paddle over the sternocostal portion of the muscle. The blood supply to that portion of the muscle was isolated from the vascular supply to the clavicular portion of the muscle. These authors noted that the blood supply to the clavicular portion was derived from the acromial, deltoid, and clavicular branches of the acromiothoracic pedicle; the pectoral branch supplies the sternocostal segment. Hence, the sternocostal portion of the muscle could be isolated, and either it could be tunneled under the clavicular portion, or the latter could be divided. In so doing, the bulk of tissue crossing the clavicle is greatly diminished to only that tissue surrounding the vascular pedicle.

The ultimate solution to the problem of muscle bulk and limited reach was proposed by Reid et al. (45) who used microvascular surgery to transfer a composite flap based on the clavicular head of the pectoralis major with a skin island and a segment of the medial clavicle. They reported the successful use of this free flap in four patients with oral cancer and one patient with a post-traumatic defect in the tibia. The thinness and mobility of the skin overlying the clavicle was particularly advantageous for intraoral restoration. In addition, the authors discussed the potential for a sensate flap through harvest of the supraclavicular sensory nerves.

FLAP DESIGN AND UTILIZATION

The enthusiasm surrounding the introduction of the pectoralis major musculocutaneous flap led to its application to most of the major reconstructive challenges that had not been adequately solved by the available techniques. The early experience

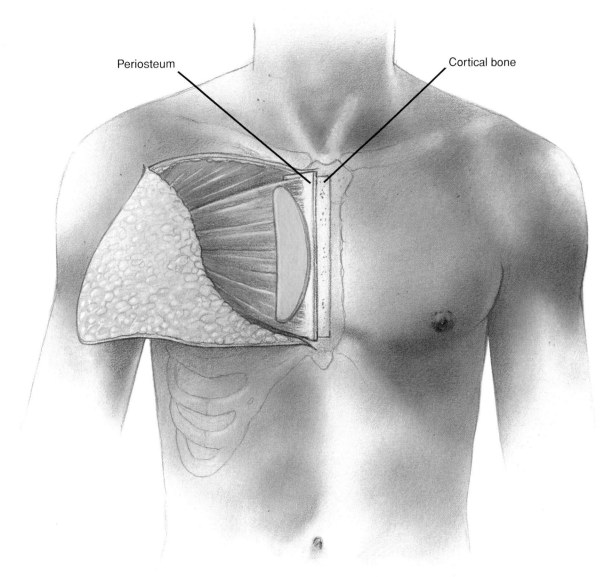

Periosteum   Cortical bone

Figure 1-8. The outer table of the sternum may be transferred as a vascularized bone composite flap. The design of a parasternal skin paddle provides a thin soft tissue component.

with this flap included the reconstruction of mucosal defects of the oral cavity and pharynx and cutaneous defects of the neck (4). Ariyan and Cuono (2) and Ariyan (1) reported the successful application of this flap to the reconstruction of skull base defects following temporal bone resection and orbitomaxillary resection. Full-thickness defects of the pharynx and cheek were easily reconstructed by any of the techniques described previously that achieve two epithelial surfaces, including the use of the ipsilateral deltopectoral flap (14). In 1970, Snyder et al. (54) described a number of techniques to transfer vascularized bone to the head and neck using regional cutaneous flaps. The use of vascularized bone for primary reconstruction of the mandible led to a flurry of activity, using the composite osteomusculocutaneous pectoralis major flap. However, advances in microvascular surgery that occurred in the latter part of the 1970s and early 1980s demonstrated that vascularized bone could be transferred from a number of distant sites to achieve a more reliable and accurate restoration of mandibular continuity (59).

The pectoralis major flap was used to restore form and function to the crippled oral cavity. Conley and Parke (15) reported its use to augment the chin following glossectomy and anterior mandibulectomy. They noted that the bulk of the soft tissue

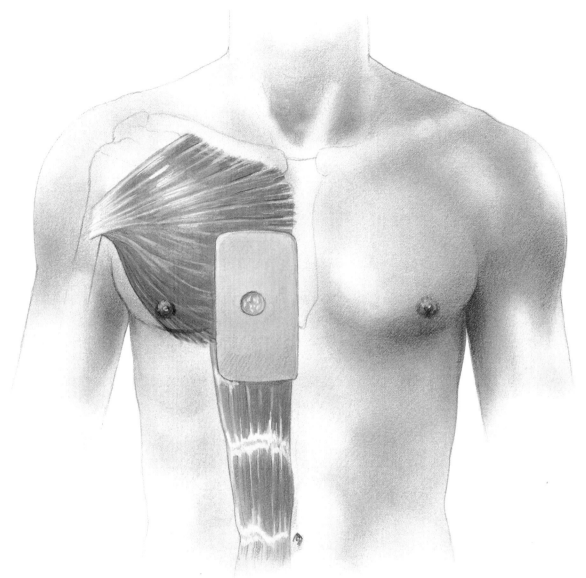

Figure 1-9. The rich vascularity of the pectoralis major flap allows it to be modified for reconstruction following ablative surgery for stomal recurrent cancer. The opening in the center of the flap is sutured to the end of the trachea and, therefore, solves the problem of the short trachea and coverage of the great vessels in the mediastinum.

component alone provided an improved external profile of the mentum but warned, that, over time, gravity would lead to a distortion of the external contour when a flap of too great dimensions was used. This could be overcome through primary or secondary mandibular reconstruction. In 1981, Conley et al. (16) reported their experience in reconstructing total glossectomy defects with the reinnervated pectoralis major musculocutaneous flap. The pectoral nerves were anastomosed to the stump of the hypoglossal nerve. Reinnervation of the muscle could be demonstrated through electromyographic recordings. However, although atrophy of the muscle could be prevented, meaningful coordinated movement of the "new tongue" could not be restored. This technique was investigated in the rat model in which a pectoralis muscle flap was reinnervated through anastomosis to the hypoglossal nerve. The restoration of contractile activity was confirmed by electromyographic recordings and the measurement of isometric contractions. The use of horseradish peroxidase confirmed that the hypoglossal nerve was the source of the central motor neuron activity (29).

Another use for the dynamic activity of the pectoralis major is in facial reanimation. Milroy and Korula (37) transferred the clavicular head of the pectoralis major in a two-stage procedure, with the first stage being the placement of a cross-facial nerve graft. The clavicular head was based on a separate neurovascular pedicle than the one supplying the sternal head of the muscle. They reported the restoration of dynamic facial reanimation by using this technique in one patient.

The problem of pharyngoesophageal reconstruction continued to plague head and neck surgeons because of the necessity for multistaged procedures when using either the tubed deltopectoral flap or the Wookey technique (7,64). In 1980, Theogaraj et al. (57) published their experience with the pectoralis major flap in seven patients of whom six underwent secondary reconstructions and one, a primary reconstruction of the pharynx and esophagus. In five cases of pharyngoesophageal stricture, the pectoralis major flap was used to augment the lumen after opening the stricture and preserving the posterior mucosal strip. Circumferential tubing of the pectoralis major musculocutaneous flap to reconstruct the total pharyngoesophageal segment was difficult because of the bulk of the subcutaneous tissue. As noted previously, Murakami et al. (39) overcame this problem by placing a skin graft on the muscle and then, at a second stage, creating a new pharyngoesophagus by tubing the skin-grafted muscle. Baek et al. (5) advised the extension of the skin paddle over the sternum to harvest thinner skin to facilitate tubing of the flap. Fabian (21) described a new technique for reconstructing the circumferential pharyngoesophageal segment by placing a skin graft along the prevertebral fascia and using a partially tubed pectoralis major flap to resurface the anterior and lateral walls. In 1988, he updated his experience in 22 patients who underwent this form of reconstruction and noted a success rate of 88%, with one flap failure and one stenosis (22). Lee and Lore (31) modified this technique by placing a dermal graft along the posterior wall of the reconstructed pharynx.

Reconstruction of the upper thoracic and lower cervical defects following ablative surgery for stomal recurrence was considered a risky procedure and fraught with complications as a result of the exposure of the great vessels. In addition, the reconstructive techniques that were used for this defect, prior to the pectoralis flap, did not obliterate the dead space in the mediastinum. In 1981, Biller et al. (10) reported the successful application of the pectoralis flap to this defect in seven consecutive patients. The skin paddle was designed with a semilunar shape when resurfacing stomal recurrences that involved the superior margin of the tracheostoma. When circumferential skin defects were created, the new stoma was formed by placing the opening in the center of the pectoralis skin paddle (Figure 1-9). By suturing the distal trachea to the opening in the skin, a portion of the depth of the new stoma was composed of the involuted pectoralis skin paddle. A redundant skin paddle was needed to accommodate the surface area required for the involuted portion. This technique not only solved the problem of the "short trachea," but it also permitted great vessel coverage and dead space obliteration. Sisson and Goldman (53) corroborated the value of this reconstructive technique for stomal recurrence in their report of seven cases in 1981.

As an extension of this technique, Fleischer and Khafif (23) described a tubed pectoralis major musculocutaneous flap to reconstruct the trachea following total laryngectomy and tracheal resection for a recurrent thyroid carcinoma. The tracheal resection left only one cartilaginous ring above the carina. One end of the pectoralis skin tube was sutured to the trachea, and the other end was sutured to the skin, creating a new stoma. This technique is particularly useful when the depth of the cut end of the trachea relative to the level of the skin and the remaining sternum, makes placement of a fenestrated pectoralis major flap difficult. The depth of the funnel that is created places additional tension on the tracheal suture line. We have used a trapezoid design of the tubed pectoralis flap. This technique creates a larger opening at the cutaneous level of the chest wall and, therefore, facilitates visualization of the depth of the airway while helping to prevent stenosis.

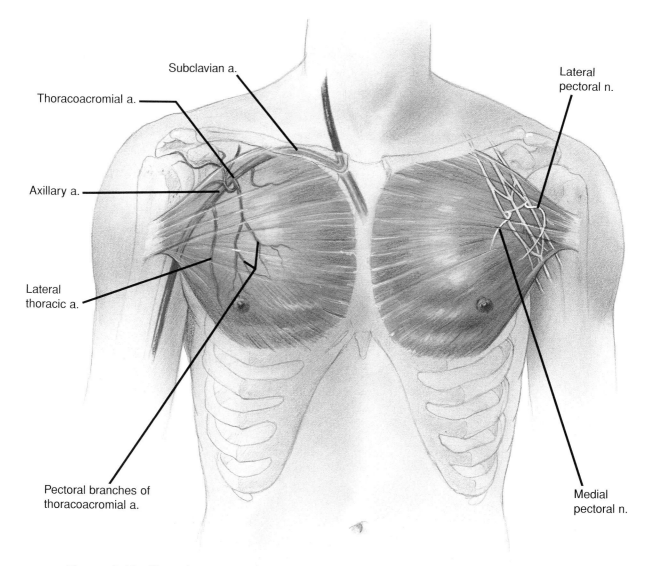

Figure 1-10. The primary vascular supply to the pectoralis major muscle arises from the thoracoacromial artery, which is a branch of the second part of the axillary artery. The lateral thoracic artery also supplies some degree of vascularity to the pectoralis muscles, the extent of which is controversial. The lateral thoracic artery is variable in size and its contribution may be completely replaced by the lateral intercostal perforators. The medial and lateral pectoral nerves supply motor innervation to different regions of the muscle. The clavicular head is primarily supplied by the lateral nerve; the sternocostal head is supplied by the medial nerve.

NEUROVASCULAR ANATOMY

According to the classification scheme of Mathes and Nahai (35), the pectoralis major is a type V muscle with one major vascular pedicle from the thoracoacromial artery and secondary segmental parasternal perforators that arise medially from the internal mammary artery. The thoracoacromial artery is a branch from the second part of the axillary artery (Figure 1-10). It commonly divides into four major branches: deltoid, acromial, clavicular, and pectoral (Figure 1-11). It is the latter branch, which descends medial to the tendon of the pectoralis minor, that supplies the pectoralis major.

The lateral thoracic artery is not commonly believed to contribute significantly to the vascularity of the pectoralis major. However, Freeman et al. (24) reported information to the contrary. In a cadaveric study in which they examined the vascular

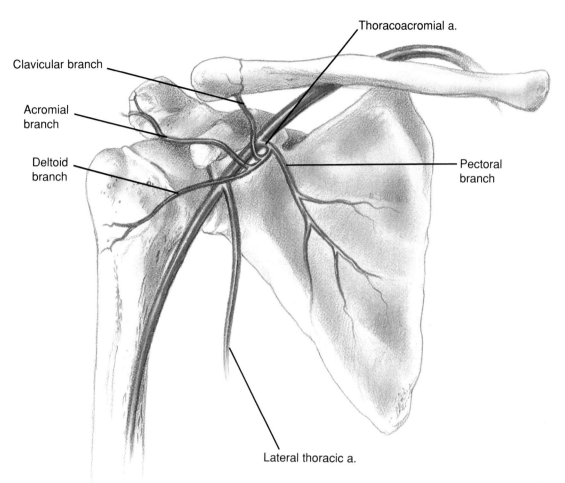

Clavicular branch

Acromial
branch

Deltoid
branch

Thoracoacromial a.

Pectoral
branch

Lateral thoracic a.

Figure 1-11. The thoracoacromial axis classically divides into four main branches: the clavicular, deltoid, pectoral, and acromial arteries. The lateral thoracic artery may also arise from this system but, more commonly, branches out separately from the axillary artery. The thoracoacromial artery commonly divides into two major branches: the pectoral and deltoid. The acromial and clavicular arteries variably arise from either division. The deltoid artery runs in the deltopectoral groove with the cephalic vein, supplying both the pectoralis major and deltoid. It gives off a cutaneous perforator in the midportion of the deltopectoral groove. The acromial branch contributes to a vascular plexus along with branches from the deltoid, suprascapular, and posterior humeral circumflex vessels. The clavicular branch runs a cephalad and medial course toward the sternoclavicular joint. The pectoral branch pierces the clavipectoral fascia and then runs a cephalocaudal course on the deep surface of the pectoralis major, which it supplies.

supply to the pectoralis major, they found that the lateral thoracic artery was present in all 17 specimens that were examined. It arose from the axillary artery and pierced the clavipectoral fascia lateral to the tendon of pectoralis minor. In its course within the muscular fascia, it provided a significant vascular contribution to the pectoralis major and the major cutaneous supply to the female breast. Through the injection of contrast material, followed by xeroradiography, the authors found that the pectoral branch of the thoracoacromial artery supplied the clavicular and upper sternal portion of the muscle; the lateral thoracic artery perfused the inferior and medial portions.

In their investigation of 10 aortic arch arteriograms and detailed dissections of 35 pectoralis major muscles, Moloy and Gonzales (38) corroborated these findings. These authors reported that, in all cases, the diameter of the lateral thoracic artery was equal to or greater than the diameter of the pectoral branch of the thoracoacromial artery. Manktelow et al. (34) reported that a branch of the lateral thoracic artery, approximately 1 mm in diameter, entered the inferior one fifth of the muscle in more than 70% of their dissections. Although the lateral thoracic artery is sacrificed by most surgeons to improve the arc of rotation of the pectoralis major musculocutaneous flap, these anatomic studies suggest that it may provide an important contribution to the vascular supply of this flap.

Reid and Taylor (44) performed the most extensive study of the vascular supply of the pectoralis major that has been reported in the literature. Their study included 50 dissections in fixed cadavers and 50 dissections in fresh cadavers. In the latter group, injections of the arterial tree included both ink and barium contrast medium. Although their study focused on the acromiothoracic axis, they reported no significant contribution from the lateral thoracic artery. They found that the pectoralis major had a regional distribution of its blood supply, with the pectoral artery supplying the sternocostal portion and the deltoid artery supplying the clavicular head. They reported only one instance of a very small pectoral branch and none of complete absence of this branch. Ink-injection studies of the pectoral artery revealed staining of the skin overlying the lateral and the sternocostal portion of the muscle. The clavicular head of the muscle was not stained until the deltoid branch of the acromiothoracic axis was injected. The deltoid muscle and its overlying skin were also stained by ink injection of the deltoid branch. There were two other interesting observations in this study. The first was that a significant zone in the medial aspect of the pectoralis major was not stained with injections of either the pectoral or deltoid branches. This zone was thought to be the primary territory of the internal mammary perforators. The second observation was that the major vessels supplying the skin in the territory of the pectoralis major were actually fasciocutaneous perforators that ran a course around the free lower and lateral border of the muscle. These fasciocutaneous vessels were considerably larger than the musculocutaneous perforators exiting from the muscle.

The superior thoracic artery provides a small vascular supply to the pectoralis major. The parasternal internal mammary perforators perfuse the medial aspect of the muscle, which allows it to be used as a turnover flap for reconstruction of midline chest wall defects.

The pectoral branch of the thoracoacromial artery and the lateral thoracic artery penetrate the clavipectoral fascia along with the medial and lateral pectoral nerves (Figure 1-12). The two arteries are both accompanied by their venae comitantes. After penetrating the clavipectoral fascia, they run in a cephalocaudal direction before entering the pectoralis major; either the pectoral branch of the thoracoacromial artery or the lateral thoracic artery supplies branches to the pectoralis minor near the clavicle. This explains the avascular plane of dissection between the pectoralis major and minor. The deltoid branch of the thoracoacromial artery accompanies the cephalic vein in the deltopectoral groove. Either the acromial or the deltoid branch gives off a direct cutaneous vessel at the most cephalad extent of the deltopectoral groove. In addition, the deltoid artery commonly gives off a cutaneous perforator in the midportion of the groove.

The application of the angiosome concept to the blood supply of the anterior chest wall helps to explain the behavior of the pectoralis major musculocutaneous flap. Taylor and Palmer (56) defined an angiosome as a segment of tissue supplied by a single source artery and vein. A system of "choke" arteries was described that connect adjacent angiosomes. Based on clinical observations and injection studies, it appears that an adjacent angiosome can be reliably "captured" after interrupting its source artery. However, when the area of tissue that is to be harvested is extended to the subsequent angiosome, or the "angiosome once removed," then necrosis becomes more likely. Taylor and Palmer surmised that this phenomenon was caused by the pressure gradient across the choke vessels that connect angiosomes. The more angiosomes that are harvested in series, the greater the reduction in pressure is.

The pectoralis major and its overlying skin can be divided into vascular territories or angiosomes. There appears to be some controversy as to whether the lateral portion of the muscle is supplied by the pectoral branch or by the lateral thoracic artery.

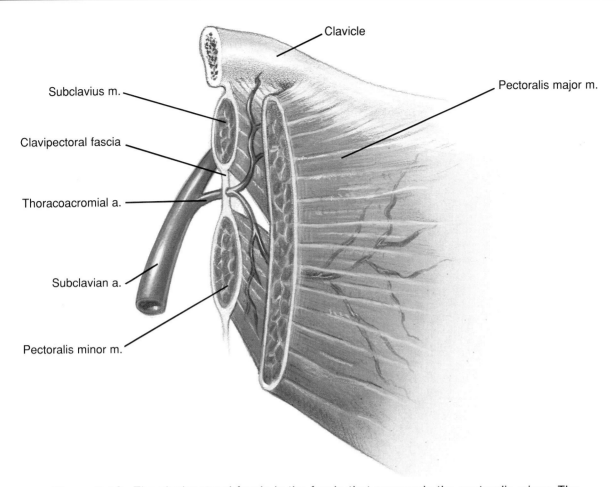

Figure 1-12. The clavipectoral fascia is the fascia that surrounds the pectoralis minor. The fascial layers from the posterior and anterior surfaces of this muscle converge to form a single fascial sheath that runs cephalad to the clavicle. Before reaching the clavicle, the clavipectoral fascia again splits to surround the subclavius muscle. The thoracoacromial artery also traverses this fascia before dividing into its terminal branches. The pectoral branch sends an artery to the pectoralis minor before forming the primary pedicle of the pectoralis major.

It seems clear, however, that the medial portion of the muscle is supplied by the internal mammary perforators. The skin overlying the rectus sheath is part of the angiosome of the superior epigastric artery and vein. It is no surprise, therefore, that capture of this skin in the upper abdomen (based on the pectoral branch) is tenuous because it is part of an angiosome that is once removed from the primary angiosome. This hypothesis maintains that the reduction of the pressure gradient from the pectoral artery, as it traverses the system of choke vessels that surround the internal mammary territory, leads to a tenuous blood supply in the skin overlying the upper abdomen. This was evident by the poor staining of skin in this region following ink injections of the pectoral artery. Reid and Taylor (44) noted the staining of a network of vessels on the surface of the rectus sheath, which gives credence to the suggestion that this layer should be harvested along with skin extensions distal to the territory of the pectoralis. These authors also advised great caution in the technique utilized when interrupting the internal mammary perforators on the undersurface of the muscle. They warned that the internal mammary branches should be either ligated or controlled with bipolar cautery. Excessive use of unipolar cautery may lead to ascending trauma of the vessels in the internal mammary angiosome, which would further jeopardize the flow across this angiosome to the distal skin (56).

The nerve supply to the pectoralis major is from the lateral (C-5 to C-7) and medial (C-8 to T-1) pectoral nerves. Manktelow et al. (34) identified multiple nerves entering different parts of the pectoralis major, which numbered from four to ten individual nerves entering the sternocostal portion of the muscle alone. This muscle has been transferred as a dynamic free flap through anastomosis of these motor nerves to recipient motor nerves (27,37).

ANATOMIC VARIATIONS

Congenital absence of the pectoralis major is rare. In a clinic population, this anomaly was observed with a frequency of approximately 1:11,000 (12). Congenital absence of the sternocostal head of the pectoralis major was first reported by Alfred Poland (43) in 1841. This anomaly was described in conjunction with ipsilateral syndactyly, and this combination bears the name Poland's syndrome or Poland's anomaly. It is reported to occur with an incidence of 1:25,000. The potential causes for this condition include abortion attempts and leukemia (8,63).

The variability in the vascular supply to the pectoralis major was studied by Moloy and Gonzales (38). They evaluated 10 aortic arch arteriograms and 35 fresh cadaver dissections. The study revealed that the lateral thoracic artery was equal to or larger in diameter to the pectoral branch of the thoracoacromial artery in 90% of cases. They found extensive collateral flow between these two vessels in all cases. There was only one instance of a nonvisualized thoracoacromial system in a patient with extensive atherosclerosis in the subclavian artery.

POTENTIAL PITFALLS

The overall reliability of the pectoralis major musculocutaneous flap is attested to by the low incidence of complete flap failure. In several large series, the incidence of total flap necrosis was reported to be 1.0% (40), 1.5% (6), 3% (51), and 7% (62). This low incidence of total flap necrosis is a reflection of the constancy of the anatomy and the ease of flap harvest. Partial flap necrosis, however, has been reported at a much greater rate. Schusterman et al. (50) noted a 14% incidence of flap loss involving greater than 50% of the skin surface area. Other large series have reported partial necrosis rates in the range of 4% (40) and 7% (6). Partial necrosis rates were probably a function of how far caudal the skin flap was harvested. Shah et al. (51) reviewed their complications in 211 pectoralis major flaps during a 10-year period. Although they reported a 29% incidence of partial flap necrosis, they did not break down this figure according to the number of skin paddles that were "placed" at the risk of partial necrosis by virtue of their caudal extension over the rectus sheath. The authors identified a number of patient-related factors that were statistically significant in their series for the development of flap necrosis as follows: age older than 70 years, female sex, overweight, albumin level less than 4 g/dl, and oral cavity defects, in particular, subtotal or total glossectomy. In addition, a variety of systemic diseases were also associated with an increased risk of necrosis. Although many of the complications in this series did not require additional surgical procedures, they did lead to prolonged hospitalization.

The potential pitfalls in harvesting the pectoralis major musculocutaneous flap begin with flap selection. The use of this donor site to resurface defects that extend more cephalad on the face or scalp calls for skin paddles designed over the more caudal aspects of the chest wall and upper abdomen. As noted previously, this may result in high rates of partial flap failure. Excessive bulk may be problematic, not only from a functional point of view, but also in terms of wound healing. In wounds that are likely to pose problems with healing as a result of prior radiation and/or poor nutrition, the effect of gravity can be extremely detrimental and may require the selection of an alternative nondependent donor site (3).

Pedicle compression may result from external causes, such as tracheostomy tapes or circumferential dressings. The creation of an inadequate tunnel for the pedicle may also cause vascular compromise. Shearing of the skin paddle and the muscle may disrupt the musculocutaneous perforators, leading to partial or complete necrosis.

Donor site problems are rare. Hematomas usually occur because of a failure to control bleeding adequately following transsection of the humeral head of the muscle.

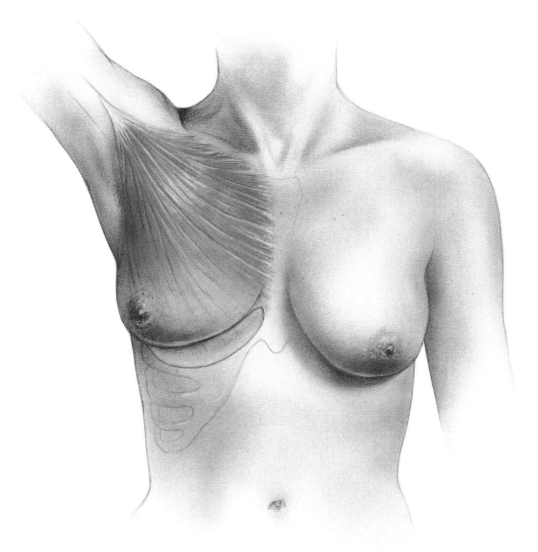

Figure 1-13. The inframammary skin paddle leads to less distortion of the female breast by avoiding medial displacement following closure.

The use of a large skin paddle may lead to excess wound tension in donor site closure. Necrosis of the skin of the chest wall may result. In theory, excess tension in closure may also lead to restrictive pulmonary disease, although this is rare. The incidence of radiologically evident and clinically significant pulmonary atelectasis was investigated by Schuller et al. (49) who selected two groups of patients with head and neck cancer who underwent ablative surgery for their disease. One group underwent reconstruction with a pectoralis major flap, and the other did not. Both groups were subdivided into patients with and without pre-existing pulmonary disease. In addition, the patients who underwent pectoralis flap reconstruction were divided, based on whether the cutaneous paddle was greater than or less than 40 cm^2. Although there was a fairly high rate of radiographic atelectasis in all patient groups, the incidence of clinically significant pulmonary complications was low. The group of patients with pre-existing pulmonary disease and flaps greater than 40 cm^2 had the highest incidence of both major radiographic signs of atelectasis and clinical pulmonary symptoms. However, no statistical analysis was reported in this study. It should be noted that the development of postoperative pulmonary complications is probably multifactorial, with the preoperative nutritional status being a potentially important factor not considered in this study. When bilateral pectoralis major flaps are harvested, it is not uncommon that closure of the second side may require a skin graft. Exposure of the costochondral cartilage may lead to serious infections, including chondritis (60).

In women, distortion of the breast following donor site closure may be minimized with an inframammary skin paddle (Figure 1-13).

The use of this donor site in male patients may lead to problems with excessive hair growth in the oral cavity or pharynx. When radiation is given postoperatively, this problem is usually remedied. Finally, Schuller (48) raised concern about the ability to detect recurrences in the neck in a timely fashion because of the bulk of the muscle pedicle. He also pointed out the significant morbidity to the shoulder when the pectoralis major is utilized on the side of a denervated trapezius. As noted previously, this parameter has not been adequately studied.

POSTOPERATIVE CARE

The use of a suction drainage system in the chest wall donor site is imperative to help avoid the formation of a seroma. Passive and active range of motion and strengthening exercises for the shoulder are instituted within a few days after surgery.

Flap Harvesting Technique

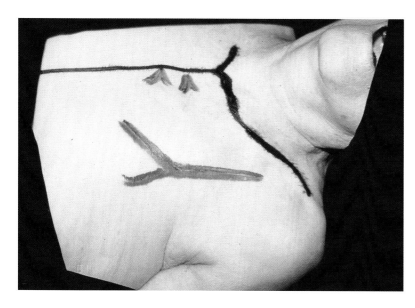

Figure 1-14. The clavicle and lateral border of the sternum are marked on the chest wall. The approximate course of the dominant vascular pedicle is marked along an axis drawn from the acromion to the xiphoid process. The parasternal perforators to the deltopectoral flap are also marked.

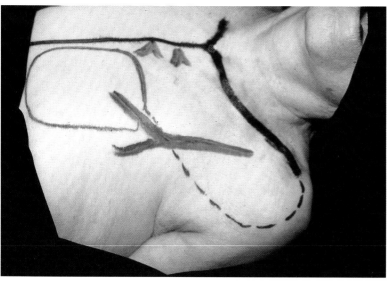

Figure 1-15. A skin paddle has been marked over the caudal medial portion of the chest wall. The upper limb of the pectoralis paddle corresponds to the lower border of the deltopectoral flap, which is preserved. Various skin paddle shapes and sizes may be harvested, depending on the requirements of the defect.

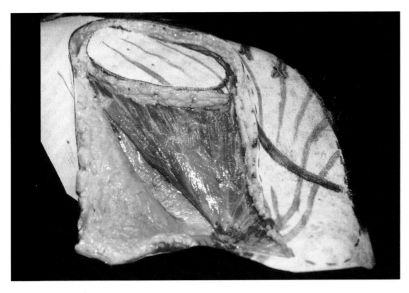

Figure 1-16. The lateral border of the pectoralis major is identified through wide undermining of the skin of the lateral chest wall. Obtaining this exposure early in the dissection allows the surgeon to evaluate the caudal extent of the muscle and, therefore, the extent of the "random" component of the skin paddle. It is evident that the skin flap that has been designed completely overlies the pectoralis major.

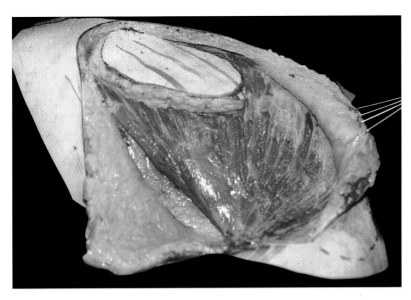

Figure 1-17. A circumferential incision around the skin paddle has been completed, along with complete exposure of the pectoralis major. The deltopectoral flap is elevated to the level of the clavicle without violating its parasternal blood supply. Although tacking sutures were originally placed between the skin and muscle to help prevent shearing forces and injury to the musculocutaneous perforators, this is no longer thought to be necessary. Care must be taken in handling this flap to prevent devascularization as a result of this factor.

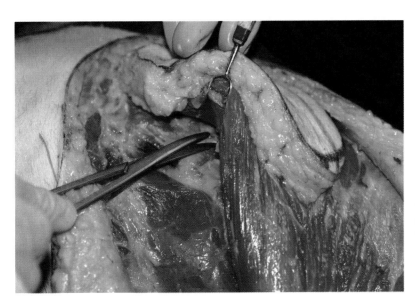

Figure 1-18. The pectoralis major is elevated off the chest wall by blunt and sharp dissection. Intercostal perforators entering the deep surface of the muscle must be ligated or coagulated. The deep plane of dissection along the intercostal muscles must be respected to prevent entry into the thoracic cavity.

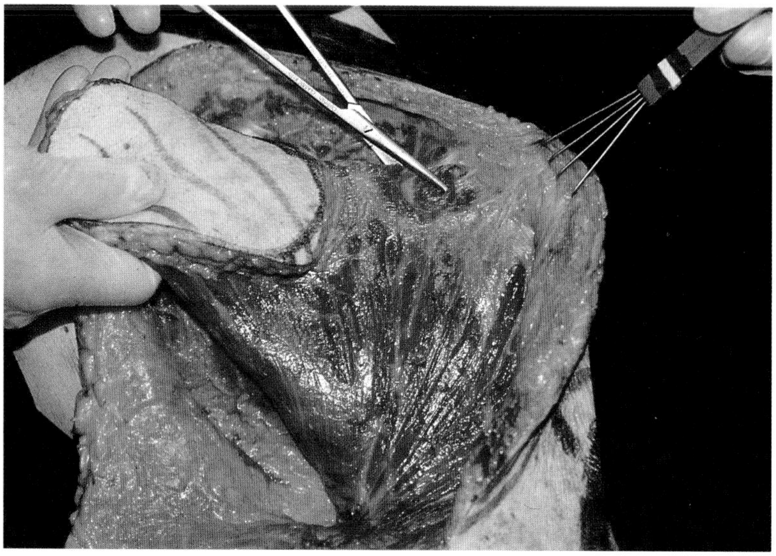

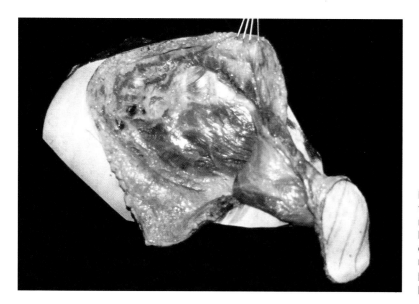

Figure 1-19. The medial attachments to the sternum are then transsected up to the level of the clavicle. Careful attention must be paid to stay lateral to the internal mammary perforators in the second and third intercostal spaces. Internal mammary perforators in the lower interspaces must be identified and controlled.

Figure 1-20. The plane of dissection between the pectoralis major and pectoralis minor is avascular, and separation can be done largely by blunt dissection. The cuff of muscle that is left attached to the sternum in the region of the second and third interspaces preserves the vascular supply to the deltopectoral flap.

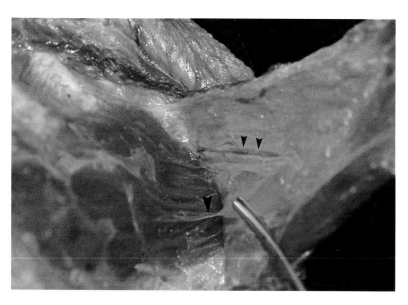

Figure 1-21. The pectoral branch of the thoracoacromial artery (*small arrows*) is easily visualized on the undersurface of the pectoralis major. The vascular pedicle is usually located along the medial aspect of the pectoralis minor. In addition, one of the pectoral nerves (*arrow*) is seen exiting the pectoralis minor and must be transsected to achieve additional mobilization of the muscle.

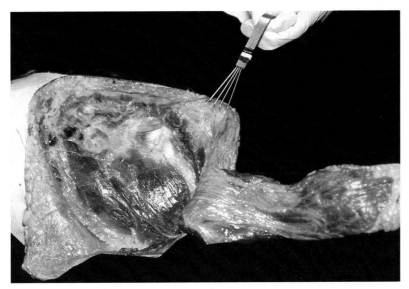

Figure 1-22. The muscular attachments to the humerus are transsected while keeping the vascular pedicle in full view to prevent injury to the nutrient supply. It is imperative to obtain good hemostasis as the lateral portion of the muscle is transsected. This is the most common location for postoperative bleeding to occur.

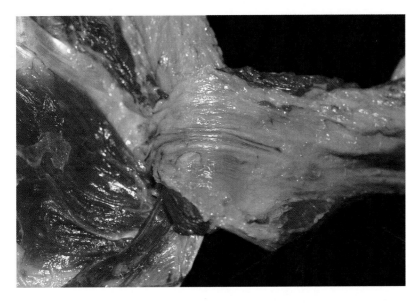

Figure 1-23. A close-up view of the under-surface of the muscle reveals the vascular pedicle and transsected muscle fibers coursing across the axilla to insert on the humerus.

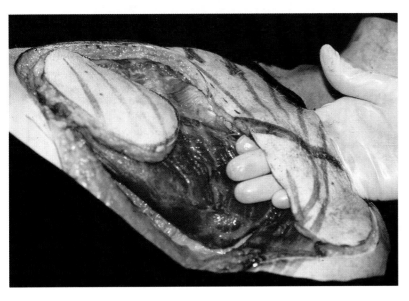

Figure 1-24. A tunnel is created for the passage of the pectoralis flap into the neck. Adequate undermining must be achieved to prevent compression of the vascular pedicle. The ability to comfortably pass four fingers into this tunnel is usually deemed adequate. A distal incision has been made in the deltopectoral flap for the purpose of delay to improve the vascular supply in the event that it is needed. A delay procedure may also be performed by elevating the deltopectoral flap without a distal incision to avoid committing it to a predetermined length.

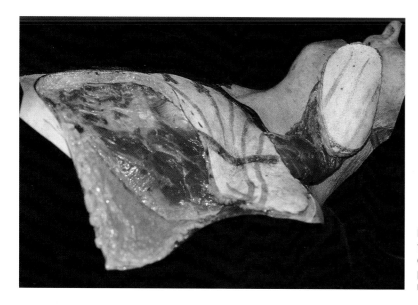

Figure 1-25. The pectoralis flap has been transferred into the neck, superficial to the clavicle. It is important to avoid twisting or placing excess tension on the pedicle in this maneuver.

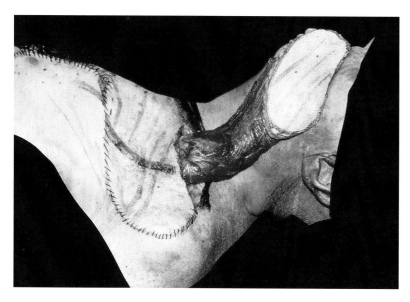

Figure 1-26. Donor site closure has been accomplished by wide undermining of the chest wall skin. Suction drains are needed to prevent seromas and hematomas.

REFERENCES

1. Ariyan S: The pectoralis major myocutaneous flap. A versatile flap for reconstruction in the head and neck. *Plast Reconstr Surg* 1979;63:73.
2. Ariyan S, Cuono C: Use of the pectoralis major myocutaneous flap for reconstruction of large cervical facial or cranial defects. *Am J Surg* 1980;140:503.
3. Aviv J, Urken ML, Lawson W, Biller HF: The superior trapezius myocutaneous flap in head and neck reconstruction. *Arch Otolaryngol Head Neck Surg* 1992;118:702.
4. Baek S, Biller HF, Krespi Y, Lawson W: The pectoralis major myocutaneous island flap for reconstruction of the head and neck. *Head Neck* 1979;1:293.
5. Baek S, Lawson W, Biller HF: Reconstruction of hypopharynx and cervical esophagus with pectoralis major island myocutaneous flap. *Ann Plast Surg* 1981;7:18.
6. Baek S, Lawson W, Biller HF: An analysis of 133 pectoralis major myocutaneous flaps. *Plast Reconstr Surg* 1982;69:460.
7. Bakamjian VA: A two-stage method for pharyngoesophageal reconstruction with a primary pectoral skin flap. *Plast Reconstr Surg* 1965;36:173.
8. Beals R, Crawford S: Congenital absence of the pectoral muscles. A review of twenty-five patients. *Clin Orthop* 1976;119:166.
9. Bell M, Barron P: The rib-pectoralis major osteomusculocutaneous flap. *Ann Plast Surg* 1981;6:347.
10. Biller HF, Baek S, Lawson W, Krespi Y, Blaugrund S: Pectoralis major myocutaneous island flap in head and neck surgery. Analysis of complications in 42 cases. *Arch Otolaryngol Head Neck Surg* 1981;107:23.

11. Biller HF, Krespi Y, Lawson W, Baek S: A one-stage flap reconstruction following resection for stomal recurrence. *Otolaryngol Head Neck Surg* 1980;88:357.
12. Bing R: Ueber angeborene Muskeldefecte. *Virchows Arch* 1902;170:175.
13. Brown R, Fleming W, Jukiewicz M: An island flap of the pectoralis major muscle. *Br J Plast Surg* 1977;30:161.
14. Bunkis J, Mulliken J, Upton J, Murray J: The evolution of techniques for reconstruction of full thickness cheek defects. *Plast Reconstr Surg* 1982;70:319.
15. Conley J, Parke R: Pectoralis myocutaneous flap for chin augmentation. *Otolaryngol Head Neck Surg* 1981;89:1045.
16. Conley J, Sachs M, Parke R: The new tongue. *Otolaryngol Head Neck Surg* 1982;90:58.
17. Cuono C, Ariyan S: Immediate reconstruction of a composite mandibular defect with a regional osteomusculocutaneous flap. *Plast Reconstr Surg* 1080;65:477.
18. Davis K, Price J: Bipedicled delay of the deltopectoral flap in raising the pectoral myocutaneous flap. *Laryngoscope* 1984;94:554.
19. De Azevedo JF: Modified pectoralis major myocutaneous flap with partial preservation of the muscle: a study of 55 cases. *Head Neck Surg* 1986;8:327–331.
20. Dennis J, Kashima H: Introduction of the Janus flap. A modified pectoralis major myocutaneous flap for cervical esophageal and pharyngeal reconstruction. *Arch Otolaryngol Head Neck Surg* 1981;197: 431.
21. Fabian R: Reconstruction of the laryngopharynx and cervical esophagus. *Laryngoscope* 1984;94: 1334.
22. Fabian R: Pectoralis major myocutaneous flap reconstruction of the laryngopharynx and cervical esophagus. *Laryngoscope* 1988;98:1227.
23. Fleischer A, Khafif R: Reconstruction of the mediastinal trachea with a tubed pectoralis major myocutaneous flap. *Plast Reconstr Surg* 1989;84:342.
24. Freeman J, Walker E, Wilson J, Shaw H: The vascular anatomy of the pectoralis major myocutaneous flap. *Br J Plast Surg* 1981;34:3.
25. Green M, Gibson J, Bryson J, Thomson E: A one-stage correction of mandibular defects using a split sternum pectoralis major osteomusculocutaneous transfer. *Br J Plast Surg* 1981;34:11.
26. Hueston J, McConchie I: A compound pectoral flap. *Aust N Z J Surg* 1968;38:61–63.
27. Ikuta Y, Kubo T, Tsuge K: Free muscle transplantation by microsurgical technique to treat severe Volkmann's contracture. *Plast Reconstr Surg* 1976;58:407.
28. Johnson M, Langdon J: Is skin necessary for intraoral reconstruction with myocutaneous flaps? *Br J Oral Maxillofac Surg* 1990;28:299–301.
29. Katsantonis G: Neurotization of pectoralis major myocutaneous flap by the hypoglossal nerve in tongue reconstruction: clinical and experimental observations. *Laryngoscope* 1988;98:1313.
30. Lam K, Wei W, Sui K: The pectoralis major costomyocutaneous flap for mandibular reconstruction. *Plast Reconstr Surg* 1984;73:904.
31. Lee K, Lore J: Two modifications of pectoralis major myocutaneous flap (PMMF). *Laryngoscope* 1986;96:363.
32. Magee W, McCraw J, Horton C, McInnis W: Pectoralis "paddle" myocutaneous flaps. The workhorse of head and neck reconstruction. *Am J Surg* 1980;140:507.
33. Maisel RH, Liston SL: Combined pectoralis major myocutaneous flap with medially based deltopectoral flap for closure of large pharyngocutaneous fistulas. *Ann Otol Rhinol Laryngol* 1982;91:98–100.
34. Manktelow R, McKee N, Vettese T: An anatomical study of the pectoralis major muscle as related to functioning free muscle transplantation. *Plast Reconstr Surg* 1980;65:610.
35. Mathes S, Nahai F: *Clinical Applications for Muscle and Musculocutaneous Flaps.* St. Louis: CV Mosby; 1991.
36. McCullough D, Fredrickson J: Neovascularized rib grafts to reconstruct mandibular defects. *Can J Otolaryngol* 1973;2:96.
37. Milroy BC, Korula P: Vascularized innervated transfer of the clavicular head of the pectoralis major muscle in established facial paralysis. *Ann Plast Surg* 1988;20:75–81.
38. Moloy P, Gonzales F: Vascular anatomy of the pectoralis major myocutaneous flap. *Arch Otolaryngol Head Neck Surg* 1986;112:66.
39. Murakami Y, Saito S, Ikari T, Haraguehi S, Okada K, Maruyama T: Esophageal reconstruction with a skin grafted pectoralis major muscle flap. *Arch Otolaryngol Head Neck Surg* 1982;108:719.
40. Ossoff R, Wurster C, Berktold R, Krespi Y, Sisson G: Complications after pectoralis major myocutaneous flap reconstruction of head and neck defects. *Arch Otolaryngol Head Neck Surg* 1983;109:812.
41. Ostrup L, Fredrickson J: Reconstruction of mandibular defects after radiation using a free, living bone graft transferred by microvascular anastomoses: an experimental study. *Plast Reconstr Surg* 1975;55: 563.
42. Pickerel KL, Baker HM, Collins JP: Reconstructive surgery of the chest wall. *Surg Gynecol Obstet* 1947;84:465.
43. Poland A: Deficiency of the pectoral muscles. *Guy's Hosp Rep* 1841;6:191.
44. Reid C, Taylor GI: The vascular territory of the acromiothoracic axis. *Br J Plast Surg* 1984;37:194.
45. Reid C, Taylor GI, Waterhouse N: The clavicular head of pectoralis major musculocutaneous free flap. *Br J Plast Surg* 1986;39:57.
46. Robertson M, Robinson J: Immediate pharyngoesophageal reconstruction. Use of a quilted skin grafted pectoralis major muscle flap. *Arch Otolaryngol Head Neck Surg* 1984;110:386.
47. Sharzer LA, Kalisma M, Silver CE, Strauch B: The parasternal paddle: a modification of the pectoralis major myocutaneous flap. *Plast Reconstr Surg* 1981;67:753–762.
48. Schuller D: Limitations of the pectoralis major myocutaneous flap in head and neck reconstruction. *Arch Otolaryngol Head Neck Surg* 1980;106:709.
49. Schuller D, Daniels R, King M: Analysis of frequency of pulmonary atelectasis in patients undergoing pectoralis major musculocutaneous flap reconstruction. *Head Neck* 1994;16:25.

50. Schusterman M, Kroll S, Weber R, Byers R, Guillamondegui O, Goepfert H: Intraoral soft tissue reconstruction after cancer ablation: a comparison of the pectoralis major flap and the free radial forearm flap. *Am J Surg* 1991;162:397.

51. Shah JP, Haribhakti V, Loree TR, Sutaria P: Complications of the pectoralis major myocutaneous flap in head and neck reconstruction. *Am J Surg* 1990;160:352–355.

52. Sisson G, Bytell D, Becker S: Mediastinal dissection—1976: indications and newer technique. *Laryngoscope* 1977;87:751.

53. Sisson G, Goldman M: Pectoral myocutaneous island flap for reconstruction of stomal recurrence. *Arch Otolaryngol Head Neck Surg* 1981;107:446.

54. Snyder C, Bateman J, Davis C, Warder G: Mandibulofacial restoration with live osteocutaneous flaps. *Plast Reconstr Surg* 1970;45:14.

55. Strelzow V, Finseth F, Fee W: Reconstructive versatility of the pectoralis major myocutaneous flap. *Otolaryngol Head Neck Surg* 1980;88:368.

56. Taylor G, Palmer J: The vascular territories (angiosomes) of the body: experimental study and clinical applications. *Br J Plast Surg* 1987;40:113.

57. Theogaraj S, Meritt W, Acharya G, Cohen I: The pectoralis major musculocutaneous island flap in single-stage reconstruction of the pharyngoesophageal region. *Plast Reconstr Surg* 1980;65:267.

58. Tobin G, Spratt J, Bland K, Weiner L: One-stage pharyngoesophageal and oral mucocutaneous reconstruction with two segments of one musculocutaneous flap. *Am J Surg* 1982;144:489–493.

59. Urken ML: Composite free flaps in oromandibular reconstruction: review of the literature. *Arch Otolaryngol Head Neck Surg* 1991;117:724.

60. Weaver A, Vandenberg H, Atkinson D, Wallace J: Modified bilobular ("Gemini") pectoralis major myocutaneous flap. *Am J Surg* 1982;144:482.

61. Wei W, Lam K, Wong J: The true pectoralis major myocutaneous island flap: an anatomical study. *Br J Plast Surg* 1984;37:568.

62. Wilson J, Yiacaimettis A, O'Neill T: Some observations on 112 pectoralis major myocutaneous flaps. *Am J Surg* 1984;147:273.

63. Wolfson R: Syndactyly, a review of 122 cases. Proceedings of the Western Orthopaedic Association. *J Bone Joint Surg [Am]* 1971;53A:395.

64. Wookey H: Surgical treatment of carcinoma of the pharynx and upper esophagus. *Surg Gynecol Obstet* 1942;75:499.

2
CHAPTER

Trapezius System

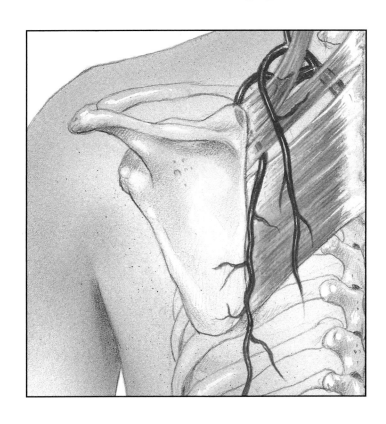

Mark L. Urken, M.D.

There are three distinct musculocutaneous flaps that can be harvested from the trapezius muscle, making it unique among the regional muscle flaps that are used in head and neck reconstruction. Conley (4), in 1972, is credited with being the first to report the use of the trapezius muscle as a carrier for skin. The skin design of this flap was similar to the one that was reported by Mutter (17) in 1842. Mutter used this cutaneous flap, which was based at the midline of the upper back and extended onto the shoulder, to release burn contractures of the neck. In 1957, Zovickian (26) reported using a "mastoid–occiput-based shoulder flap" to close pharyngeal fistulas. He staged these cutaneous flaps by putting a skin graft on the undersurface for lining, and a skin graft on the recipient bed to close the donor defect. The flap was staged one more time prior to transfer. Conley (4) reported using the same skin design but incorporated the trapezius muscle in a nondelayed flap. In addition, he reported that the trapezius muscle could be used as a vehicle to transfer a segment of vascularized clavicle to the maxillofacial skeleton. Ariyan (1) and McCraw and Dibbell (16) popularized the flap design that we now refer to as the superior trapezius flap, which is an extension of Conley's (4) original work. The superior trapezius flap, based on the paraspinous perforators, is a highly reliable flap, although limited in its utility because of its short arc of rotation.

In 1978, Demergasso (6) reported a bipedicle trapezius flap based on both the paraspinous perforators and the transverse cervical artery (TCA) and vein (TCV). In the subsequent year, at the international meeting of the American Academy of Facial Plastic and Reconstructive Surgery, both Demergasso (6,7) and Panje (21) introduced the unipedicle lateral island trapezius flap, based solely on the TCA and TCV. This musculocutaneous flap was useful but limited because of its short arc of rotation and variable vascular anatomy, which precludes the transfer of this flap in a significant percentage of patients.

The third musculocutaneous flap, the lower trapezius island musculocutaneous flap (LTIMF), was introduced by Baek et al. (3) in 1980. The transfer of a skin island overlying the lower portion of the muscle provides an increased arc of rotation, which is independent of the variable vascular anatomy of the TCA and TCV in the posterior triangle of the neck. However, the need to place the patient in the lateral decubitus position for harvest has limited the widespread use of the LTIMF.

MUSCLE ANATOMY

The trapezius muscle is a broad thin triangular muscle that covers much of the upper back and posterior neck (Figure 2-1). Its major action is to raise the lateral angle of the scapula, which is important for adduction of the arm. It is helpful to divide this muscle into three functional and anatomic units. The cephalad unit arises from the superior nuchal line, external occipital protuberance, and ligamentum nuchae. The upper fibers insert into the lateral third of the clavicle, defining the lateral boundary of the posterior triangle of the neck. The function of the upper trapezius fibers is to elevate the tip of the shoulder.

The middle portion of the trapezius muscle takes its origin from the seventh cervical and the upper six thoracic vertebrae. These muscle fibers have a transverse orientation and insert into the acromion and the upper border of the scapular spine. The major activity of the midportion of the muscle is retraction of the shoulder.

The caudal fibers of the trapezius muscle originate from the lower six thoracic vertebrae and course in an oblique cephalad direction to insert into the medial aspect of the scapular spine. This portion of the trapezius muscle overlaps the upper medial border of the latissimus dorsi muscle. The caudal portion of the trapezius assists in the functional activity of the upper portion by its downward pull on the root of the scapular spine, which helps in the rotation of the scapula.

NEUROVASCULAR ANATOMY

The blood supply to the trapezius muscle is probably the most confusing of any of the regional flaps. Mathes and Nahai (13) classified the vascular pattern to the trapezius as a type II muscle with a dominant TCA and TCV and with minor pedicles from the occipital artery and vein and the perforating posterior intercostal vessels of the cervical and thoracic regions. However, this classification does not recognize the

Figure 2-1. The trapezius is a broad thin muscle that arises from the superior nuchal line, the external occipital protuberance, the ligamentum nuchae, and the spinous process of the vertebrae of C-7 through T-12. The insertions of the trapezius muscle are to the lateral third of the clavicle, the medial border of the acromion, and the entire length of the scapular spine. There is some variability in the cephalad and caudal extent of the origin of the trapezius muscle, with the upper part failing to reach the skull and the lower part arising from the vertebrae from T-8 to L-2. The muscles lying deep to the trapezius include the levator scapulae, rhomboid minor, and rhomboid major. In its lateral extent, the trapezius also overlaps the supraspinatus and infraspinatus. The upper portion of the trapezius muscle is supplied by the TCA, which exits the posterior triangle superficial to the levator scapulae. The DSA supplies the caudal portion of the trapezius muscle. It emerges between the rhomboid major and minor muscles or less commonly between the rhomboid minor and levator scapulae (*dotted line*). Additional arterial supply to the trapezius muscle is derived from the occipital artery and the intercostal perforating arteries, which emerge in the paraspinous region.

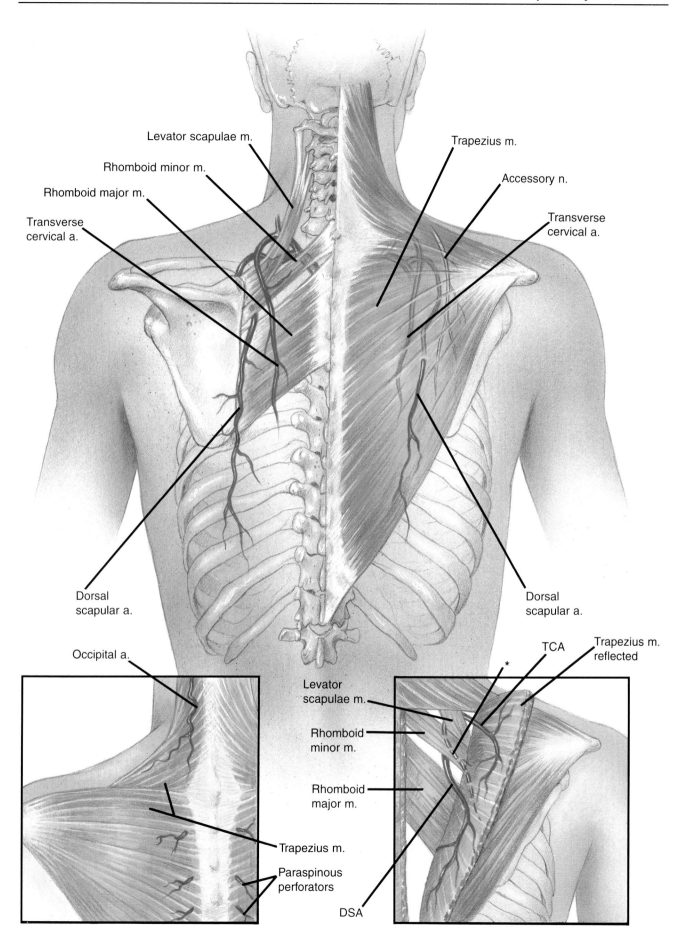

Levator scapulae m.

Rhomboid minor m.

Rhomboid major m.

Transverse cervical a.

Trapezius m.

Accessory n.

Transverse cervical a.

Dorsal scapular a.

Dorsal scapular a.

Occipital a.

TCA

Trapezius m. reflected

*

Levator scapulae m.

Rhomboid minor m.

Rhomboid major m.

Trapezius m.

Paraspinous perforators

DSA

contributions to the distal muscle from the dorsal scapular artery (DSA). Even though the DSA and the TCA commonly arise from the same parent vessel, they usually enter the muscle at separate locations; their separate contributions to different regions of the muscle have been described (Figure 2-1) (19). In reporting the "potential pitfalls" of the trapezius musculocutaneous flap, Nichter et al. (20) described a case in which an "accessory vessel," arising at the level of the scapular spine, was ligated to achieve greater mobilization of the muscle. However, the distal portion of the muscle and overlying skin showed signs of ischemia and became necrotic soon after interruption of this blood supply, despite the fact that the TCA and TCV were intact. In an effort to clarify this situation, it is easiest to begin by providing the classic description of the anatomy of these vessels before diverging into the numerous variations.

As classically described, the TCA arises from the thyrocervical trunk and courses along the posterior triangle of the neck toward the trapezius muscle (Figure 2-2). The TCA divides into a superficial branch, which passes over the levator scapulae to run on the undersurface of the trapezius muscle, and a deep branch, which passes under the levator scapulae, descending along the medial aspect of the scapula, deep to the rhomboid muscles (Figure 2-1). The superficial branch of the TCA divides into descending and ascending branches. The former runs a caudal course on the undersurface of the muscle, and the latter runs a more cephalad course, supplying the upper portions of the trapezius along with the occipital artery. The deep branch of the TCA, which we will refer to as the DSA, sends a significant branch to the caudal aspect of the trapezius muscle, which emerges between the rhomboid major and minor and less commonly between rhomboid minor and levator scapulae (Figure 2-1).

Variations in the origin of the TCA and the DSA are the rule, rather than the exception (Figure 2-2). Both branches may arise independently from the second or third part of the subclavian artery. The importance of this variation is that the vessels may then run a circuitous course, intertwined in the brachial plexus, before passing out of the posterior triangle either over (TCA) or under (DSA) the levator scapulae. This variation has no bearing on the superior trapezius flap or the LTIMF. However, the utility of the lateral island flap depends greatly on the complete mobilization of the TCA and TCV, which is impossible when the artery courses through the brachial plexus.

Netterville and Wood (19) studied the relationship between the TCA and DSA in supplying the trapezius muscle. They found that, in most cases, there was a reciprocal relationship between these two vessels, with either one or the other being dominant. In 50% of their dissections, the DSA was dominant, and the TCA was a branch of the DSA. In 30% of the dissections, the TCA was dominant, and the DSA was a branch of the TCA. In the remaining 20% of cases, the DSA and TCA appeared to be of equal dominance and size and had a separate takeoff from the subclavian artery. In addition, ink-injection studies of the TCA and the DSA revealed that the former supplied the skin overlying the trapezius above the rhomboid minor and the latter

Figure 2-2. The anatomy of the TCA and the DSA in the posterior triangle is highly variable. **A:** The TCA is classically described as arising from the thyrocervical trunk and running across the posterior triangle of the neck. It divides into a superficial branch, which crosses over the levator scapulae, and a deep branch, which runs deep to the levator scapulae. The superficial branch divides into an ascending branch and a descending branch, which supply the upper and lower portions of the trapezius muscle, respectively. The deep branch of the TCA runs deep to levator scapulae and then gives rise to a superficial branch that arises between either the levator scapulae and rhomboid minor or, more commonly, between the rhomboid major and minor, supplying the distal portion of the trapezius muscle. **B:** A common anatomic variation is shown in which the DSA arises separately from the second or third part of the subclavian artery. The TCA may also arise directly from the subclavian artery. **C:** In some cases, the DSA and the TCA may run a course below or intertwined in the brachial plexus. This variation is most important to identify when harvesting a lateral island trapezius flap in which mobilization of the TCA is critical to achieving an adequate arc of rotation.

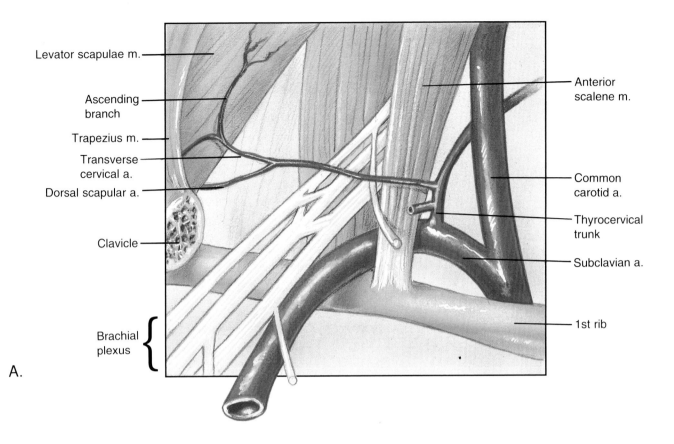

Levator scapulae m.

Ascending branch

Trapezius m.

Transverse cervical a.

Dorsal scapular a.

Clavicle

Brachial plexus

Anterior scalene m.

Common carotid a.

Thyrocervical trunk

Subclavian a.

1st rib

A.

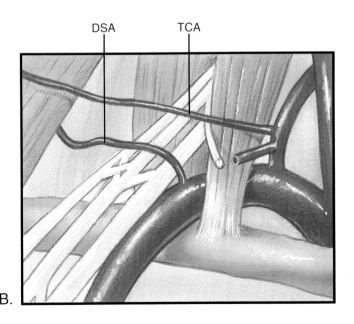

DSA   TCA

B.

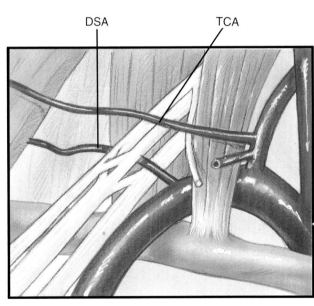

DSA   TCA

C.

supplied the skin below the rhomboid minor. These findings conflict with the results of selective intra-arterial injections of prostaglandin E_1 by Maruyama et al. (11). Following selective catheterization of the transverse cervical artery, the authors reported that injection of prostaglandin E_1 led to flushing of the skin over the entire territory of the trapezius muscle. These findings can be explained by assuming that the DSA was a branch of the TCA, and therefore, both the proximal and distal blood supplies were probably injected in Maruyama's study.

The venous anatomy is equally variable. Goodwin and Rosenberg (9) identified three major patterns of TCV anatomy. In the majority of cases, the TCV is a single vessel, but it may be a dual system. The TCV exits the trapezius muscle on its deep surface, close to the point of entry of the TCA, which is 2 to 5 cm above the clavicle. Although the TCA always runs deep to the omohyoid muscle, the TCV may be superficial in 25% of cases. In 60% of cases, the authors found that the TCV traveled with the TCA; in 15%, it followed a course under or through the brachial plexus. In the remaining 25%, the TCV ran a more caudal course beneath the clavicle, terminating in the subclavian vein. In the majority of cases the TCV enters the medial subclavian vein. It can enter the lower portion of the external jugular vein in one third of cases.

The accessory nerve, cranial nerve XI, provides motor innervation to the trapezius muscle after supplying innervation to the sternocleidomastoid muscle. There are contributions to the nerve supply of the trapezius from C-2 through C-4, but the exact nature of this additional innervation is uncertain.

SUPERIOR TRAPEZIUS FLAP

The superior trapezius flap is an extremely reliable source of coverage for defects of the posterolateral portion of the neck that extend no further medially than the midline. In our review of the literature on this flap, we found no instances of total flap failure. We have found it extremely reliable, with no instances of either partial or total necrosis in more than 30 cases (2).

This flap is usually transferred as a peninsula of skin and muscle, which is based at the midline of the back. However, an island of skin, overlying the lateral aspect of the muscle, may also be transferred. The primary blood supply to this flap is derived from the paraspinous perforators, with some contribution from the occipital artery. This flap is unique among the trapezius flaps in that its blood supply is unaffected by a prior radical neck dissection with transsection of the transverse cervical vessels. In fact, the vascularity of the distal portion of this flap may be enhanced through a delay phenomenon when the transverse cervical vessels have been previously interrupted.

The rationale for this hypothesis is based on the angiosome concept. Taylor et al. (24) proposed that the delay phenomenon is caused by the opening up of choke vessels between angiosomes located in series as a result of interrupting the source artery in an adjacent angiosome. Under normal circumstances, without a delay, it was hypothesized that only one adjacent angiosome could be captured, but not an angiosome once removed. This hypothesis can be applied to the superior trapezius flap by

Figure 2-3. Angiosomes of the superior trapezius flap. The superior trapezius flap is primarily supplied by the paraspinous perforators that exit in the posterior cervical region. The primary angiosome (I) is shown in yellow; the adjacent angiosome (II), supplied by the transverse cervical artery, is shown in blue. Finally, the third angiosome (III) in the series, the angiosome once removed, is supplied by a branch of the thoracoacromial system, which is the primary blood supply to the deltoid. Interruption of the TCA leads to a delay phenomenon of the skin overlying the deltoid by opening up the choke vessels that separate these three angiosomes. The third angiosome in the series, can be more reliably captured by improving the hemodynamic pressure gradient across the middle zones.

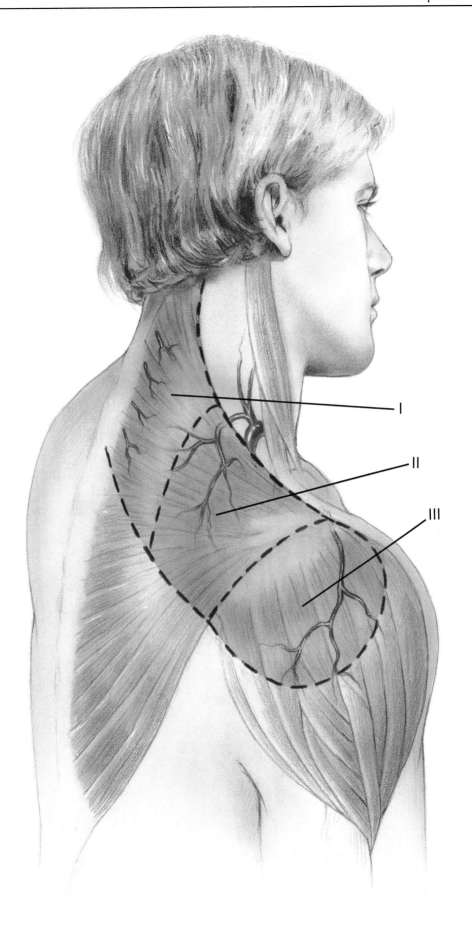

dividing it into its component angiosomes. The primary angiosome, which has its base at the midline posteriorly, is supplied by the paraspinous perforators. The adjacent angiosome overlying the lateral aspect of the muscle is supplied by the transverse cervical vessels. Finally, the third angiosome in line, or the angiosome once removed, which overlies the deltoid muscle, is supplied by a branch of the thoracoacromial artery (Figure 2-3). Following interruption of the transverse cervical vessels during radical neck dissection, the choke system of vessels between the three angiosomes becomes dilated, allowing a more favorable pressure gradient by which the skin overlying the deltoid can be reliably captured by the medial angiosome supplied by the paraspinous perforators (2,24).

The major use for this flap is to resurface cutaneous defects of the posterior and lateral aspects of the neck. Following a radical neck dissection, the transfer of this flap is not only safe, but it also causes no further functional deficit because the muscle is already denervated. It is especially advantageous for the coverage of heavily irradiated wounds, including those in which the carotid artery is exposed. It is unique among the regional musculocutaneous flaps in that it is superiorly based; therefore, gravity does not cause the flap to pull away from the recipient bed as readily as is the case with other regional flaps with dependent muscles. The success of this flap in the "problem wound" is enhanced by inserting the flap along its entire path to the site of the defect, even if intervening skin must be excised to do so. The poorer aesthetic result of wrapping the flap around the neck is counterbalanced by the increased chances of successful wound healing. More often than not, a skin graft is required for closure of the donor site. Secondary correction of the "dog-ear" deformity below the auricle is often necessary.

LATERAL ISLAND TRAPEZIUS FLAP

The lateral island trapezius flap is the least reliable of the three musculocutaneous flaps because its arc of rotation is dependent on favorable anatomy and meticulous mobilization of the TCA and TCV. Preliminary exploration of the posterior triangle of the neck is essential to assess the suitability of these vessels. Because the musculocutaneous island is completely isolated on the nutrient vascular pedicle, there are no alternative effluent routes through secondary venous channels, such as might occur in a musculocutaneous flap in which the muscle is not completely detached. It is therefore imperative that a patent TCV is present along with the artery. The likelihood of both vessels being present following radical neck dissection is small, and therefore, both the lateral island flap and the LTIMF should not be selected in such patients.

The primary use of the lateral island flap is for external defects of the lateral and anterior neck. It may also be used for mucosal defects of the pharynx and oral cavity. Panje (21) described an extension of the lateral island flap, which he classified as the trapezius musculocutaneous island paddle flap. In this design, a small island of muscle is used as a carrier for an extended island of skin that is harvested well beyond the lower lateral border of the muscle in the direction of the axilla. The proposed advantage of this flap is the large area of thin skin that can be harvested, which improves the arc of rotation without completely interrupting shoulder function (18).

Ryan et al. (23) described a novel use of the lateral island trapezius flap to achieve dynamic facial reanimation in a variety of situations that led to facial paralysis. The surgical technique involved the transfer of an innervated and vascularized segment of the trapezius muscle to the paralyzed side of the face. The muscle was inset into the corner of the mouth and the temporalis fascia. In some cases, the vascular pedicle was not long enough to reach the defect, and the pedicled muscle flap was converted to a free muscle flap. This technique was also used for composite cheek defects by transferring an innervated musculocutaneous flap. By maintaining the accessory nerve intact, there was no chance for denervation atrophy to occur. However, the disadvantage of this technique is that facial movement requires a conscious effort by the patient to tense the ipsilateral shoulder.

LOWER TRAPEZIUS ISLAND MUSCULOCUTANEOUS FLAP

The skin paddle of the LTIMF is designed over the inferior aspect of the trapezius muscle between the vertebrae and the medial border of the scapula. The harvest of this flap is facilitated by placing the patient in the lateral decubitus position with adduction and internal rotation of the ipsilateral arm to increase the space between the medial edge of the scapula and the midline of the back. The lower extent of the flap design is somewhat controversial; some authors report reliable skin vascularity up to 15 cm below the inferior border of the scapula (22).

The angiosome concept provides some insight into what the safe caudal extent of this skin flap should be. The blood supply to the trapezius muscle allows it to be divided into three separate angiosomes. The TCA supplies the angiosome of the lateral cephalad portion of the muscle; the cervical paraspinous perforators supply the medial cephalad angiosome. The lower portion of the trapezius is supplied by the dorsal scapular artery, which enters the deep surface of the muscle at the upper border of the rhomboid major. The flaps that extend below the lower border of the trapezius muscle fall into the angiosome of the latissimus dorsi which, in this region, is supplied by the intercostal arteries (Figure 2-4) (24).

By applying the principles of the angiosome concept to the LTIMF, the safe lower border of this skin paddle becomes readily apparent. When the skin paddle extends beyond the lower border of the scapula, into the medial angiosome of the latissimus dorsi, then this inferior portion of the skin is in the angiosome immediately adjacent to the one supplied by the DSA. The skin overlying the latissimus dorsi angiosome should be readily captured if the dorsal scapular vessels are preserved. Attempts to capture the skin of an angiosome once removed, without a delay, are often met with complications. However, we and others have transferred distal skin paddles with success, despite the increased incidence of ischemia. Alternatively, a skin island that does not extend beyond the confines of the trapezius muscle can be reliably transferred on the TCA–TCV pedicle alone, through capture of the adjacent angiosome of the DSA and dorsal scapular vein (DSV) (24).

In routine cases in which the skin paddle is confined to the territory of the TCA and DSA angiosomes, we do not preserve the DSA pedicle. However, if a large DSA is encountered, then temporary occlusion of the DSA may be accomplished with a microvascular clamp. Observation of the color and quality of the dermal bleeding in the distal skin allows the surgeon to decide about the necessity of preserving the DSA pedicle (25). Because preservation of the DSA severely limits the arc of rotation, this pedicle can be mobilized by cutting a cuff of rhomboid minor on either side of the vessel to improve the arc of rotation. When this maneuver is performed, the distal portion of the DSA must be ligated (Fig. 2-20).

The tremendous arc of rotation of the LTIMF makes it the most versatile of the three trapezius musculocutaneous flaps. Mobilization of the entire muscle may be achieved by pedicling of it solely on the TCA and TCV in the posterior triangle of the neck, similar to the lateral island flap. We have not found such extensive dissection to be necessary in the routine application of this flap to defects of the lateral skull, the midface, the neck, and the oral cavity. The primary advantages of this flap, aside from the arc of rotation, are the thinness and pliability of the tissue compared with that of the other regional musculocutaneous flaps. The donor defect is also minimal. Preservation of the function of the upper trapezius muscle fibers can often be accomplished by mobilizing only that portion of the muscle needed to transfer the skin to the defect (12). The major disadvantage of the LTIMF is the necessity to place the patient in a lateral decubitus position. This flap is most useful in patients who require reconstruc-

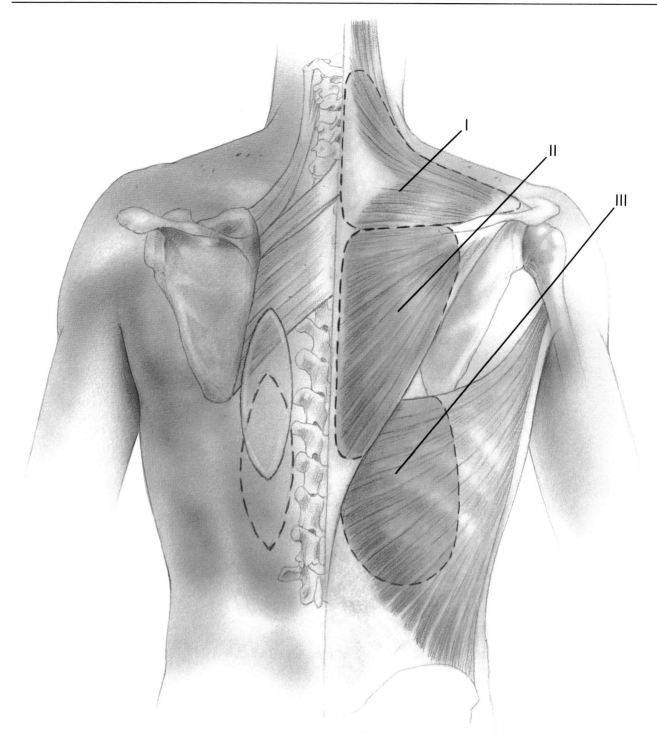

Figure 2-4. Trapezius angiosomes. The primary angiosomes of the trapezius muscle are divided between the TCA (I) and the DSA (II). The primary angiosome of the TCA is shared by the paraspinous perforators, which enter the muscle in its medial cephalad region. The division between angiosomes I and II is signified by the underlying division between rhomboid minor and rhomboid major through which the contribution from the DSA enters the undersurface of the trapezius muscle. In harvesting the LTIMF, the position of the skin paddle may extend caudal to the lower border of the trapezius muscle into the area of the latissimus muscle (III). The third angiosome in the series, which is supplied by the paraspinous perforators entering the latissimus dorsi, may be reliably captured by the trapezius flap by incorporating the dorsal scapular blood supply. However, if the dorsal scapular vessels are interrupted and the flap is based solely on the TCA, then the third angiosome in the series may be less reliable. This explains some of the variability that we have encountered in harvesting this flap and the questionable reliability of this skin paddle that has been reported in the literature. On the left hand side, two

tion of lateral skull and cheek defects in which the ablative procedure can also be performed in the lateral decubitus position.

TRAPEZIUS OSTEOMUSCULOCUTANEOUS FLAP

Although Conley (4) and Dufresne et al. (8) reported the transfer of a portion of the clavicle with the trapezius flap, the most commonly transferred segment of bone is the spine of the scapula. Cadaveric injection studies indicated that the TCA provides a periosteal circulation to the spine. Approximately 10 to 14 cm of bone can be harvested while preserving the acromion to minimize shoulder and upper arm dysfunction (15). The scapular spine is most effectively transferred with the lateral island flap design. The transfer of bone with the superior trapezius flap, although feasible, is limited in its reach and the flexibility of positioning the skin relative to the bone. The quality of the blood supply to the scapular spine is probably comparable to the vascularity of the rib transferred with the pectoralis major flap.

Bone-containing composite free flaps offer several distinct advantages that favor their use for oromandibular reconstruction as follows: (a) a rich vascular supply to the bone; (b) a flexible relationship of the soft tissue to the bone, allowing a more accurate restoration of normal anatomy and function; and (c) a complete freedom to position the bone for the restoration of defects involving the symphysis and contralateral body.

POTENTIAL PITFALLS

Each of the three trapezius flaps has its own potential problems, which may cause an unsuccessful outcome. The superior trapezius flap is probably the least problematic if its limited arc of rotation is respected and the extent of the defect for closure does not cross the midline anteriorly.

The lateral island flap is technically easy to harvest, but it is imperative that the posterior triangle be carefully explored to ensure that the anatomy of the TCA and TCV is favorable. Failure to identify and carefully isolate both an artery and vein will lead to inevitable failure. Particular attention must be taken in preserving the TCV, which may be in jeopardy because of its course superficial to the posterior belly of the omohyoid and its entry into the external jugular vein. Both of these venous patterns must be sought when dissecting in this region to avoid inadvertent injury (9).

The most common error performed in harvesting the LTIMF is the failure to raise the trapezius muscle in the plane superficial to the rhomboid major and minor muscles. This is best accomplished by identifying the lateral border of the caudal portion of the trapezius muscle. Meticulous dissection in the plane deep to the trapezius muscle allows the surgeon to identify the fibers of the rhomboid major muscle that run in a more transverse orientation and insert into the medial border of the scapula. Krespi et al. (10) described the combined rhombotrapezius flap, which reportedly enhanced vascularity to the overlying skin, provided added bulk, and allowed transfer of vascularized bone from the medial border of the scapula. The additional vascularity is

---

◄ ──────────────────────────────────────

different skin paddles are drawn. The *solid line* denotes a skin paddle that would be theoretically readily captured by the transverse cervical artery because of the fact that it lies entirely within the territory of the adjacent angiosome (11). The *dotted line* indicates a skin paddle that partially overlies the lower portion of the trapezius and extends into the territory of the latissimus dorsi. The more caudal skin island has a greater arc of rotation. However, the reliable transfer of this more caudal segment of skin would require preservation of the DSA. The disadvantage of this approach is that it requires the harvest of a cuff of the rhomboid minor muscle to achieve an adequate arc of rotation. The advantage is that it preserves the upper fibers of the trapezius muscle, which helps to stabilize the shoulder and preserve its function. Our usual approach to harvesting skin paddles that extend more than 5 cm below the scapular border is to place a temporary microvascular clamp on the dorsal scapular vessels and to observe the blood supply of the skin paddle to determine whether interruption is safe.

undoubtedly a result of including the dorsal scapular system by dissecting in the plane deep to the rhomboids. However, the harvest of the rhomboid major is not critical to achieving this end. The bulk that is obtained by incorporating the thin rhomboid muscles is minimal after denervation atrophy occurs. Finally, the medial border of the scapula is a thin bone that is not suitable for functional mandibular reconstruction. The morbidity of a winged scapula that results from total disruption of the medial muscle group outweighs the limited benefits of this flap design.

The LTIMF has been labeled an unreliable reconstructive technique, with complication rates caused by partial or total flap necrosis ranging from 0% (14) to 57% (5) among the larger series of cases that used this donor site (24). The interpretation of these complications must be placed in the context of the flap designs that were utilized in each series. Mathes and Stevenson (14) reported a 0% rate of complications when using the LTIMF for the repair of 13 posterior neck and skull defects. Although these authors divided the dorsal scapular pedicle, the arc of rotation to the defects of the posterior neck and skull allowed the skin paddle to be placed over the distal muscle. Significant mobilization of the muscle was not required. Cummings et al. (5) reported a 57% incidence of flap necrosis. Although these authors noted that they extended the distal skin paddle beyond the lower border of the muscle in some patients, they did not analyze their complications with this variable in mind.

In the largest series of 45 LTIMFs reported by Urken et al. (25), there was a 6.5% incidence of major complications defined as a greater than 20% flap loss. There was similarly a 6.5% incidence of minor (20%) flap loss. In no case in this series was the dorsal scapular pedicle preserved. The lower border of the skin paddle was not extended beyond 5 cm below the scapular border in most patients. Of note was the fact that all but one case of flap necrosis occurred in patients who underwent flap transfer on the side in which a prior neck dissection had been performed. It is evident from this finding that a prior radical neck dissection should be considered a contraindication to harvesting an ipsilateral LTIMF.

Donor site problems are rarely significant. However, seroma formation is common, and long-term suction drainage is recommended.

Flap Harvesting Technique
Superior Trazepius Flap

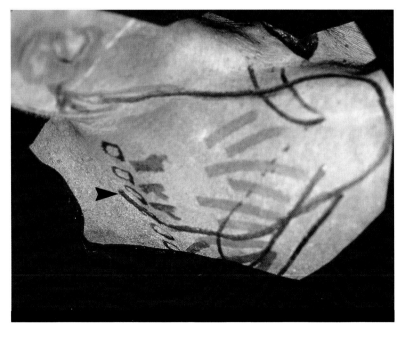

Figure 2-5. The superior trapezius flap is based on the paraspinous perforators of the lower cervical region. The flap is outlined over the upper portion of the trapezius muscle with the anterior incision of the flap placed along the anterior border of the trapezius muscle. The posterior border of the flap is a transverse incision parallel to the anterior incision. The width of the flap is determined in part by the width of the defect and by the necessity to incorporate several perforators. The arc of rotation of this flap is limited by the posterior inferior attachment (*arrow*). This rotation may be improved slightly by extending the incision across the midline in a cephalad direction. This modification was introduced by Panje (21) and helps to add additional length to this flap. The distal portion of the skin paddle may extend several centimeters beyond the acromion process. In our experience, this flap is extremely reliable, and up to 8–10 cm of random skin beyond the distal lateral extent of the trapezius muscle may be safely incorporated.

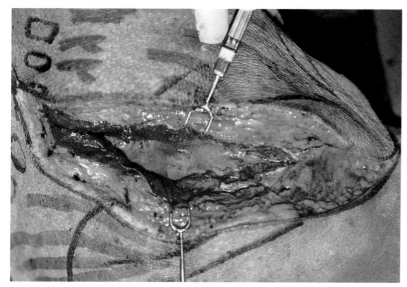

Figure 2-6. The posterior incision is made through the skin and through the trapezius muscle. The firm attachments of the trapezius to the spine of the scapula must be incised to maintain the proper depth of dissection. The TCA and TCV are encountered in this portion of the dissection and must be ligated and transsected. The deep plane of dissection is between the trapezius and supraspinatus. In the medial aspect of the dissection, the trapezius is elevated off the levator scapulae and the rhomboid minor.

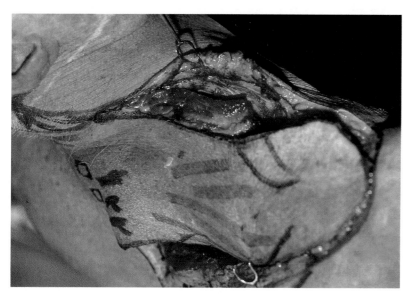

Figure 2-7. The incisions along the anterior border of the flap are made to coincide with the anterior border of the trapezius muscle. The distal portion of the skin paddle is elevated along the plane just superficial to the deltoid fascia. On reaching the lateral aspect of the trapezius muscle, the plane of dissection is then deepened to incorporate that muscle. The TCA and TCV must be ligated and transsected when encountered in the dissection along the anterior border.

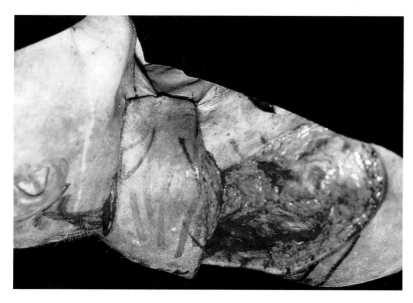

Figure 2-8. Rotation of the superior trapezius flap is demonstrated. This flap can be used to close defects that do not extend beyond the midline of the neck anteriorly. Closure of the donor site is achieved by wide undermining. In most cases, a skin graft is needed to cover the wound. The area of skin grafting may be reduced by using retention sutures to lessen the area of the defect.

Lateral Island Trapezius Flap

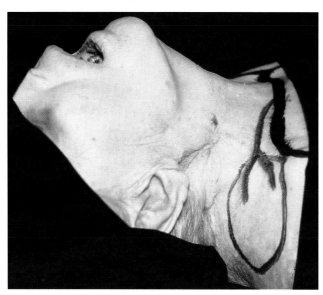

Figure 2-9. The lateral island trapezius flap is designed as an island of skin overlying the lateral aspect of the cephalad portion of the trapezius muscle where it inserts into the clavicle and the acromion process of the scapula. The anterior border of the trapezius muscle is marked at its insertion on the distal one third of the clavicle. The skin island may be designed over the approximate boundaries of the trapezius muscle and with random portions extending more distally. The dimensions of the flap are limited by the redundancy of the tissue in this region, which would permit primary closure of the defect.

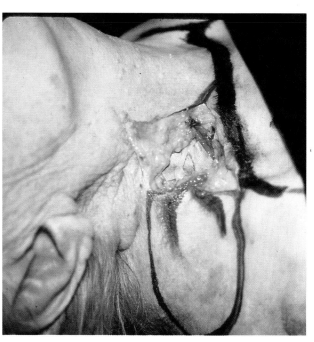

Figure 2-10. The dissection begins by exposure of the inferior aspect of the posterior triangle. The supraclavicular fossa is carefully dissected to identify the transverse cervical artery and vein. When a neck dissection is performed at the same time as a lateral island flap, particular attention must be paid to preserving the TCV.

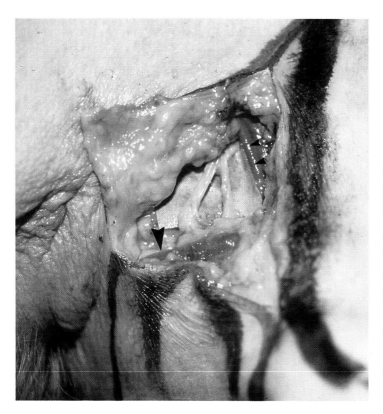

Figure 2-11. The anterior border of the trapezius (*large arrow*) has been identified. The posterior belly of the omohyoid has also been isolated (*small arrows*). The TCA runs along the floor of the posterior triangle. The TCV may run a more superficial course relative to the omohyoid and the artery. The incisions around the skin paddle are made after the anatomy of the vessels has been determined and the surgeon has ensured that the TCA and TCV are not intertwined with the roots of the brachial plexus. Variations in the entry site of the TCA and TCV along the anterior border of the trapezius may cause the skin paddle to be altered so that it is centered on the vascular pedicle. After the skin paddle is outlined, the incisions are made circumferentially through the skin, subcutaneous tissue, and trapezius muscle.

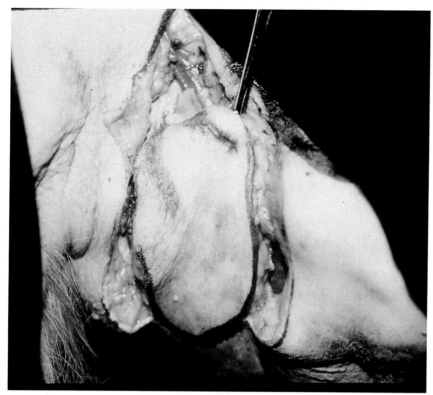

Figure 2-12. Mobilization of the lateral island flap has been completed. Ligation of the distal TCA and TCV, as they descend along the more caudal aspect of the trapezius muscle, must be accomplished when the distal incision through the flap is made. The DSA may arise as a branch of the TCA. Because of its course deep to the levator scapulae muscle, the DSA must be ligated and transsected.

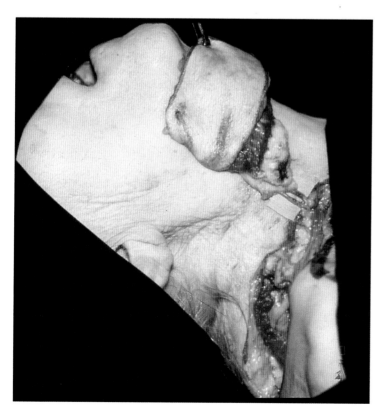

Figure 2-13. Transposition of this flap into the recipient site is now completed. Greater mobilization of this flap can be achieved by dissection along the vessels in the medial aspect of the posterior triangle. Wide undermining followed by layered closure is required to manage the donor site defect.

Lower Trapezius Island Musculocutaneous Flap

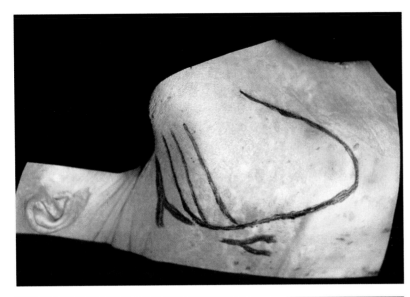

Figure 2-14. The approximate position of the scapula is outlined on the back along with that of the TCA, which courses over the shoulder on the undersurface of the trapezius muscle. The DSA enters the deep surface of the trapezius along the medial scapular border. Adduction and internal rotation of the ipsilateral arm is helpful to lateralize the scapula and open up the space between the scapula and the midline of the book.

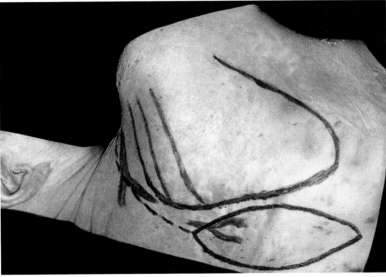

Figure 2-15. A skin paddle has been outlined between the medial border of the scapula and the midline of the back. The inferior extent of the skin paddle may be reliably placed up to 5 cm below the inferior border of the scapula.

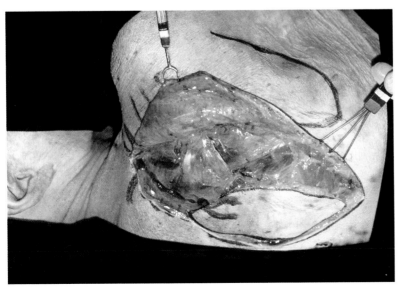

Figure 2-16. The dissection begins by incising the skin paddle and a vertical line drawn from the proximal tip of the skin paddle toward the posterior triangle of the neck. This incision is carried down to the level of the trapezius muscle, and then, skin flaps are elevated both medially and laterally to expose the full extent of the trapezius muscle.

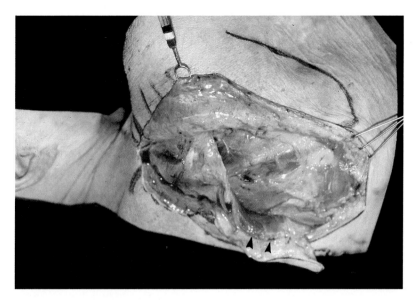

Figure 2-17. The lateral border of the trapezius (*arrows*) muscle has been identified and elevated, with the overlying skin paddle, in the plane between the trapezius and rhomboid muscles.

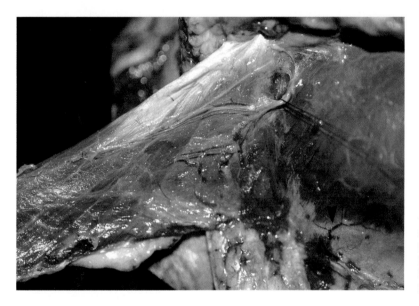

Figure 2-18. The muscle attachments to the midline vertebrae are then transsected sharply to mobilize the muscle distally to proximally. Paraspinous perforators (*arrow*) must be ligated and transsected. A suture has been placed around the dorsal scapular pedicle.

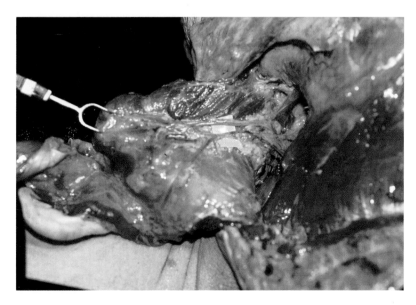

Figure 2-19. At the junction of the rhomboid major and rhomboid minor, the DSA and DSV are identified as they enter the undersurface of the trapezius muscle.

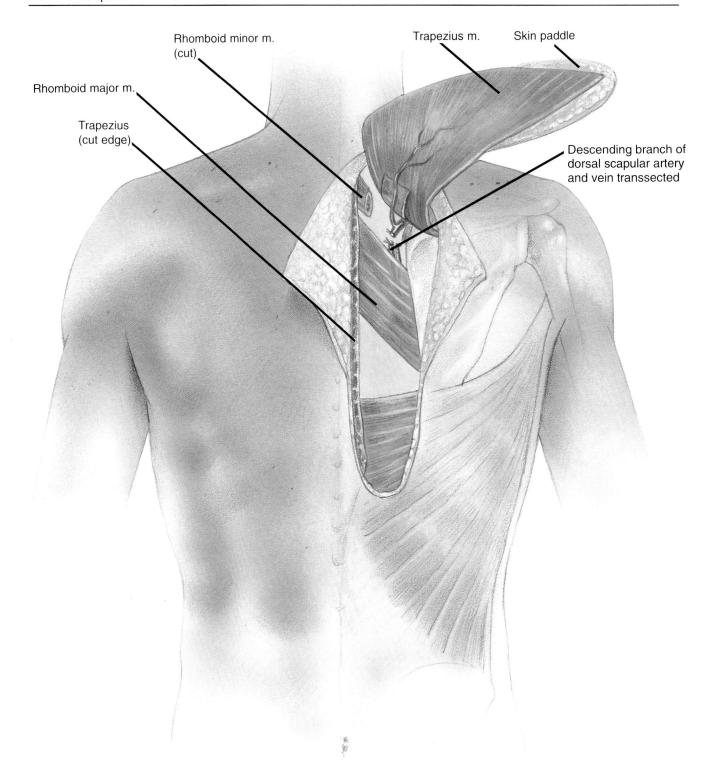

Figure 2-20. If the DSA and DSV are to be preserved and further mobilization of the trapezius muscle is required to reach the donor site, then dissection deep to the rhomboid muscles must be carried out to transsect the distal branches of the dorsal scapular pedicle. A cuff of rhomboid minor must be taken to allow the DSA and DSV to be mobilized.

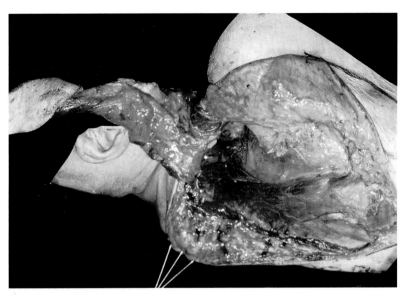

Figure 2-21. The DSA has been preserved through harvest of the cuff of the rhomboid minor muscle. With more proximal dissection, the TCA and TCV are identified on the undersurface of the trapezius muscle. Preservation of both of these pedicles to ensure vascularity to the distal portion of the muscle may be carried out, depending on the location of the recipient defect. If a temporary microvascular clamp applied to the DSA reveals no disturbance in the circulation to the distal skin paddle, then the DSA can be ligated and transsected. The arc of rotation is enhanced by transsecting the insertions of the trapezius muscle along the scapular spine and the medial attachments to the vertebrae. The flap has been completely mobilized. The cephalad extent to which the skin paddle can be used is evident by its position relative to the auricle. Wide undermining is critical for closure of the donor defect. A suction drain must be placed with an exit site along the midaxillary line.

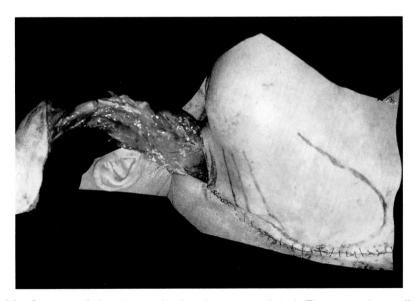

Figure 2-22. Closure of the donor site has been completed. The muscular pedicle may be tunneled under the intervening skin to provide access to the recipient defect. In select situations, exteriorization of the trapezius muscle may be preferable. The second stage transsection of the muscle must then be carried out in approximately 2 to 3 weeks.

REFERENCES

1. Ariyan S: One-stage repair of a cervical esophagostome with two myocutaneous flaps from the neck and shoulder. *Plast Reconstr Surg* 1979;63:426.
2. Aviv J, Urken ML, Lawson W and Biller HF: The superior trapezius myocutaneous flap in head and neck reconstruction. *Arch Otolaryngol Head Neck Surg* 1992;118:702.
3. Baek SM, Biller HF, Krespi YP, Lawson W: The lower trapezius island myocutaneous flap. *Ann Plast Surg* 1980;5:108–114.
4. Conley J: Use of composite flaps containing bone for major repairs in the head and neck. *Plast Reconstr Surg* 1972;49:522.
5. Cummings C, Eisele D, Coltrera M: The lower trapezius myocutaneous island flap. *Arch Otolaryngol Head Neck Surg* 1989;115:1181.
6. Demergasso F: The lateral trapezius flap. Presented at the Third International Symposium of Plastic and Reconstructive Surgery, New Orleans, Louisiana, April 29–May 4, 1979.
7. Demergasso F, Piazza M: Colgajo cutaneo aislada a pediculo muscular en cirugia reconstruction por cancer de cabeza y cuello: tecnica original. The 47th Congreso Argentine de Cirugia Forum de Investigaciones. *Rev Argent Chir* 1977;32:27.
8. Dufresne C, Cutting C, Valouri F, Klim M, Colen S: Reconstruction of mandibular and floor of mouth defects using the trapezius osteomyocutaneous flap. *Plast Reconstr Surg* 1987;79:687.
9. Goodwin WJ, Rosenberg G: Venous drainage of the lateral island trapezius musculocutaneous island flap. *Arch Otolaryngol Head Neck Surg* 1982;108:411.
10. Krespi Y, Oppenheimer R, dud Flanyer J: The rhombotrapezius myocutaneous and osteomyocutaneous flaps. *Arch Otolaryngol Head Neck Surg* 1988;114:734.
11. Maruyama Y, Nakajima H, Fujino T, Koda E: The definition of cutaneous vascular territories over the back using selective angiography and the intra-arterial injection of prostaglandin E_1: some observations on the use of the lower trapezius myocutaneous flap. *Br J Plast Surg* 1981;34:157.
12. Mathes S, Nahai F: Muscle flap transposition with function preservation: technical and clinical considerations. *Plast Reconstr Surg* 1980;66:242.
13. Mathes S, Nahai F: *Clinical Applications for Muscle and Musculocutaneous Flaps.* St. Louis: CV Mosby; 1982:50.
14. Mathes S, Stevenson T: Reconstruction of posterior neck and skull with vertical trapezius musculocutaneous flap. *Am J Surg* 1988;156:248.
15. Maves M, Phillippsen L: Surgical anatomy of the scapular spine in the trapezius-osteomuscular flap. *Arch Otolaryngol Head Neck Surg* 1986;112:173.
16. McCraw JB, Dibbell DG: Experimental definition of independent myocutaneous vascular territories. *Plast Reconstr Surg* 1977;60:212.
17. Mutter J: Cases of deformities of burns, relieved by operation. *Am J Med Sci* 1842;4:66.
18. Netterville J, Panje W, Maves M: The trapezius myocutaneous flap: dependability and limitations. *Arch Otolaryngol Head Neck Surg* 1987;113:271.
19. Netterville JL, Wood D: The lower trapezius flap: vascular anatomy and surgical technique. *Arch Otolaryngol Head Neck Surg* 1991;117:73.
20. Nichter L, Morgan R, Harman D, et al.: The trapezius musculocutaneous flap in head and neck reconstruction: potential pitfalls. *Head Neck* 1984;7:129.
21. Panje WR: The island (lateral) trapezius flap. Presented at the Third International Symposium of Plastic and Reconstructive Surgery, New Orleans, Louisiana, April 29–May 4, 1979.
22. Rosen H: The extended trapezius musculocutaneous flap for cranio-orbital facial reconstruction. *Plast Reconstr Surg* 1985;75:318.
23. Ryan R, Waterhouse N, Davies D: The innervated trapezius flap in facial paralysis. *Br J Plast Surg* 1988;41:344.
24. Taylor GI, Palmer JH, McManamny D: The vascular territories of the body (angiosomes) and their clinical applications. In: McCarthy JG, ed. *Plastic Surgery.* vol. 1. Philadelphia: WB Saunders; 1990:329.
25. Urken ML, Naidu R, Lawson W, Biller HF: The lower trapezius island musculocutaneous flap revisited. Report of 45 cases and a unifying concept of the vascular anatomy. *Arch Otolaryngol Head Neck Surg* 1991;117:502.
26. Zovickian A: Pharyngeal fistulas: repair and prevention using mastoid-occiput based shoulder flaps. *Plast Reconstr Surg* 1957;19:355.

3
CHAPTER

Sternocleidomastoid

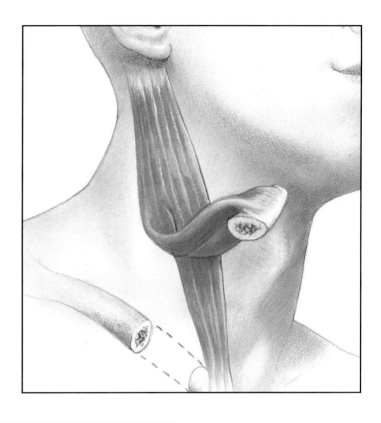

Mark L. Urken, M.D., and
Hugh F. Biller, M.D.

The first reported use of the sternocleidomastoid (SCM) muscle in head and neck reconstruction was by Jiano (19) in 1908 in which it was transposed to a paralyzed face to restore dynamic reanimation. Schottstaedt et al. (32) used the SCM to replace the masseter muscle in a child who had developed paralysis in the distribution of the trigeminal nerve, which resulted from poliomyelitis. Additional cases were reported by Dingman et al. (10) and Hamacher (14) who transferred a segment of the SCM muscle with its intact motor nerve and vascular supplies for replacement of the congenitally absent or paralyzed masseter. Owens (28), in 1955, is credited with being the first to report a musculocutaneous flap based on the SCM. He transferred a superiorly based flap but maintained a broad cutaneous attachment of the skin in the region of the mastoid (Figure 3-1). Owens incorporated the platysma and the SCM to enhance the blood supply to the skin. Bakamjian (4) modified Owens flap by extending the skin territory below the level of the clavicle. Littlewood (23) reported additional experience in using the extended SCM flap and identified the contributions of the occipital and posterior auricular arteries to the vascular supply of the muscle. O'Brien (27) is credited with being the first to transfer an island of skin overlying the caudal aspect of the neck with the SCM pedicled superiorly (Figure 3-2). Finally, Ariyan (2,3) identified the inferior vascular supply from the thyrocervical trunk and successfully transferred an inferiorly based flap (Figure 3-3).

The SCM flap has been extensively studied but not widely used. It has been criticized on oncologic grounds, which are related to the safety of preserving this muscle when there are regional lymphatic metastases. The limited size of the musculocuta-

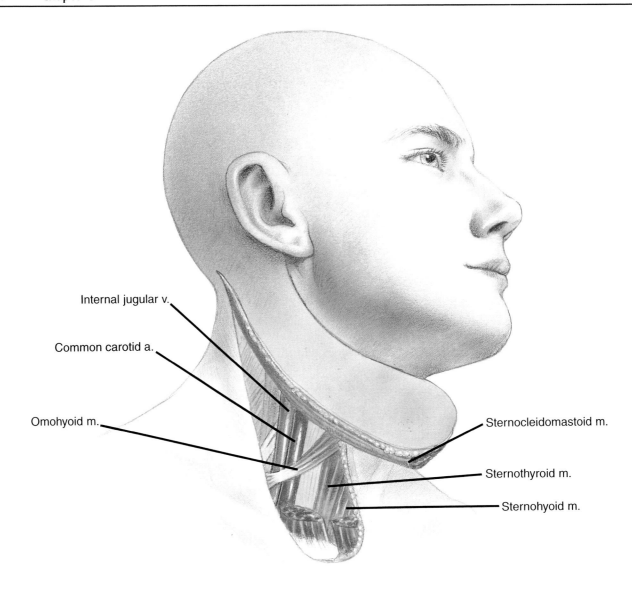

Internal jugular v.

Common carotid a.

Omohyoid m.

Sternocleidomastoid m.

Sternothyroid m.

Sternohyoid m.

Figure 3-1. The original SCM musculocutaneous flap described by Owens (28) had a broad attachment superiorly at the level of the mastoid and included the SCM and the platysma muscles. Bakamjian (4) modified this design by extending the skin paddle below the clavicle.

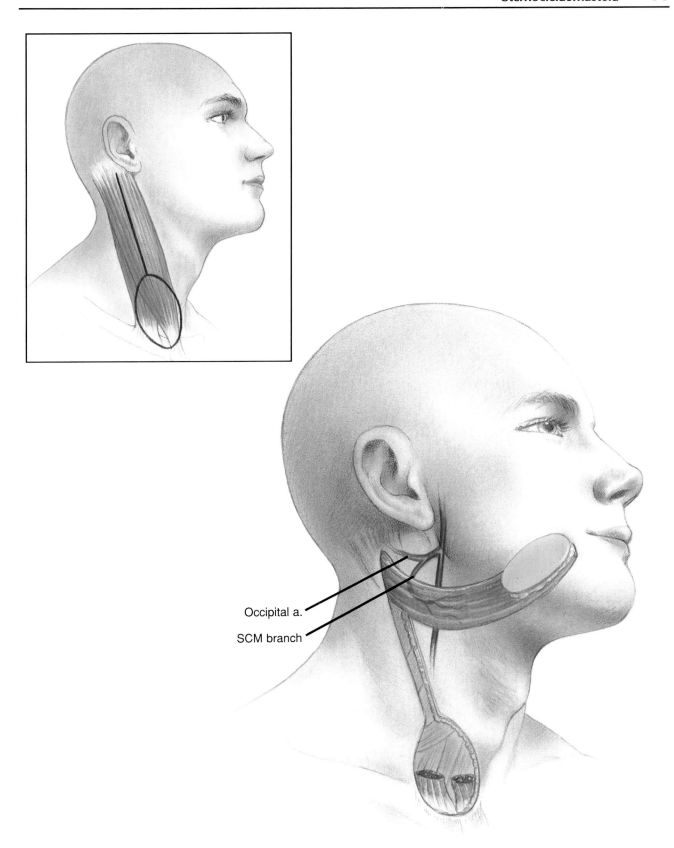

Occipital a.

SCM branch

Figure 3-2. The superiorly based SCM island musculocutaneous flap transfers skin from the caudal aspect of the neck that overlaps the distal third of the muscle and the medial portion of the clavicle. The primary blood supply to this flap arises from the posterior auricular, occipital, and the superior thyroid arteries.

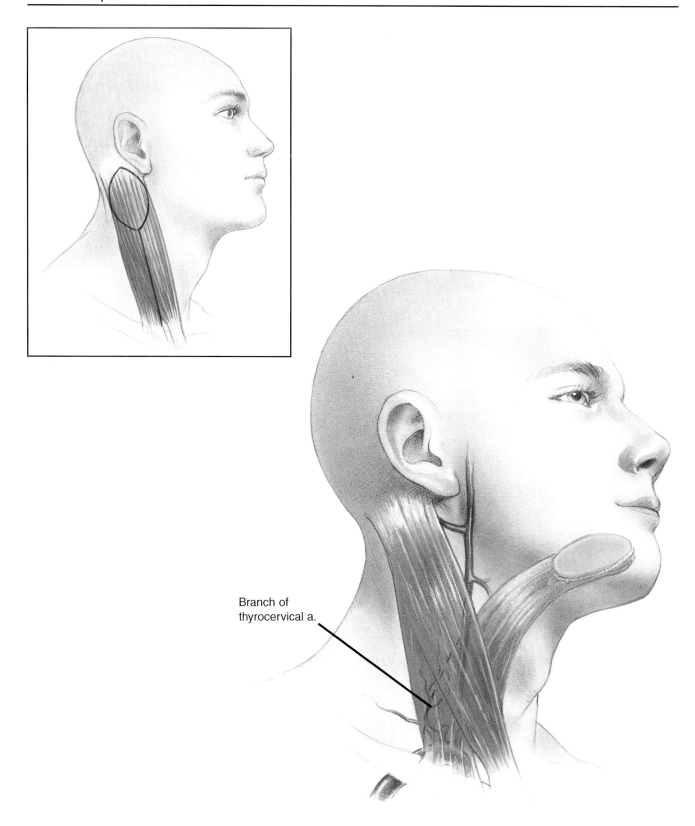

Branch of
thyrocervical a.

Figure 3-3. The inferiorly based SCM island musculocutaneous flap transfers a segment of skin overlying the upper third of the SCM muscle. The primary blood supply to this flap arises from the thyrocervical trunk and the superior thyroid artery.

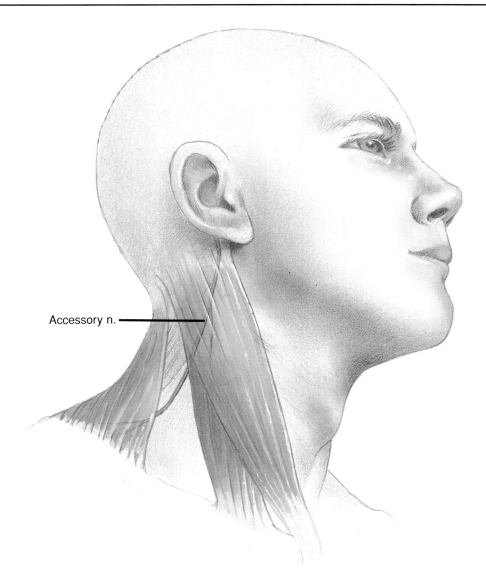

Accessory n.

Figure 3-4. The SCM muscle originates from the manubrium and the medial aspect of the clavicle. It inserts into the mastoid process and the superior nuchal line. The accessory cranial nerve supplies the innervation to the SCM and the trapezius muscles.

neous flap restricts its use to small defects. Finally, this flap has been criticized for the unreliability of the skin paddle and for the contour deformity in the neck following flap transfer. These issues are addressed in this chapter.

The SCM is a round muscle that originates from the manubrium and the medial aspect of the clavicle. It runs an oblique course in the neck to insert on the mastoid process and the superior nuchal line (Figure 3-4). Contraction of the SCM leads to tilting of the head, bringing the ipsilateral ear closer to the shoulder. The superficial layer of the deep cervical fascia splits to provide coverage of the SCM on both its deep and superficial surfaces (16).

FLAP DESIGN AND UTILIZATION

The evolution in flap design since the introduction of the broad superiorly based musculocutaneous flap of Owens (28) was outlined in the introduction to this chapter. The superiorly based and inferiorly based island musculocutaneous flaps are presently the most commonly used SCM flaps. Although Bakamjian (4) and Littlewood (23) extended the skin territory below the clavicle with the superiorly based "peninsular" flap, there has been little reported that substantiates such maximum dimensions when the flap is harvested as an island of skin. In addition to transfer of the musculocutaneous unit, there have been numerous reports of using the SCM to transfer clavicular periosteum (12,36,37) and segments of the clavicular bone for reconstruction of the mandible (5,35).

The problem of the donor site contour deformity was addressed by Alvarez et al. (1) who reported the use of the split SCM musculocutaneous flap in 1983. Transposition of the entire belly of the SCM produced an objectionable bulge in the midneck and a concavity in the lower neck. Alvarez et al. described a series of cases in which either the sternal head or the clavicular head of the muscle was transferred to the recipient site. They cautioned that this longitudinal split could only be carried through approximately two thirds of the muscle's belly in its longitudinal direction.

The ability to transfer the SCM with the preservation of its vascular and neural supply led to the application of this flap to reconstructive problems requiring dynamic activity. The early report by Jiano (19) in restoring mimetic activity to the paralyzed face was one such example. O'Brien (27) used the SCM to reconstruct a total lower lip defect, with the skin island providing the inner lining. The dynamic activity of the SCM was preserved and believed to have functional value in restoring oral competence. In the introduction, it was noted that this flap was also applied to the problem of dynamic restoration of the masticator muscle sling (10,14,31). Finally, Matulic et al. (26) reported the combination of the SCM muscle flap with a forehead cutaneous flap to reconstruct the oral cavity following glossectomy. The forehead flap provided the inner lining, and the SCM was transposed to provide dynamic tongue activity. As in many reconstructive techniques that purport to restore motion, the documentation by electromyography of motor activity does not necessarily translate into coordinated functional activity. An exception to this statement is in facial reanimation in which muscle transposition has been shown to be an effective means of restoring mimetic activity. The SCM has been supplanted by the temporalis and masseter muscles because of the improved axis of pull of the latter two muscles in producing a symmetric smile.

The SCM muscle flap has also been used to restore a normal lateral facial contour following parotidectomy and mandibular reconstruction. Hill and Brown (15) transposed a superiorly based muscle flap over a free iliac bone graft to achieve a more satisfactory lower facial contour in secondary mandibular reconstruction. Bugis et al. (7) reported their experience with the use of the SCM muscle flap to restore the facial contour in 31 patients following parotidectomy. In addition, they reported the successful application of this flap in two patients who had postoperative salivary fistulas. Despite these findings, the SCM muscle flap was not found to be an effective method to prevent Frey's syndrome in an extensive series of patients reported by Kornblut et al. (20,21). A group of 35 patients who underwent parotidectomy and SCM muscle transposition into the parotid bed were compared with a control group of 35 patients who underwent comparable ablative procedures but no muscle transposition. The rationale for transposing the muscle was to interfere with the presumed mechanism of Frey's syndrome, which is the misdirection of auriculotemporal secretomotor fibers from their normal end organ, which is the salivary tissue. It is thought that the transsected nerves are rerouted to the sweat glands of the overlying skin, thereby producing "gustatory sweating." Kornblut et al. reported no difference in the incidence of Frey's syndrome in the two study groups.

The SCM musculocutaneous flap has been used for oral and pharyngeal mucosal defects since Bakamjian's (4) initial report of the use of this flap to reconstruct the palate following radical maxillectomy. As noted previously, Bakamjian used an extended peninsular skin muscle flap that was transferred through the posterior oral cavity. At a second stage, the flap's pedicle was transsected, with closure of the orostoma. Ariyan (3) reported 14 cases of either superior or inferior musculocutaneous flaps used in the oral cavity or pharynx. He noted "partial epithelial loss" in seven cases, but only one developed a salivary fistula. Re-epithelialization of the denuded areas of the oral cavity was reported, and biopsies from the healed reconstructed site demonstrated preservation of the dermal layer. In this report, Ariyan also described primary closure of the donor site defect through cutaneous advancement flaps rather than by application of a skin graft. Additional reports on the SCM musculocutaneous flap cited varying degrees of skin viability. Sasaki (31) used four inferiorly based and one superiorly based flap to reconstruct the floor of the mouth and tonsillar regions. The skin of the superiorly based flap underwent total necrosis; partial skin necrosis was reported in two of the remaining inferiorly based flaps. Despite these complications, there were no cases of salivary fistulas, which Sasaki attributed to the viability of the underlying SCM muscle. Marx and McDonald (24) reported a more favorable experience with the superiorly based flap in eight patients in whom they noted distal skin necrosis 2 cm from the tip of the flap. These 8 cases of oral cavity reconstruction represented a subset of the 16 reported cases of SCM flaps also used for a variety of other indications. These authors emphasized the necessity of maintaining the vascular contributions from the superior thyroid artery and vein. The importance of this contribution from the superior thyroid pedicle is discussed later in detail. Finally, Ariyan (2) reported closure of a cervical esophagostoma by using a superiorly based SCM flap for inner lining followed by a superior trapezius flap for outer cutaneous coverage.

The use of vascularized segments of the clavicle supplied by adjacent soft tissue was introduced in the early 1970s as a solution to the frustrating problem of restoring bone continuity following segmental mandibulectomy. Siemssen et al. (35) referred to two of the earliest reports that used portions of the clavicle to reconstruct the mandible, which dated back to the beginning of the 20th century. They credited Rydygier (30) with being the first to transfer an osteocutaneous flap containing a portion of the clavicle. This was followed by Blair's (6) description of composite flaps containing clavicle and rib. Snyder et al. (36) is credited with reviving this concept with a report issued in the current era in which vascularized bone was used to restore bony defects of the maxillofacial skeleton. They reported several cases of vascularized bone transfer based on regional cutaneous flaps. They transferred either full- or split-thickness segments of clavicle with the overlying skin in a two-stage procedure. This publication was followed by Conley's (9) report in 1972 of a series of 50 regional bone-containing flaps for mandibulofacial reconstruction. Included in this series were a variety of different composite flaps, including the deltopectoral acromion flap, the trapezius–scapular flap, the temporalis–calvarial flap, and the SCM–clavicular flap. Although Conley reported three complete flap failures in this series, there were few details regarding the actual techniques used for each of these donor sites. He warned about the potential shoulder morbidity associated from segmental defects of the clavicle and advised that a sagittal split be performed to transfer only the outer cortex.

Siemssen et al. (35) reported on a series of 18 patients who underwent mandibular reconstruction with either split or segmental segments of the clavicle pedicled on the clavicular head of the SCM. Although seven bone flaps were transferred in the primary setting, internal lining was achieved with either a forehead or deltopectoral flap. There were significant complications in the group of five patients in this series who underwent split clavicle transfers, with fractures occurring at both the donor and recipient sites. In the remaining patients in this series, a full segment of the clavicle was harvested anterior to the attachment of the trapezius muscle (Figure 3-5). The authors reported little to no shoulder morbidity in these patients. In addition, the clavicle was pedicled on the clavicular head of the SCM and passed under the sternal head to avoid a contour deformity in the neck. Finally, they speculated about the possibility of reconstructing a near-total mandibular defect by transferring the anterior portions of both clavicles with an intervening segment of the manubrium pedicled on both SCM muscles. There was only one total flap necrosis in this series.

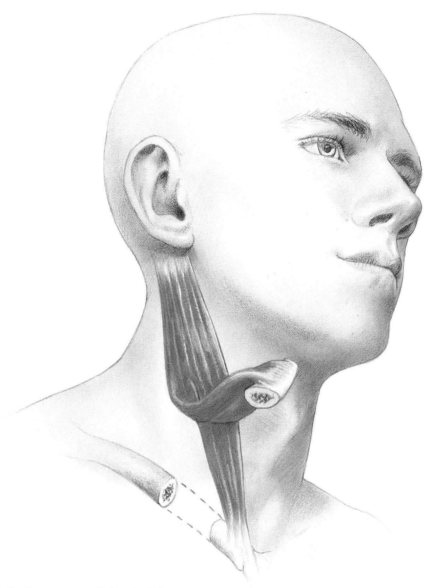

Figure 3-5. A segment of the clavicle a pedicled on the clavicular head of the SCM may be transferred as a vascularized bone graft.

Barnes et al. (5) reported a similar favorable experience with the use of this musculoclavicular flap in four primary and one delayed mandibular reconstruction. The viability of the neomandible was confirmed with postoperative technetium scans.

The SCM musculoclavicular flap has also been used for rigid support in laryngotracheal reconstruction for the correction of stenotic segments. Schuller and Parrish (33) reported the successful use of vascularized split clavicle grafts to provide rigid support of the cervical airway. Approximately one half the circumference of the clavicle was harvested and "hollowed out" with a bone curette to create a rigid lumen. The bony shell was then lined with a free mucosal graft. Alternatively, Tovi and Gittot (37) described a myoperiosteal flap to achieve a similar result (Figure 3-6). The clavicular periosteum, pedicled on the SCM, was used to repair noncircumferential defects of the larynx and trachea in three patients. A stent was placed in one patient. All three patients were successfully decannulated, and at the time of follow-up endoscopy, the reconstructed portion of the airway was relined with normal-appearing respiratory epithelium. Friedman et al. (12) examined the SCM myoperiosteal flap in dogs who underwent tracheal reconstruction. The growth of new bone from the transplanted periosteum was documented at the 6- and 9-month follow-ups. In addition, the patency of the lumen was preserved.

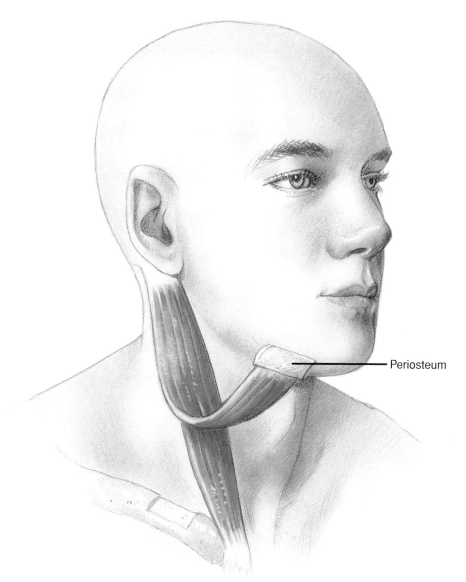

Periosteum

Figure 3-6. The SCM myoperiosteal flap transfers vascularized periosteum for use in airway reconstruction.

An alternative technique for the repair of laryngotracheal stenoses was described by Eliachar and Moscona (11) who used a SCM island musculocutaneous flap. This flap was used to augment the lumen after resection of the stenotic framework. A T-tube with a laryngeal stent were kept in place for 4 to 6 weeks after surgery.

NEUROVASCULAR ANATOMY

The vascular supply to the SCM muscle and its overlying skin is arguably the most confusing of any flap used in head and neck reconstruction. This is one explanation why this flap has not been embraced with a significant amount of enthusiasm. The SCM has a type II vascular supply, according to the classification scheme of Mathes and Nahai (25). There is one dominant pedicle arising superiorly from the occipital artery and vein and three minor pedicles: a branch of the posterior auricular artery and vein, a branch of the superior thyroid artery and vein, and a branch of the thyrocervical trunk (Figure 3-7). As noted previously, the segmental nature of the vascular supply allows this muscle to be pedicled either superiorly or inferiorly. The motor supply to the SCM is from a branch of the accessory nerve, which continues across

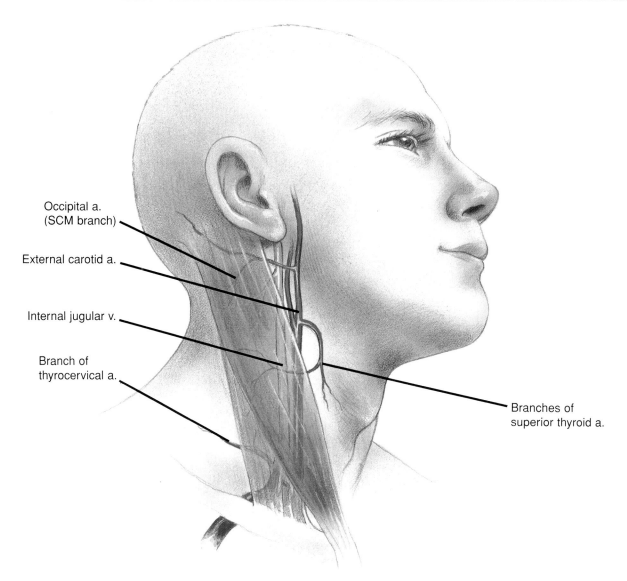

Occipital a.
(SCM branch)

External carotid a.

Internal jugular v.

Branch of
thyrocervical a.

Branches of
superior thyroid a.

Figure 3-7. The dominant arterial supply to the SCM muscle is from the occipital artery. Minor vascular contributions arise from branches of the posterior auricular artery, the superior thyroid artery, and the thyrocervical trunk.

the posterior triangle of the neck to innervate the trapezius muscle as well. There remains some controversy as to whether the contribution to the SCM's innervation from C-2 and C-3 is motor or sensory.

The successful transfer of skin as a musculocutaneous flap requires preservation of the vascular supply to the muscle and capture of the musculocutaneous perforators that exit the superficial surface of the muscle. The relationship of the SCM to the overlying cervical skin varies, depending on whether the caudal aspect of the neck or the region below the mastoid tip is regarded. The reason for this difference is the presence of the platysma muscle, which is a sheetlike muscle of varying thickness that runs in the superficial fascia of the neck (Figure 3-8). It arises below the clavicle from the muscular fascia overlying the pectoralis major and the deltoid. It courses obliquely across the neck at right angles to the SCM to blend with the muscles inserting on the lower lip. The paired platysma muscles are deficient in the midline of the neck; laterally, they overlap the SCM only to approximately the midlevel of the neck. Therefore, the caudal half of the SCM is separated from the overlying skin by a layer of platysma; the cephalad half has no such intervening layer. This difference can readily be felt by assessing the relative mobility of the lower neck skin compared with the tightly adherent skin of the upper neck.

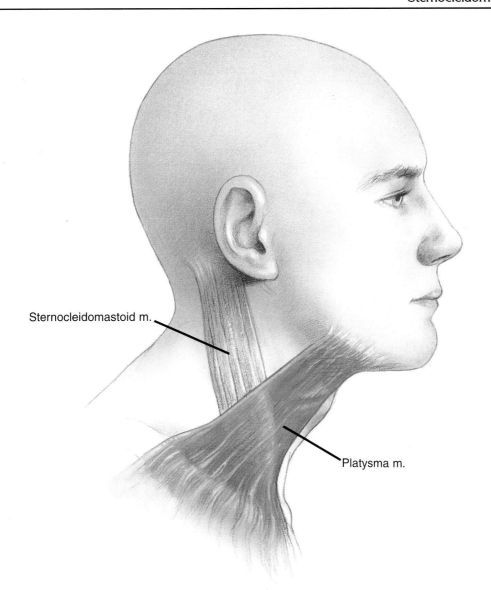

Sternocleidomastoid m.

Platysma m.

Figure 3-8. The platysma muscle originates from the muscular fascia overlying the pectoralis major and runs an oblique course across the neck. It completely overlaps the caudal aspect of the SCM muscle.

The platysma muscle is a vestige of the panniculus carnosus in lower animals. The skin is tightly adherent to this muscle, and it has long been recognized that cervical skin flaps are more viable when the platysma is included. The platysma has been successfully used as a carrier of cervical skin, as introduced by Futrell et al. (13) in 1978. The platysma is primarily supplied by the submental branch of the facial artery. The platysma musculocutaneous unit has been shown to be reliable in subsequent reports (8).

What is unique about the superiorly based SCM island flap is that a successful outcome requires capture by a deeper muscle (SCM) of a more superficial musculocutaneous unit (platysma). There is no other flap used in the head and neck or perhaps elsewhere in the body in which the blood supply to the skin must traverse two distinct muscle layers. The cephalad portion of the muscle appears to be a more favorable donor site to harvest skin because of the lack of the intervening muscle layer. However, the inferiorly based flap is at a disadvantage as a result of the smaller vascular pedicle entering the caudal aspect of the muscle.

Studies that have investigated the vascular supply to the cervical skin are helpful in shedding light on this problem. One of the earliest reports that looked at the vascular contributions from the SCM to the cervical skin was by Jabaley et al. (18) In a series of cadaver dissections, these investigators reported an extreme paucity of musculo-cutaneous perforators arising from the lower two thirds of the SCM. They did, however, identify a direct cutaneous branch from the transverse cervical artery that penetrates the platysma to supply the supraclavicular skin.

Two publications from the University of Pittsburgh reported on a series of fresh cadaveric studies that also examined the blood supply to the cervical skin. A summary of the findings in these two studies is enlightening (17,29). These investigators corroborated the observations of Jabaley et al. (18) that there are few musculocutaneous perforators from the SCM and those that were present are extremely small. Direct cutaneous perforators were identified from a number of sources, including the occipital, posterior auricular, and superior thyroid arteries, which were the most consistent. These three branches of the external carotid artery, therefore, supply feeders to the SCM muscle and direct perforators to the skin. In 80% of the cadaver dissections, a large cutaneous vessel from the superior thyroid artery was identified coursing around the anterior border of the SCM, which supplied the platysma and skin of the midneck. It is likely that the success reported by Marx and McDonald (24) in their series of superiorly based SCM flaps was directly related to the preservation of the superior thyroid branches. Ink-injection studies of the cutaneous branch of the superior thyroid artery caused staining of the skin of the middle and lower cervical regions. In one dissection, the direct cutaneous branch from the superior thyroid system traveled on the undersurface of the SCM and then entered the platysma and the overlying skin between the sternal and clavicular heads of the SCM (29).

This review of the vascular anatomy points out potential pitfalls in regard to both the superiorly and the inferiorly based island flaps. The superiorly based flap preserves the dominant blood supply to the muscle but is problematic because of the intervening layer of platysma. The inferiorly based flap relies on the nondominant contributions to the muscle from the caudal aspect of the neck after transsecting the dominant cephalad muscular branches. However, the skin overlying the cephalad portion of the SCM appears to be more favorably related to the muscle because of the absence of the platysma. The peninsular skin flap, as described by Owens (28), should have an excellent chance of viability because of the preservation of the dominant blood supply to the muscle and direct cutaneous feeders to the skin entering from the occipital and posterior auricular branches. Muscle only or muscle plus periosteum, with or without clavicle, also appear to be reliable flaps.

POTENTIAL PITFALLS

Many of the potential complications of this donor site have been discussed in this chapter. The viability of the skin of either a superiorly or an inferiorly based flap is questionable. However, the experience of Marx and McDonald (24), suggests that preservation of the superior thyroid artery may be extremely important, for the reasons mentioned. It may be possible to mobilize the superior thyroid pedicle to enhance the arc of rotation.

One of the other major criticisms of this donor site is its intimate relationship to the region of most common nodal metastases from the head and neck primaries. The necessity for a formal radical neck dissection eliminates this flap as a surgical option. Modified neck dissections may allow preservation of the SCM, but its vascular supply is placed in jeopardy. Transfer of a SCM flap from the contralateral neck may be feasible. Arguments against violating a potential site of regional metastases have been raised (22). However, the opposing point of view in this controversy is that, in raising the SCM, the posterior fascial layer does not need to be violated and, therefore, the envelope of deep cervical fascia that encloses the lymph node-bearing tissue can be preserved.

The largest published series of SCM flaps was reported by Sebastian et al. in 1994 (34). A total of 121 superiorly based SCM flaps were utilized in 120 patients with clinically N0 necks. The branches to the SCM muscle arising from the occipital artery were preserved. Total flap loss occurred in 7.3% of patients while superficial skin loss was reported in 22.7%. Orocutaneous fistulas were noted in 11.8% of patients. The authors noted a significantly higher incidence of flap complications in patients who were previously irradiated. Finally, nodal recurrence occurred in 5.7% of ipsilateral necks that were pathologically N0 and in 17.4% of ipsilateral necks that demonstrated pathologically positive nodes.

Flap Harvesting Technique

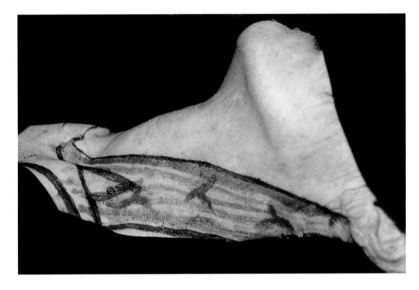

Figure 3-9. The left sternocleidomastoid muscle is outlined over the left neck with the approximate positions of the superior, middle, and inferior blood supplies.

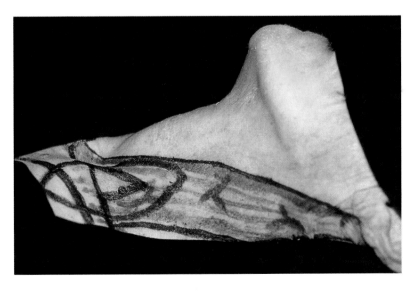

Figure 3-10. The skin paddle of a superiorly based island flap is outlined over the caudal aspect of the muscle.

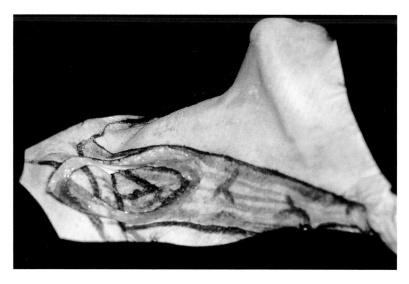

Figure 3-11. An incision is made around the perimeter of the skin flap. The caudal aspect of the flap overlies the clavicle. The incision is carried through the skin, subcutaneous tissue, and platysma muscle to expose the superficial layer of the deep cervical fascia, which encompasses the SCM.

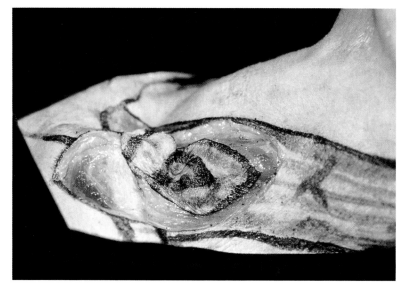

Figure 3-12. The random caudal extension of the skin is elevated off the clavicular periosteum. The inferior attachments of the SCM to the clavicle are transsected. Care must be taken to avoid causing any shearing forces between the skin and the underlying SCM. If a segment of the clavicle is to be harvested, osteotomies would be made at this time.

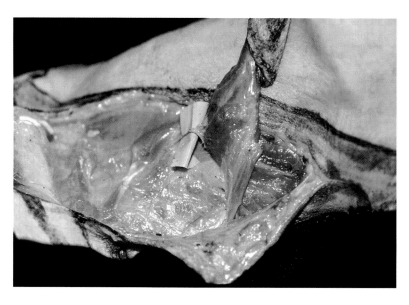

Figure 3-13. A vertical incision has been made to expose the cephalad portion of the SCM. The inferior blood supply from the thyrocervical trunk has been transsected. The middle blood supply from the superior thyroid artery and vein is shown entering the deep surface of the SCM just above the omohyoid muscle.

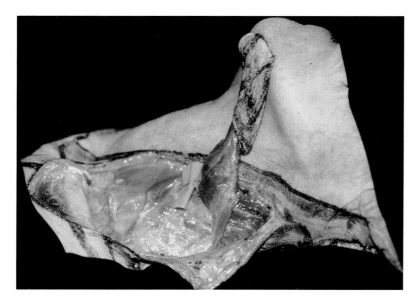

Figure 3-14. Preservation of the superior thyroid pedicle limits the arc of rotation but improves the vascular supply to the superiorly based SCM flap.

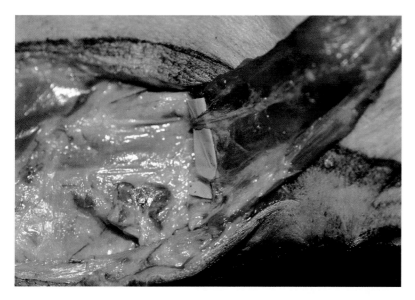

Figure 3-15. The dominant superior blood supply arising from either the occipital artery or directly from the external carotid artery has been isolated. This branch usually runs a course cephalad to the hypoglossal nerve.

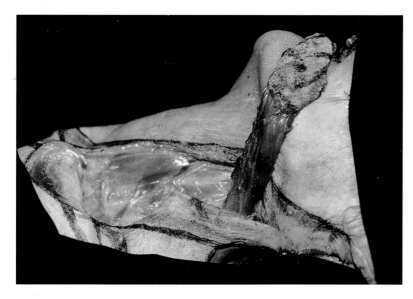

Figure 3-16. By transsecting the caudal and middle blood supply, the arc of rotation is greatly improved. This flap can be used for intraoral, facial, and pharyngeal defects.

REFERENCES

1. Alvarez G, Escamilla J, Carranza A: The split sternocleidomastoid myocutaneous flap. *Br J Plast Surg* 1983;36:183–186.
2. Ariyan S: One-stage repair of a cervical esophagostoma with two myocutaneous flaps from the neck and shoulder. *Plast Reconstr Surg* 1979;63:426–429.
3. Ariyan S: One stage reconstruction for defects of the mouth using a sternomastoid myocutaneous flap. *Plast Reconstr Surg* 1979;63:618–625.
4. Bakamjian V: A technique for primary reconstruction of the palate after radical maxillectomy for cancer. *Plast Reconstr Surg* 1963;31:103–117.
5. Barnes D, Ossoff R, Pecaro B, Sission G: Immediate reconstruction of mandibular defects with a composite sternocleidomastoid musculoclavicular graft. *Arch Otolaryngol Head Neck Surg* 1981;107: 711–714.
6. Blair VP: *Surgery and Diseases of the Mouth and Jaws*. St. Louis: CV Mosby; 1918.
7. Bugis S, Young J, Archibald S: Sternocleidomastoid flap following parotidectomy. *Head Neck* 1990;12:430–435.
8. Coleman J, Jurkiewicz M, Nahai F, Matthes S: The platysma musculocutaneous flap: experience with 24 cases. *Plast Reconstr Surg* 1983;72:315–321.
9. Conley J: Use of composite flaps containing bone for major repairs in the head and neck. *Plast Reconstr Surg* 1972;49:522–526.
10. Dingman RO, Grabb WC, O'Neal RM, Ponitz RJ: Sternocleidomastoid muscle transplant to masseter area: case of congenital absence of muscles of mastication. *Plast Reconstr Surg* 1969;43:5–12.
11. Eliachar I, Moscona AR: Reconstruction of the laryngotracheal complex in children using the sternocleidomastoid myocutaneous flap. *Head Neck* 1981;4:16–21.
12. Friedman M, Grybaieskas V, Skolnick E, Toriumi D, Chilis T: Sternomastoid myoperiosteal flap for reconstruction of the subglottic larynx. *Ann Otol Rhinol Laryngol* 1987;96:163–169.
13. Futrell J, Johns M, Edgerton M, Cantrell R, Fitz-Hugh GS: Platysma myocutaneous flap for intraoral reconstruction. *Am J Surg* 1978;136:504–507.
14. Hamacher E: Sternocleidomastoid muscle transplants. *Plast Reconstr Surg* 1969;1:1–4.
15. Hill H, Brown R: The sternocleidomastoid flap to restore facial contour in mandibular reconstruction. *Br J Plast Surg* 1978;31:143–146.
16. Hollinshead WH: *Anatomy for Surgeons: The Head and Neck*. New York: Harper and Row; 1982: 446.
17. Hurwitz D, Rabson J, Futrell JW: The anatomic basis for the platysma skin flap. *Plast Reconstr Surg* 1983;72:302–314.
18. Jabaley M, Heckler F, Wallace W, Knott L: Sternocleidomastoid regional flaps: a new look at an old concept. *Br J Plast Surg* 1979;32:106–113.
19. Jiano J: Paralizie faciale dupa extriparea unei tumori a parotidee trata prin operatia dlui gomoue. *Bull Mem Soc Clin Bucharest* 1908;vol:22.
20. Kornblut A, Westphal P, Michlke A: The effectiveness of a sternomastoid muscle flap in preventing post-parotidectomy occurrence of the Frey syndrome. *Acta Otolaryngol (Stockh)* 1974;77:368–373.
21. Kornblut A, Westphal P, Michlke A: A re-evaluation of the Frey syndrome following parotid surgery. *Arch Otolaryngol Head Neck Surg* 1977;103:258–261.
22. Larson DL, Goepfert H: Limitations of the sternocleidomastoid musculocutaneous flap in head and neck cancer reconstruction. *Plast Reconstr Surg* 1982;3:328–335.
23. Littlewood M: Compound skin and sternomastoid flaps for repair in extensive carcinoma of the head and neck. *Plast Reconstr Surg* 1967;20:403–419.
24. Marx RE, McDonald DK: The sternocleidomastoid muscle as a muscular or myocutaneous flap for oral and facial reconstruction. *J Oral Maxillofac Surg* 1985;213:155–162.
25. Mathes S, Nahai F: *Clinical Applications for Muscle and Musculocutaneous Flaps*. St. Louis: CV Mosby; 1982:38–39.
26. Matulic Z, Bartovic M, Mikolji V, Viras M: Tongue reconstruction by means of the sternocleidomastoid muscle and a forehead flap. *Br J Plast Surg* 1978;31:147–151.
27. O'Brien B: A muscle-skin pedicle for total reconstruction of the lower lip: case report. *Plast Reconstr Surg* 1970;45:395–399.
28. Owens N: A compound neck pedicle designed for the repair of massive facial defects: formation, development, and application. *Plast Reconstr Surg* 1955;15:369–389.
29. Rabson J, Hurwitz D, Futrell J: The cutaneous blood supply of the neck: relevance to incision planning and surgical reconstruction. *Br J Plast Surg* 1985;38:208–219.
30. Rydygier LR: Zum Osteoplastischen ersatz nach Unterkieferresektion. *Zentralbl Chir* 1908;36:1321.
31. Sasaki C: The sternocleidomastoid myocutaneous flap. *Arch Otolaryngol Head Neck Surg* 1980;106: 74–76.
32. Schottstaedt E, Larsen L, Bost F: Complete muscle transposition. *J Bone Joint Surg* 1955;37:897–919.
33. Schuller D, Parrish RT: Reconstruction of the larynx and trachea. *Arch Otolaryngol Head Neck Surg* 1988;114:278–286.
34. Sebastian P, Cherian T, Ahamed I, Jayakumar K, Sivaramakrishnan P: The sternomastoid island myocutaneous flap for oral cancer reconstruction. *Arch Otolaryngol Head Neck Surg* 1994;120:629.
35. Siemssen S, Kirkby B, O'Connor T: Immediate reconstruction of a resected segment of the lower jaw using a compound flap of clavicle and sternomastoid muscle. *Plast Reconstr Surg* 1978;61:724–735.
36. Snyder C, Bateman J, Davis C, Warden G: Mandibulofacial restoration with live osteocutaneous flaps. *Plast Reconstr Surg* 1970;45:14–19.
37. Tovi F, Gittot A: Sternocleidomastoid myoperiosteal flap for the repair of laryngeal and tracheal wall defects. *Head Neck* 1983;5:447–451.

REGIONAL FLAPS
Muscle and Musculocutaneous Flaps

Temporalis

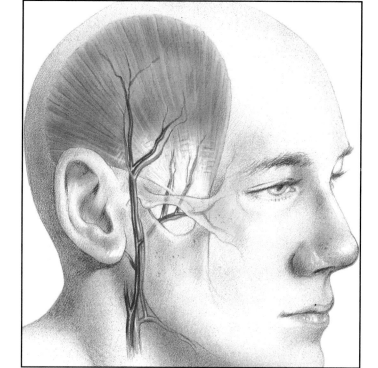

Mack L. Cheney, M.D.

Because of its anatomical proximity to the midface and its ease of transfer, the temporalis muscle has been used for a variety of reconstructive problems in the maxillofacial region (4,6,12,15,18,19,21,24,28). Described in 1898 by Golovine (12), the temporalis flap is one of the earliest reported muscle flaps (16). It was initially reported for use in obliterating the dead space following orbital exenteration owing to the bulk and proximity of the temporalis muscle to the orbit (3,8,12,23,24,31). In the 1930s, Gillies (11) introduced the use of the temporalis as a method of rehabilitation of the paralyzed face. Sheehan (30) also added to the early development of this flap by describing the reduction or removal of the zygomatic arch to increase the arc of rotation and to improve the problem of excessive bulk in the midface. In 1951, Anderson modified the Gillies technique by using temporalis fascia, instead of the fascia lata, to reconstruct the eyelids in patients with facial paralysis (28). In the 1970s and 1980s, May (19–21), McKenna et al. (22), Rubin et al. (29), Rubin (28), and Edgerton et al.(9) added substantially to the usefulness of this flap by their reports advocating the use of temporalis muscle in the management of the paralyzed face. Rubin et al. (29) and Rubin (26–28) also clarified the application of this flap in oral commissure reanimation by carefully categorizing human smile patterns and detailing the anatomic relationship between the orbicularis oris and the facial muscles. These reports established the temporalis as a logical option for reanimation of the paralyzed face. Further refinements in the transfer of the temporalis increased its clinical usefulness in managing contour defects following maxillofacial resections (3,4,25) and in eyelid (14) and intraoral reconstruction (5).

FLAP DESIGN AND UTILIZATION

The temporalis flap has gained acceptance for a variety of clinical purposes, including the augmentation of regional tissue deficiencies and the elimination of scar contractures. It may also serve as a vascular surface for free skin grafting, as protection for the carotid artery, as a myo-osseous flap, and provide dynamic rehabilitation of the paralyzed face (6,9,19–22,27–29).

The temporalis may be transferred in its entirety or in part, depending on the reconstructive challenge. The dimensions of the muscle vary with the thicker aspect of the muscle located in the anterior third of the temporal fossa; the middle and posterior thirds of the muscle are consistently thinner and slightly longer. The length of the muscle in the middle third makes this portion ideal for use in the rehabilitation of the paralyzed face. Although some authors have relied on the muscle for ocular and midfacial rehabilitation, it has been our experience that the independent reconstruction of these two important functional zones of the face improves the overall outcome. This approach allows the surgeon to limit the amount of the muscle transferred into the midface, thereby minimizing the degree of contour irregularity over the zygomatic arch.

The temporalis has established itself as an important technique for the reconstruction of the paralyzed face (Figure 4-1). Although criticized by many because of its lack of spontaneous facial movement, the transferred temporalis allows for immediate reanimation of the paralyzed face and may be used when potential facial nerve recovery exists. The muscle has many anatomical characteristics, which make it desirable for use in facial rehabilitation. It is relatively short (3 to 5 cm) and thin (2 to 3 mm) and has a contraction capability of 1 to 1.5 cm. The midportion of the muscle has sufficient strength to adequately mobilize the face and resist the forces of soft tissue contracture (21,22). An additional advantage when using this muscle is the fact that it is innervated in a segmented pattern by the branches of the trigeminal nerve (branch V2). This allows for independent segments of the muscle to be designed for use in the orbit and midface. For a muscle transfer to be functional, it must have an origin and a point of insertion. The zygomatic arch can be used effectively to provide the transferred muscle with a fixed point of origin after it is transposed into the midface.

Although the temporalis is firmly attached to the coronoid process and ramus, the surgeon can vary the point of attachment of the distal transposed end of the muscle. This flexibility has been noted by Renner et al. (25), Rubin et al. (29), and Rubin (26,27) and allows the vectors of muscle contracture to be varied in an attempt to individualize the procedure to the particular characteristics of the patient's smile, as analyzed on the normal side (6,22,25–26).

There have been several limitations noted when the temporalis is used for facial reanimation. Muscle contracture is initiated by the fifth cranial nerve and is therefore not mimetic with the contralateral face. This drawback can be improved by early and regular physical therapy. The other common concern with this technique has been the management of the donor site. When the muscle is transferred over the zygomatic arch, the contour of the temporoparietal scalp and the midface can become distorted. By limiting the amount of muscle that is transferred to a 2-cm width from the middle third of the body of the muscle, the amount of bulk over the zygoma is minimized. The segmental neurovascular supply allows the muscle to be safely divided in this fashion. The secondary depression in the infratemporal fossa has conventionally been managed with synthetic implants. However, these implants have an unnatural feel and are susceptible to extrusion. As an alternative solution to this problem, we have elevated an independent temporoparietal fascial flap, based on the superficial temporal artery and vein, and used this flap to reliably re-establish the scalp contour of this region (6).

Cranial nerve injury is a common consequence of skull base procedures. Although the sensory function of the fifth cranial nerve is commonly affected, the motor com-

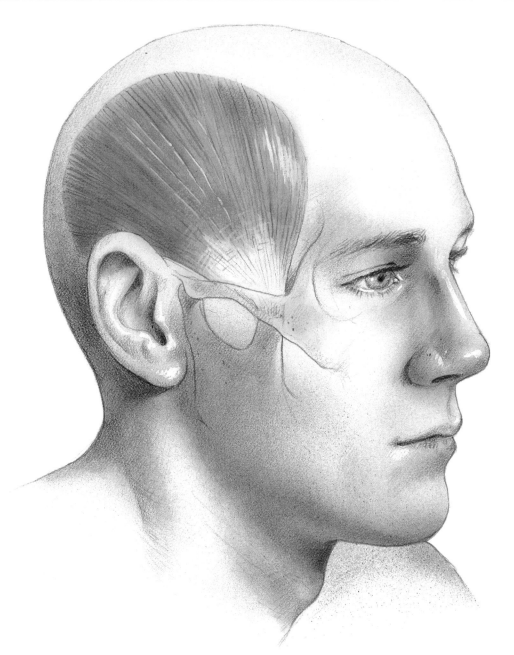

Figure 4-1. The temporalis originates from the surface of the calvarium on the lateral aspect of the skull. The superior attachment forms a gentle arc that is referred to as the inferior temporal line. The temporalis occupies the entire temporal fossa and inserts into the coronoid process and the anterior aspect of the mandibular ramus. The temporalis is covered by a thick fascial layer, the temporalis muscular fascia, which is described as being a second point of origin of the muscle. The temporalis fascia is adherent to the skull at the superior temporal line where it is continuous with the pericranium that covers the remainder of the skull. Inferiorly, the temporalis muscular fascia splits into a deep and superficial layer approximately 2 cm cephalad to the arch. These two layers merge with the periosteum of the medial and lateral surfaces of the zygomatic arch, respectively. The superficial layer of the deep muscular fascia is continuous with the masseteric muscular fascia.

ponent of this nerve is rarely involved. The temporalis muscle is, therefore, a viable option for the reconstruction of the paralyzed face when other cranial nerve–muscle units may not be available.

The temporalis has been used to reconstruct a variety of midfacial defects by designing it as a turnover flap, with the point of rotation based at the zygomatic arch. Because the flap has a rotational radius of 8 cm, it is possible to cover defects of the mastoid, cheek, pharynx, and palate. The muscle is longer and thinner than the masseter, and therefore, it can be placed throughout the midface, which allows muscle bulk to be transferred to anatomic locations that are not within the rotational range of other regional muscle flaps (7,13). The arc of rotation can be improved by passing the temporalis deep to the zygomatic arch, a maneuver that is often made simpler by osteotomies to remove and then replace the bone. An additional advantage of the temporalis is that it readily accepts split-thickness skin grafts. This feature may be useful in managing full-thickness defects of the middle third of the face.

Although temporalis transposition has been used primarily for rehabilitation of the paralyzed face, it can also be considered for the reconstruction of full-thickness defects in the midface. It provides adequate bulk to obliterate full-thickness defects of the orbit and lateral oral cavity (15). Orbital cavity defects may be managed by a variety of techniques. The temporalis should be a primary consideration because it will completely or partially fill the cavity without the problem of limited excursion, and it also creates a favorable milieu for later prosthetic placement. The muscle has also been successfully used in the closure of oroantral fistulas and for reconstruction of the lateral maxilla and skull base (5).

Craniofacial surgical procedures often produce a communication between the anterior cranial fossa and the nasal or paranasal sinus cavities. Separation of these two regions is critical to minimize complications such as cerebrospinal fluid leaks, epidural abscess, and meningitis. The temporalis has been successfully used for this purpose (18,25). It should be noted that this muscle may be harvested without interfering with the vascular supply to the scalp when using a coronal incision for exposure for the craniotomy.

The temporalis may also be used as a carrier of vascularized outer calvarial bone (2,10,18). This technique utilizes the temporalis and its distal pericranial extension to provide a vascular basis for this myo-osseous flap. The thinness and contour of unicortical calvarial bone grafts makes this compound flap useful for palatal (10), orbital rim, and orbital floor reconstruction. Although described for use in segmental defects of the lateral mandible, the limited bone stock of this donor site pales in comparison with the bone stock of other donor sites currently in use for oromandibular reconstruction. Vascularized calvarial bone grafts have also been used extensively as onlay bone grafts for contour deformities of the maxillofacial skeleton resulting from congenital deformities, trauma, or ablative surgery (18).

The disadvantages of this flap are primarily related to the inability to transfer overlying skin with the muscle and the relatively short arc of rotation, which limits the usefulness of this technique when reconstruction requires extension beyond the nasolabial crease. To improve the distal excursion of the transfer, the zygomatic arch may be removed, allowing an additional 2 to 3 cm of muscle length. The muscle flap may be skin grafted on both the medial and lateral surfaces when required. However, contracture of the skin graft in the midface often leads to surface contour deformities, although it may provide a satisfactory replacement of the inner mucosal defects. In addition to the limits encountered with the transfer of this muscle, the management of the secondary contour deformity of the donor site is also an important issue that has been discussed earlier.

NEUROVASCULAR ANATOMY

The temporalis is broadly based, arising from the inferior temporal line. It fills the entire temporal fossa and narrows as it inserts onto the coronoid process of the man-

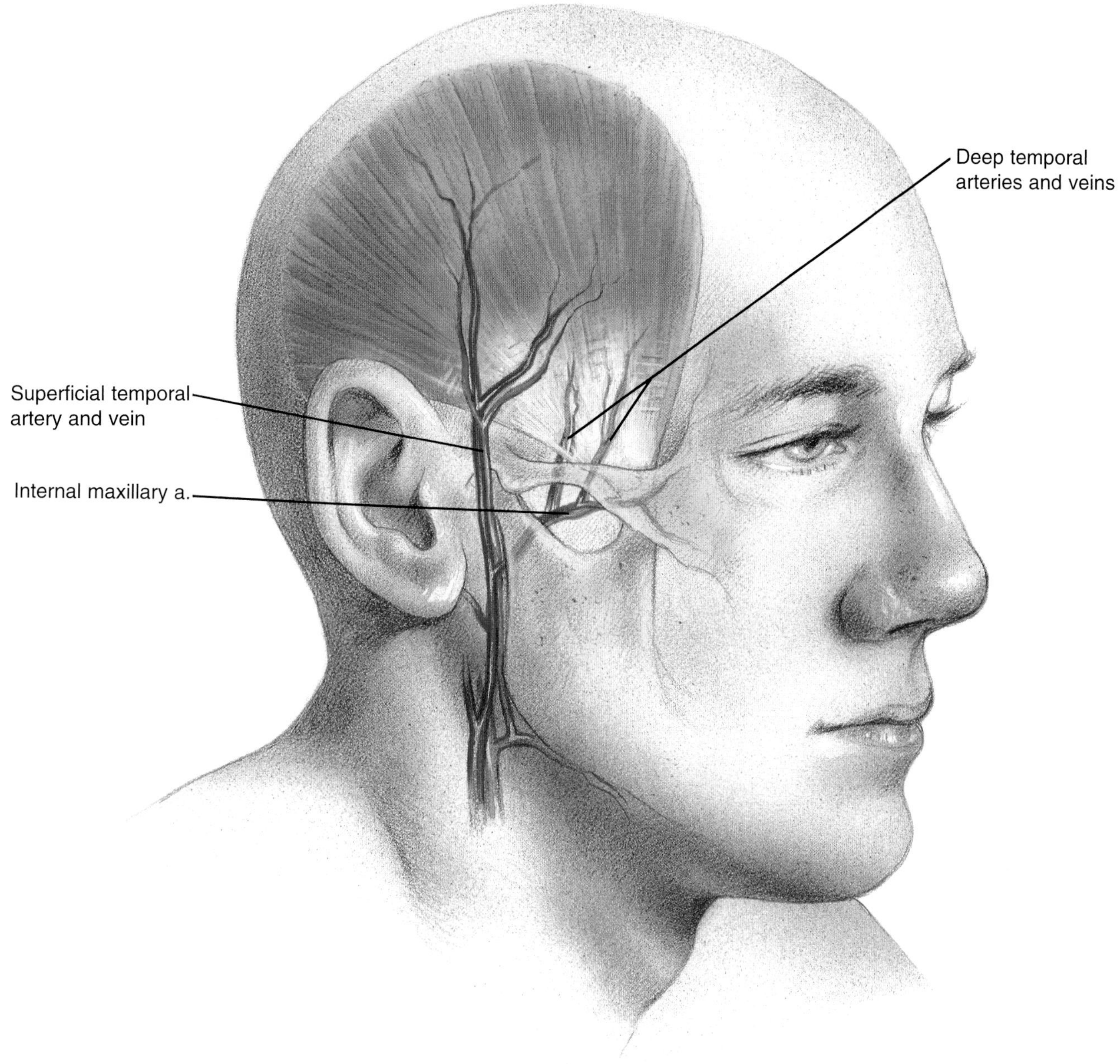

Figure 4-2. The temporalis is supplied by the anterior and posterior deep temporal arteries, which arise from the internal maxillary artery and enter the muscle anterior and posterior to the coronoid process, respectively. These two vessels enter the muscle on its deep aspect. The anterior artery tends to enter the muscle at a more caudal point than the posterior artery does, but both vessels usually enter the substance of the muscle by the upper edge of the zygomatic arch. The nerves to the temporalis also enter on its deep surface and are typically three but, sometimes, four in number. The temporal nerves run between the superior and inferior heads of the lateral pterygoid muscle, crossing over the superior head along with the deep temporal arteries, to enter the temporalis.

dible (Figure 4-1). It is covered by the temporalis muscular fascia (deep temporal fascia) superficially. The temporalis functions in mastication, in conjunction with the masseter and pterygoid muscles, to elevate and retract the mandible. The vascular supply to the temporalis is the deep temporal artery and vein, which arise from the internal maxillary system deep to the zygomatic arch. The deep temporal vessels penetrate the undersurface of the temporalis, providing a segmental vascular pattern (Figure 4-2) (15). The muscle is classified as having a type III pattern of circulation (two dominant vascular pedicles), as described by Mathes and Nahai (17). An additional arterial supply to the muscle arises from the middle temporal artery, which sends minor branches through the superficial aspect of the muscle. The middle temporal artery arises from the superficial temporal artery and crosses over the zygomatic arch to provide a separate vascular supply to the temporalis muscular fascia.

The temporalis muscular fascia inserts on the superior temporal line. In its caudal extent, it divides into two leaves, approximately 2 cm above the zygomatic arch. The deep and superficial muscular fascial layers insert on the medial and lateral aspects of the arch and are separated by a layer of fat. The muscular fascia fuses with the periosteum of the arch to form a very dense fibrous layer. The temporal and zygomatic branches of the facial nerve cross the zygomatic arch in the layer of the temporoparietal fascia, which is superficial to the muscular fascia–periosteal layer. The fatty plane that separates the two layers of the temporalis muscular fascia may be used by the surgeon to protect the facial nerve branches. By starting at the root of the zygomatic arch and incising the superficial layer of the temporalis muscular fascia, the fatty plane is entered. If this incision is made at a 45-degree angle in the anterosuperior direction and the zygomatic arch is uncovered in a subperiosteal plane, the facial nerve branches can be protected by reflecting this fascial–periosteal layer in an anterior and inferior direction (1).

POTENTIAL PITFALLS

The use of the temporalis in midfacial reconstruction is a dependable technique; however, there are a number of features of this flap that pose potential problems. As mentioned previously, the muscle transfer relies heavily on capturing an adequate neural and vascular supply. In patients who have undergone extensive skull base or neck surgery, interruption of the neurovascular supply can result in a muscle that is not suitable for transfer.

Another concern when transferring this flap in conjunction with the temporoparietal fascial flap is secondary alopecia of the overlying scalp. This problem is of particular concern for patients who have undergone regional radiation therapy and/or in whom a scalp incision has been used to gain access to the skull base. It has been our experience that patients who have undergone occipital approaches to the skull base utilizing temporal incisions around the auricle are not good candidates for the use of the temporoparietal fascial flap because partial devascularization of the auricle occurs in a significant percentage of patients.

The frontal branch of the facial nerve is located in the temporoparietal fascia. Above the zygomatic arch, it runs approximately 2.0 cm lateral to the lateral aspect of the eyebrow. Its course may be outlined by drawing a line from the tragus to a point 2.0 cm above the lateral eyebrow. This nerve branch should be identified in this location and avoided during the anterior dissection and elevation of the muscle. The auriculotemporal nerve, a branch of the third division of the trigeminal nerve, courses under the zygomatic arch and then runs in a cephalad direction posterior to the superficial temporal artery and vein. It supplies sensation to the anterior auricle, the external auditory meatus, and the scalp of the temporal region, and this nerve must be identified and preserved if sensation of the temporoparietal area is to be maintained.

PREOPERATIVE ASSESSMENT

Prior to surgery, it is imperative for the temporalis muscle to be examined by asking patients to clench their teeth to ensure that the muscle exhibits normal strength and tone. This is particularly important in patients who have undergone prior skull base procedures in which the viability of the fifth cranial nerve may be in question. Asymmetric wasting of the temporal fossa is a telltale sign of denervation atrophy of the temporalis. It is also important to establish the patency of the superficial temporal artery and vein to assess the viability of the temporoparietal fascia if this fascia is to be used to obliterate the donor site defect that results from the harvest of this muscle (6).

POSTOPERATIVE WOUND CARE: MANAGEMENT OF THE DONOR SITE

Numerous techniques have been advocated for the management of the donor site created after temporalis transposition. Alloplastic implants have become less popular in recent years because of the significant incidence of secondary infection, extrusion, and implant mobility. In an attempt to reestablish adequate contour with autogenous tissue, we have used vascularized temporoparietal fascia, with satisfactory results. This fascial flap is elevated prior to harvesting the temporalis and is mobilized laterally during the elevation and transfer of the muscle segment. It is then used to obliterate the temporal defect created after all or part of the temporalis is transposed into the midface. At the completion of the procedure, a suction drain is placed in the temporoparietal scalp for 24 to 36 hours. A bulky compressive dressing is used for the first 24 hours postoperatively to prevent hematoma formation and reduce facial swelling.

Flap Harvesting Technique follows on page 72.

Flap Harvesting Technique

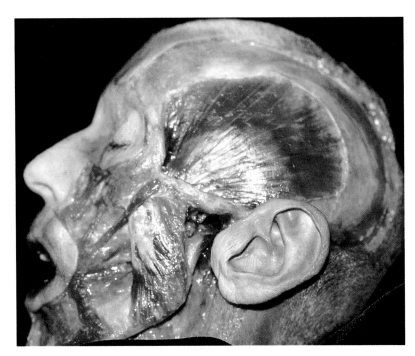

Figure 4-3. A lateral view of the face demonstrates the relationship between the mimetic muscles and the temporalis and masseter muscle bodies. It is interesting when reviewing this dissection to note the key characteristics of the facial muscles. These muscles have a bony origin with a soft tissue or muscular insertion, which allows them to move the overlying integument of the face and, therefore, produce changes in facial expression.

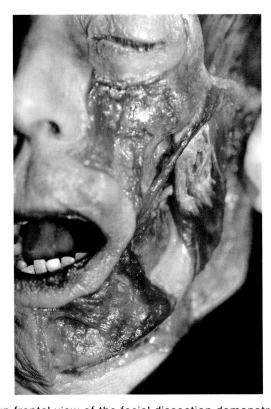

Figure 4-4. A close-up frontal view of the facial dissection demonstrates the position of the midfacial mimetic musculature. The importance of the orbicularis oris to facial expression is evident because the mimetic muscles insert into or adjacent to this circular sphincteric muscle. The small and delicate nature of the mimetic muscles in the midface is also evident in this dissection.

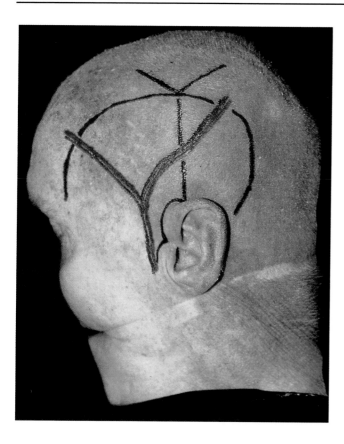

Figure 4-5. The approach to the temporalis is made through a scalp incision that has a vertical component that extends from the midportion of the superior auricular helix to approximately 2 cm above the superior temporal line. This incision allows full exposure of the muscle and its overlying fascia. The incision can be extended into the preauricular crease to gain exposure of the superficial temporal artery and vein. Preservation of the vascular pedicle to the temporoparietal fascia allows this fascia to be elevated as a separate pedicle flap to be used for donor site obliteration.

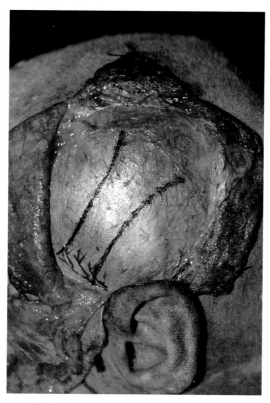

Figure 4-6. The deep muscular fascia is exposed by elevating scalp flaps approximately 6 cm anteriorly and posteriorly. The width and the orientation of the portion of the temporalis transfer is determined. We usually use a 2- to 3-cm strip harvested from the midportion of the muscle region. This segment of the muscle provides adequate length and exhibits active contractual properties that are ideal for temporalis transfer in facial reanimation. If a larger portion of the muscle is required for reconstruction of a midface or an oral cavity defect, then the incisions can be modified to elevate as much of the muscle as needed.

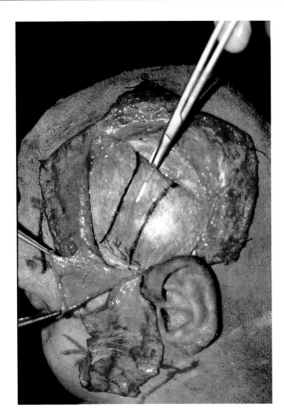

Figure 4-7. Elevation of the muscle is started by incising the deep muscular fascia along the superior temporal line. A Freer elevator is used for blunt elevation along the plane of the temporal skull. As shown in this dissection, the deep muscular fascia can be elevated as a separate soft tissue flap by dissecting in the plane between the muscle and fascia.

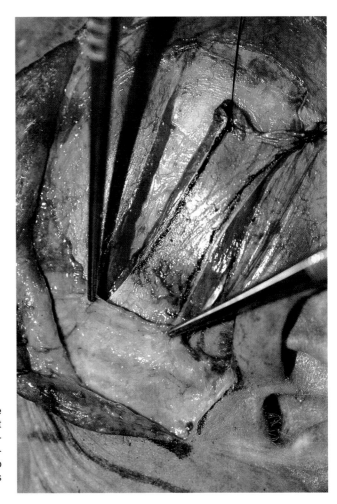

Figure 4-8. The temporalis and its overlying fascia are raised down to the zygomatic arch. In the caudal aspect of this dissection, the neurovascular supply is in jeopardy, and therefore, blunt dissection in this region is required. Avoidance of electrocautery is also advised to prevent injury to the neurovascular pedicle as it enters the undersurface of the muscle.

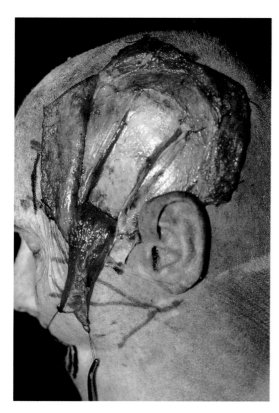

Figure 4-9. In preparation for muscle transfer, a subcutaneous tunnel is created, extending from the zygomatic arch to the oral commissure. A vermilion incision is made at the oral commissure, that extends approximately 1 to 1.5 cm along both the upper and lower lip. The lateral aspect of the orbicularis oris is identified using the full extent of this vermilion incision. The orbicularis oris may be atrophic, depending on the duration of facial paralysis. After the facial flap is fully elevated, the surgeon should be able to place both index fingers comfortably from the zygomatic arch to the vermilion border. The muscle and overlying fascia can then be passed through this tunnel and secured to the lateral border of the orbicularis oris.

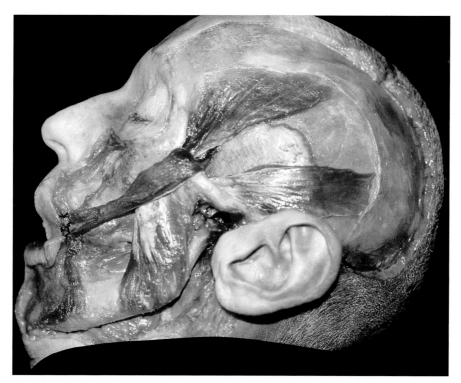

Figure 4-10. Permanent sutures are used to secure the temporalis to the lateral border of the orbicularis oris. Direct contact between the two muscles is thought to be important to enhance postoperative facial movement. Over time, the transposed temporalis tends to stretch, and this factor must be accounted for when establishing the resting position of the lateral oral commissure. To achieve the desired symmetry at rest of the oral commissure and the nasolabial fold on the paralyzed side of the face, the pull of the temporalis must be exaggerated at the time of surgery so that the second or third molar of the upper dental arch is exposed. The normal vermilion border is characteristically slightly elevated. To mimic this feature, the vermilion incision is closed using a horizontal mattress suture technique.

REFERENCES

1. Al-Kayat A, Bramley P: A modified preauricular approach to the temporomandibular joint and malar arch. *Br J Oral Surg* 1978;17:91–103.
2. Antonyshyn O, Colcleugh RG, Hurst LN, Anderson C: The temporalis myo-osseous flap: an experimental study. *Plast Reconstr Surg* 1986;77:406.
3. Antonyshyn O, Gruss JS, Birt BD: Versatility of temporal muscle and fascial flaps. *Br J Plast Surg* 1988;41:118.
4. Bakamjian V, Souther S: Use of the temporal muscle flap for reconstruction after orbito-maxillary resections for cancer. *Plast Reconstr Surg* 1975;56:171.
5. Bradley P, Brockbank J: The temporalis muscle flap in oral reconstruction. A cadaveric, animal and clinical study. *J Maxillofac Surg* 1981;9:139.
6. Cheney ML, McKenna MJ, Ojemann RG, Nadol JB: Management of facial paralysis after acoustic tumor surgery. *Arch Otolaryngol Head Neck Surg* 1994;[*in press*].
7. Conley J, Patow C: *Flaps in Head and Neck Surgery.* New York: Thieme; 1989.
8. Deitch RD, Callahan A: Temporalis muscle transplant for tissue defects about the orbit. *Am J Ophthalmol* 1964;58:849.
9. Edgerton MT, Tuerk DB, Fisher JC: Surgical treatment of Moebius syndrome by platysma and temporalis muscle transfers. *Plast Reconstr Surg* 1975;55:305.
10. Ewers R: Reconstruction of the maxilla with a double musculoperiosteal flap in connection with a composite calvarial bone graft. *Plast Reconstr Surg* 1988;3:431.
11. Gillies HD: Experience with fascia lata grafts in the operative treatment of facial paralysis. *Proc R Soc Med* 1934;27:1372.
12. Golovine SS: Procede de cloture plastique de l'orbite apres l'exenteration. *J Fr Ophtalmol* 1898;18:679.
13. Habel G, Henscher R: The versatility of the temporalis muscle flap in reconstructive surgery. *Br J Oral Maxillofac Surg* 1986;24:96.
14. Hallock GG: Reconstruction of a lower eyelid defect using the temporalis muscle. *Ann Plast Surg* 1984;13:157.
15. Hollinshead WH: *Textbook of Anatomy.* 3rd ed. Hagerstown, MD: Harper and Row; 1974.
16. Holmes AD, Marshall KA: Uses of the temporalis muscle flap in blanking out orbits. *Plast Reconstr Surg* 1979;63:336.
17. Mathes S, Nahai F: *Clinical Applications for Muscle and Musculocutaneous Flaps.* St. Louis: CV Mosby Yearbook; 1982:40.
18. Matsuba HM, Hakki AR, Little JW, Spear SL: The temporal fossa in head and neck reconstruction: twenty-two flaps of scalp, fascia and full thickness cranial bone. *Laryngoscope* 1988;98:444.
19. May M: Muscle transposition for facial reanimation. *Arch Otolaryngol* 1985;110:184.
20. May M: Facial reanimation after skull base trauma. *Am J Otol* 1985;(Nov. Suppl.):62–67.
21. May M: *The Facial Nerve.* New York: Thieme; 1986.
22. McKenna MJ, Cheney ML, Borodic G, Ojemann RG: Management of facial paralysis after intracranial surgery. *Contemp Neurol* 1991;13:519.
23. Naquin HA: Orbital reconstruction utilizing temporalis muscle. *Am J Ophthalmol* 1956;41:519.
24. Reese AB, Jones IS: Exenteration of the orbit and repair by transplantation of the temporalis muscle. *Am J Ophthalmol* 1961;51:217.
25. Renner G, Davis WE, Templer J: Temporalis pericranial muscle flap for reconstruction of the lateral face and head. *Laryngoscope* 1984;94:1418.
26. Rubin LR: *Reanimation of the Paralyzed Face: New Approaches.* St. Louis: Mosby Yearbook; 1977.
27. Rubin LR: The anatomy of a smile: its importance in the treatment of facial paralysis. *Plast Reconstr Surg* 1974;53:384.
28. Rubin LR: *The Paralyzed Face.* St. Louis: Mosby Yearbook; 1991.
29. Rubin LR, Mishiki Y, Lee G: Anatomy of the nasolabial fold: the keystone of the smiling mechanism. *Plast Reconstr Surg* 1989;83:1.
30. Sheehan JE: The muscle nerve graft. *Surg Clin North Am* 1935;15:471.
31. Tessier P, Krastinova D: La transposition du muscle temporal dans l'orbite anophtalme. *Ann Chir Plast Esthet* 1982;27:212.

REGIONAL FLAPS
Muscle and Musculocutaneous Flaps

Masseter

Mack L. Cheney, M.D., and
Mark L. Urken, M.D.

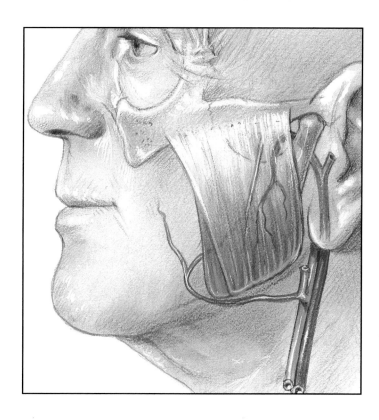

Lexer and Eden (5) are credited with being the first to use the masseter muscle for reconstructive purposes in 1911. They reported using two slips of the anterior half of the muscle, transposed into the upper and lower lip, to reanimate the paralyzed face. The early reports on masseter transfers showed this technique to be unreliable in a significant percentage of cases (7). A review of the description of early harvesting techniques indicates that surgical violation of the neural supply of the transposed muscle may have contributed to secondary atrophy and lack of coordinated movement in these early reports.

The masseter has maintained its popularity in reanimation of the mouth in patients with facial paralysis (8). In addition, it has been used for reconstruction of postablative mucosal defects of the posterior oral cavity. This muscle has a number of advantages, including its ease of surgical transfer, its dependable neurovascular supply, and the fact that it can be used to depress the paralyzed lower lip.

FLAP DESIGN AND UTILIZATION

The most common application of the masseter transposition flap has been for facial reanimation in traumatic, congenital, or postablative paralysis (3,8). It may be harvested through either an intraoral or extraoral approach for transposition to the oral commissure. Baker and Conley (1) advocated the harvest of the periosteal attachment of the masseter to provide additional length and to provide better purchase for fixation of the masseter to the lateral commissure of the mouth.

In patients with total hemifacial paralysis, rehabilitation of the eye requires the introduction of other techniques, which include gold weights, eyelid springs, and tarsal tightening. The masseter transposition flap is only useful to restore motion to the lower face. The dynamic activity produced by the masseter is triggered by the patient initiating a biting motion and not by the involuntary emotional expression produced through the facial nerve.

In this respect, both the temporalis and masseter are similar in their common trigeminal nerve innervation. The direction of pull with the masseter muscle is oriented more posteriorly than what is normally produced by the temporalis. May (6) commented on the additional bulk in the cheek that is caused by transposition of the masseter, which may be advantageous in cases of tumor ablation where added bulk may improve the final facial contour. Transposition of the temporalis muscle is also associated with a contour deformity resulting from the bulk of that muscle over the zygoma and the secondary concavity in the temporal fossa.

The masseter has been used for a variety of other purposes following ablative surgery of the oral cavity and pharynx. Conley and Gullane (2) described several applications of this muscle flap following composite resections in which the hemimandible was removed. They described suturing the masseter to the hyoid bone to assist in laryngeal elevation during swallowing. They also reported using the muscle to cover the upper portion of the internal carotid artery. The masseter has also been transposed into the nasopharynx and covered with a split-thickness skin graft to close mucosal defects that extended to this region. The application of the masseter for these reconstructive purposes is only feasible when the ramus of the mandible has been resected and not replaced.

The reconstruction of small defects of the posterior lateral oral cavity and, in particular, the retromolar trigone region can be problematic when the mandible is left intact. Regional musculocutaneous flaps may not be easily transferred because of excess bulk. Violation of the tongue to form a split-tongue transposition flap should be condemned because of the interference in lingual function. The palatal island flap is a reasonable alternative option, but it leaves a raw surface of palatal bone for closure by secondary intention and is not advisable following radiation therapy. The masseter may be used to cover these mucosal defects by mobilizing the entire muscle, except for its superior attachments to the zygoma. It is important to perform this mobilization in a subfascial plane of dissection to avoid injury to the facial nerve. The masseteric fascia is elevated with the cheek flap to expose the entire muscle, which is then freed from its attachments to the angle of the mandible. The muscle should not be mobilized above the condylar notch to avoid injury to the neurovascular pedicle. The muscle is then transposed over the mandible and sutured to the pharyngeal constrictors, mylohyoid, and digastric muscles (9).

A split-thickness skin graft may be placed on this muscle bed if mucosal approximation is not possible. Tiwari and Snow (10) reported using this technique in 24 patients with small posterolateral oral defects. One patient developed an orocutaneous fistula and a second patient required lysis of a fibrous band that developed in the retromolar trigone region and limited oral opening.

Zoller et al. (11) described a modification of this technique in which the masseter muscle flap was combined with a superiorly based cheek transposition flap. The combination of the muscle and mucosal flaps provided a reliable two-layer closure of posterior oral cavity defects. The secondary defect resulted in exposed buccinator muscle, which was allowed to close by secondary intention.

NEUROVASCULAR ANATOMY

The masseter is divided into deep and superficial bellies. The former arises from the anterior two thirds of the zygomatic arch; the latter arises from the inner surface of the arch at its posterior third. Both bellies of the muscle insert into the lateral

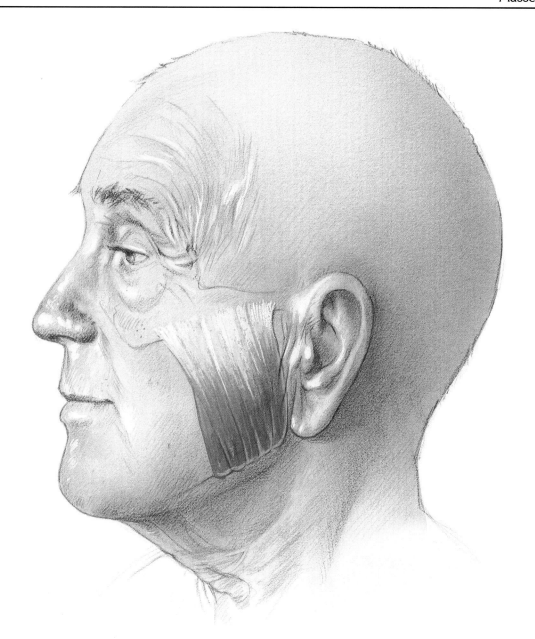

Figure 5-1. The masseter arises from the zygomatic arch and inserts into the lateral surface of the mandibular ramus. The primary action of the masseter is to close the mandible, and it also plays a minor role in protraction of the mandible, causing it to deviate to the opposite side.

surface of the ramus extending from the lower portion of the coronoid process to the mandibular angle (Figure 5-1). The major action of the masseter muscle is to close the mandible. Because of the downward posterior orientation of the muscle fibers, the masseter assists the lateral pterygoid in protraction of the mandible.

The neurovascular pedicle to the masseter enters the deep surface of the muscle through the mandibular notch. The masseteric artery arises from the internal maxillary artery. Part of the venous outflow from the masseter goes to the facial vein and part enters the pterygoid plexus and, ultimately, the internal maxillary vein. The masseteric nerve is a branch of the mandibular nerve that arises from the trigeminal nerve.

Correia and Zani (4) carefully documented the course of the nerve and advised that the safest way to preserve the innervation was to transfer the entire muscle as a unit. They also recommended that any attempt to divide the muscle with an inferiorly

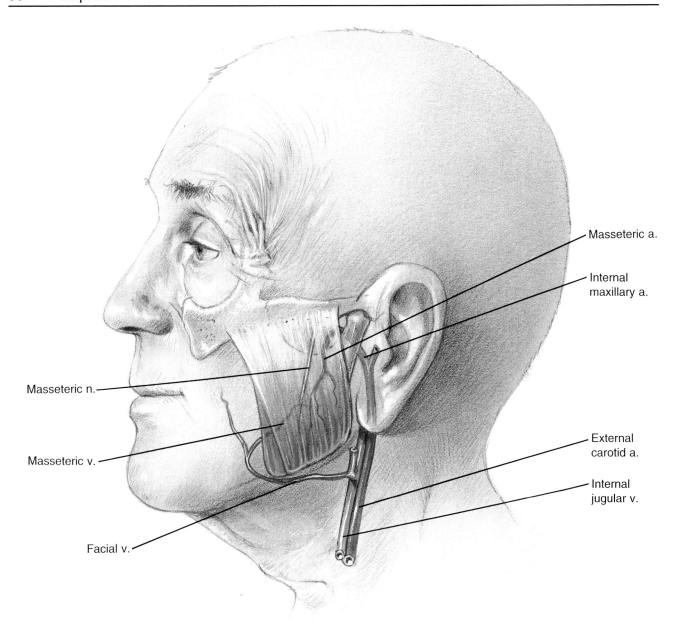

Masseteric a.

Internal
maxillary a.

Masseteric n.

External
carotid a.

Masseteric v.

Internal
jugular v.

Facial v.

Figure 5-2. The primary arterial supply to the masseter muscle arises from the internal maxillary artery. The venous drainage is through the facial vein and the pterygoid plexus.

based longitudinal split should not exceed 3.5 cm. This division should begin at the inferior border of the muscle at the junction of the anterior two thirds and the posterior third. A more cephalad division risks injury to the nerve.

ANATOMIC VARIATIONS

In a series of 25 cadaver dissections, Correia and Zani (4) found the dissection of the masseter nerve to be difficult. They were able to dissect the nerve and its branches, however, by approaching it from a posterosuperior direction, where it crosses the mandibular notch. Examination of the specimens resulted in the classification of the muscle into two groups, according to its length. A long muscle was found in 17 cases (68%) and a short muscle, in 8 cases (32%). In the short masseter type, the nerve was found to run obliquely forward and downward across the rectangle of the muscle toward its anterior inferior quadrant. The nerve was found to end in diverging branches. In the long masseter type, the course of the nerve was found to run obliquely forward and downward. As it travels downward, the nerve tends to approach the anterior border, extending to a more inferior level than the nerve of the short masseter type. In the long masseter type, the nerve most often ends in the anteroinferior segment of the muscle and exhibits a very limited branching pattern.

POTENTIAL PITFALLS

Although contour defects may result there is little other donor site morbidity following transposition of the masseter muscle. It has been our experience that this secondary defect is variable and dependent on the regional muscle anatomy of the individual.

Additional problems in the transfer of the masseter may occur if the muscle's neurovascular pedicle is not adequately visualized. This can be particularly troublesome when the muscle is approached through an intraoral incision. This may lead to an inability to obtain adequate hemostasis and also a failure to identify carefully and preserve the neural supply to the muscle.

PREOPERATIVE ASSESSMENT

Preoperative assessment of the masseter relies on the clinical demonstration of active contraction of the muscle. Prior to surgery, the patient should be examined to be sure that the muscle has normal strength and tone. This is particularly important in patients who have undergone previous skull base procedures in which the viability of the fifth cranial nerve may be in question. Careful review of prior operative reports is critical to be certain that the vascular supply has not been compromised.

POSTOPERATIVE WOUND CARE

After the muscle is transferred, the face is secured with a bulky compressive dressing. This can be reinforced by the use of Steri-Strips around the orbicularis oris to add additional support and immobilization to this area. It may be advisable to use nasogastric feeding during the immediate postoperative period to eliminate additional motion caused by mastication.

Flap Harvesting Technique follows on page 82.

Flap Harvesting Technique

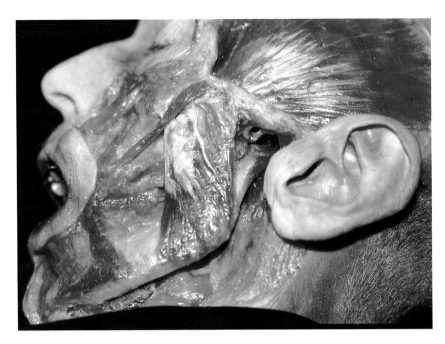

Figure 5-3. The masseter may be transposed by an extraoral or an intraoral approach. The extraoral approach is performed through a preauricular incision with a Blair extension. The muscle can be identified at the angle of the mandible and then mobilized from a posteroinferior approach. Extreme care must be exercised when mobilizing the masseter to prevent injury to the neurovascular pedicle entering the muscle at the mandibular notch.

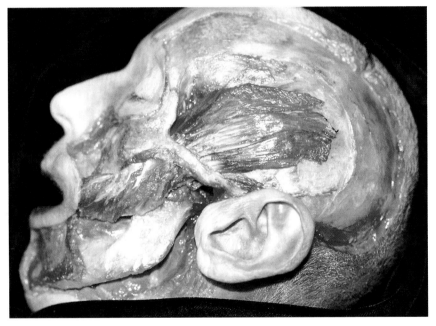

Figure 5-4. The masseter has been transposed to the lateral commissure for dynamic reanimation of the corner of the mouth. A subcutaneous tunnel is created that permits transfer of the muscle to the lateral commissure. At the lateral commissure, the masseter is longitudinally incised to allow 2 separate muscle slips to be passed into the upper and lower lids. A secondary incision at the commissure facilitates the placement of permanent anchoring sutures. Meticulous dissection of the inferior insertion of the masseter, being certain to include the tendon, helps to provide a better purchase for these critical sutures. The creation of two muscle slips to be transferred to the upper and lower lip is performed by carefully cutting the muscle in a caudal to cephalad direction for only 2 to 3 cm. It is imperative to overcorrect the pull on the lateral commissure at the time of suturing the muscle to the orbicularis oris muscle. Protection of these sutures for a period of 1 week is achieved by feeding the patient with a nasogastric tube. Oral nutrition is then resumed by instituting a liquid diet for another 1-week period. Chewing is gradually begun as is training on how to initiate and control facial movements.

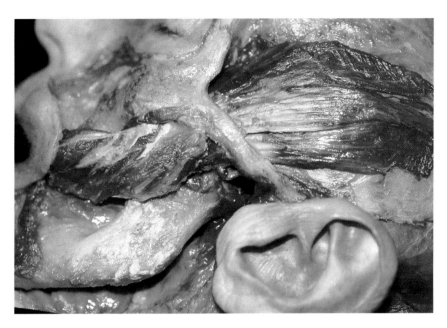

Figure 5-5. The direction of pull of the transposed masseter is slightly more horizontal than that of the temporalis. The secondary contour deformity of the cheek, at the angle of the mandible, is accentuated by the bulge in the mid-cheek caused by the transposed masseter.

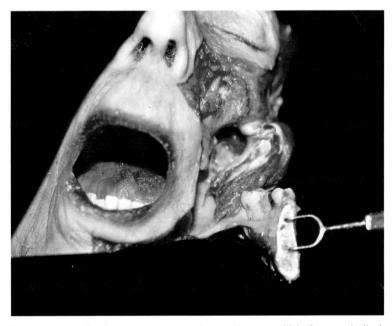

Figure 5-6. The masseter is shown transposed over the mandible for use in limited defects of the retromolar trigone. It is elevated through an intraoral approach or through a median mandibulotomy, as shown here. A major difference between the harvest of the masseter in this setting and in facial reanimation is that here the branches of the facial nerve are intact and must be protected. When raising the cheek flap for exposure, the plane of dissection must be just superficial to the fascia overlying the muscle.

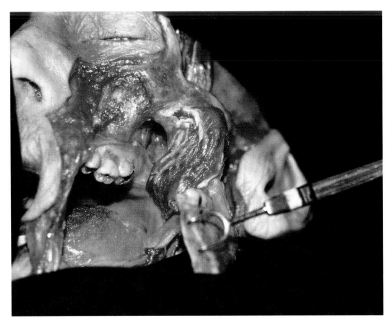

Figure 5-7. The masseter crossover flap is sutured to the mylohyoid muscle. The posterior belly of the digastric may be detached from the mastoid, transposed to the inner table of the mandible, and also sutured to the masseter. The bare muscle may be covered with a skin graft or allowed to remucosalize.

REFERENCES

1. Baker DC, Conley J: Regional muscle transposition for rehabilitation of the paralyzed face. *Clin Plast Surg* 1979;6:317–330.
2. Conley J, Gullane PJ: The masseter muscle flap. *Laryngoscope* 1978;88:605–612.
3. Conway H: Muscle plastic operations for facial paralysis. *Ann Surg* 1958;147:541.
4. Correia P, Zani R: Masseter muscle rotation in the treatment of inferior facial paralysis. *Plast Reconstr Surg* 1973;52:370–373.
5. Lexer E, Eden R: Uber die chirurgische Behandlung der peripheren Facialislahmung. *Beitr Klin Chir* 1911;73:116.
6. May M: *The Facial Nerve.* New York: Thieme; 1986.
7. Owens N: Surgical correction of facial paralysis. *Plast Reconstr Surg* 1947;2:25.
8. Rubin L: *Reanimation of the Paralyzed Face.* St. Louis: CV Mosby; 1977.
9. Tiwari R: Masseter muscle cross over flap in primary closure of oral-oropharyngeal defects. *J Laryngol Otol* 1987;101:172–178.
10. Tiwari R, Snow G: Repair of intraoral defects with masseter crossover flap after cancer surgery. *Head Neck* 1988;10:S30.
11. Zoller J, Maier H, Herrman A: The combined masseter muscle/intraoral cheek transposition (IOCT) flap for primary reconstruction of the dorsal oral cavity. *Otolaryngol Head Neck Surg* 1992;106:326–331.

6

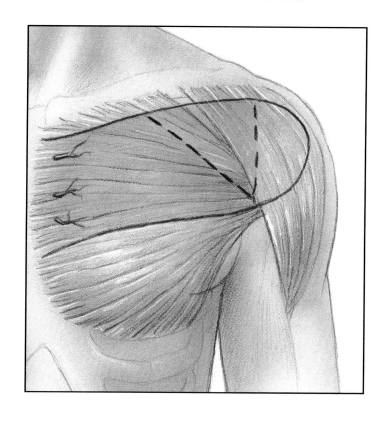

Deltopectoral

Mark L. Urken, M.D., and
Hugh F. Biller, M.D.

The medially based deltopectoral flap, also referred to as the Bakamjian flap, was a major advance in head and neck surgery when it was popularized in the early 1960s by V. Y. Bakamjian (2) as a solution to the problem of pharyngoesophageal reconstruction. The design of this flap, with its pedicle based at the sternum, represented a divergence from the commonly held belief that the midline of the body was a relatively avascular territory (19). There remains some controversy as to whether the flap reported in 1917 by Aymard (1) for nasal reconstruction was the first description of the deltopectoral flap. This flap was again described by Joseph (14) in the 1930s in his book on plastic surgery. Joseph referred to Manchot's description of the vascular territories of the body and clearly understood the nature of the blood supply to this flap (10). For approximately 40 years, the deltopectoral flap remained essentially dormant in the medical literature until Bakamjian (2,3) described its versatility and wide application in head and neck reconstruction. Along with the forehead flap introduced by McGregor (18), it was the primary method for resurfacing cutaneous and mucosal defects until the late 1970s when musculocutaneous flaps were introduced. It remains a useful tool in the reconstructive surgeon's armamentarium, although it has primarily been relegated for use in reconstructing external cutaneous defects of the neck. The major disadvantages of this flap include the requirement, in most cases, for a skin graft to close the donor site, and the unreliability of the distal portions of this flap when extended over the deltoid region.

The deltopectoral flap is a fasciocutaneous flap based on the perforating branches of the internal mammary artery. Although originally described as having a pedicle based on the first three perforators, it is now most commonly based on the second and third. When a clearly dominant perforator is present, the entire flap could probably be based on that single vascular pedicle. Primary transfer of the deltopectoral flap may be performed with a high degree of reliability provided that it does not extend into the territory overlying the deltoid muscle. Distal flap necrosis occurs with significant frequency when a flap extending onto the shoulder is raised without prior delay. Flap vascularity and the reliability of different flap designs are discussed in detail later.

FLAP DESIGN AND UTILIZATION

A variety of different flap designs have been described to reconstruct many different defects in the head and neck. Greater length and greater diversity can be achieved when a delay procedure is instituted. The body habitus of the patient greatly influences the arc of rotation of the medially based flap. The optimal situation is a patient with broad shoulders and a short neck.

There are several different ways to transfer this flap to the recipient site. The bridging portion of the flap can be tubed over the clavicle and neck skin. A staged secondary procedure is required to either return or excise the tubed component. Alternatively, the intervening skin between the defect and the clavicle may be excised to allow a one-stage insertion of the entire length of the flap. Finally, an island flap can be created by de-epithelializing the proximal portion of the flap, which is then buried beneath the cervical skin ·between the defect and the clavicle. When buried in this fashion, a secondary procedure is not required (Figure 6-1) (13).

Krizek and Robson (17) described the vertically split flap in which an incision is made through the distal end of the skin paddle creating two separate segments for restoration of the inner and outer lining (Figure 6-2). This design places less stress on the vascularity to the tip than de-epithelializing a segment and folding the flap on itself. A transverse fold in the tip of the flap allows the distal portion to be used for the internal lining of composite defects. However, this technique requires that a longer flap be harvested, and the distal fold occurs in the least viable portion. Bakamjian et al. (5) described the L-shaped design of the deltopectoral flap, with the short limb of the L extending downward along the upper arm. This flap design was used to obtain an inner lining by using a two-stage procedure. In the initial delay procedure, the upper arm extension was folded under the deltoid component to produce a buried skin flap. The two epithelial surfaces were then transferred at the time of the second procedure. An alternative solution to the requirement for a double epithelial surface is the use of a skin graft on the undersurface of the flap. The graft may be buried at the time of an initial delay procedure (22).

East et al. (8) described the placement of a fenestration in the distal portion of the deltopectoral flap for reconstruction of a tracheostoma. Although we would be wary of causing tip necrosis with this technique, the authors advised that the short arc of rotation required to reach the tracheostoma allows the design of a short flap, and therefore, the fenestra can be placed in a relatively well-vascularized portion of the flap.

The length of the deltopectoral flap that can be safely transferred without a delay is somewhat controversial. Kirkby et al. (15) reported that the end of the flap could be safely extended to the tip of the shoulder. When additional length was required, these authors recommended the creation of a back cut from the inferior limb of the flap across the sternum and then in a cephalad direction lateral to the contralateral internal thoracic perforators (Figure 6-3). However, the efficacy of this maneuver is somewhat controversial in light of the contention of McGregor and Jackson (19) that the arc of rotation of a deltopectoral flap is more limited by the upper limb of the flap than by the inferior limb, as is most commonly believed. The rationale for this contention is that the skin of the anterior axillary fold is intrinsically more redundant than is the skin of the superior limb of this flap, which is located parallel and just

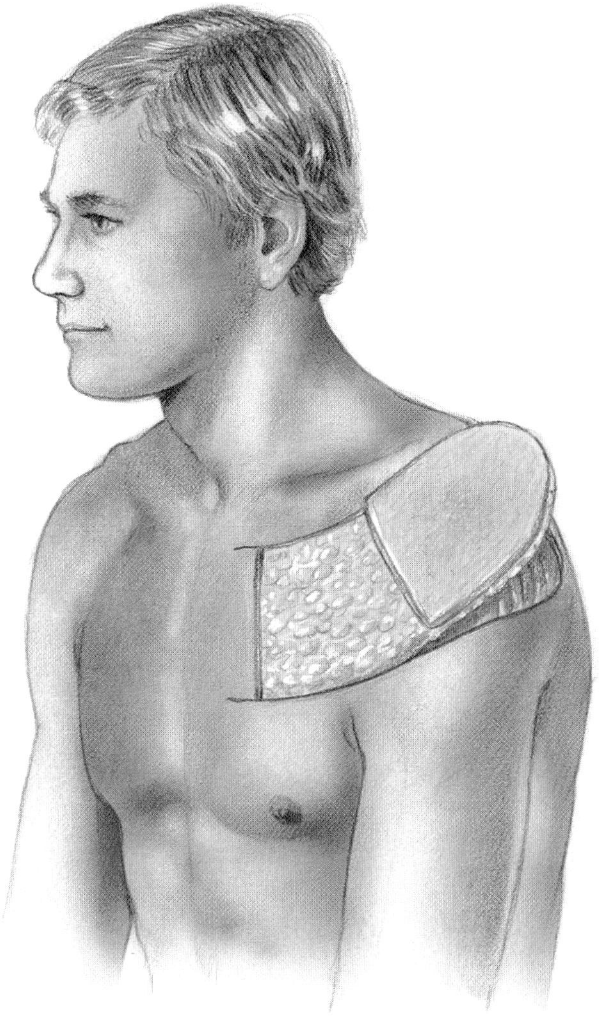

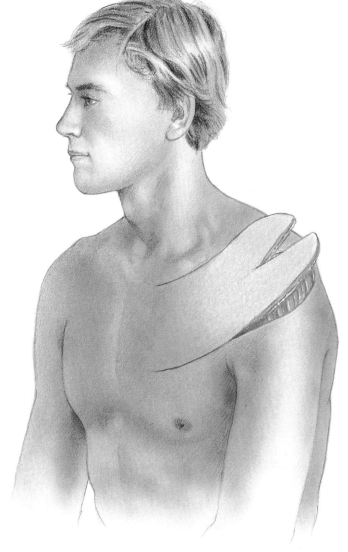

Figure 6-1. A modified design of the deltopectoral flap with the proximal portion de-epithelialized and buried beneath the intervening bridge of skin. The fasciocutaneous nature of this flap ensures that this maneuver will not impede vascularity to the distal portion.

Figure 6-2. The vertically split deltopectoral flap provides two epithelial surfaces. This design is probably safer than de-epithelializing a horizontal strip and folding the tip to achieve an inner lining.

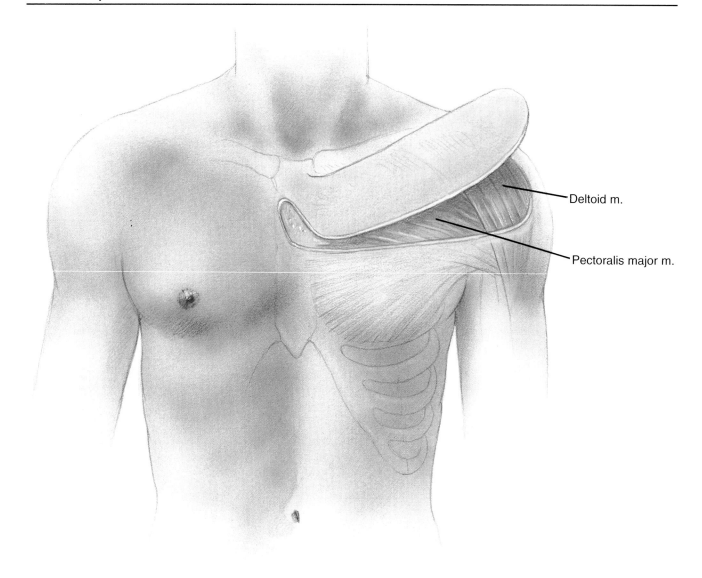

Deltoid m.

Pectoralis major m.

Figure 6-3. The desire to improve the arc of rotation of the deltopectoral flap has led to a number of modifications, including the use of a back cut on the contralateral side of the sternum.

inferior to the clavicle. It is easy to demonstrate the relative redundancy of the skin in the anterior axillary fold by raising an arm above the head. Bilateral deltopectoral flap transfers have been reported for complex reconstructions or recurrent cancers (15).

The deltopectoral flap was transferred as a microvascular free flap, as first reported by Harii et al. (12) in 1974 and then by Fujino et al. (9) in the following year. Fujino et al.'s publication described the transfer of a de-epithelialized dermis–fat flap for augmentation of contour deformities of the head and neck. Percutaneous Doppler sonography was used to localize the dominant perforator on which to base the flap. The free flap is usually harvested on the second internal mammary perforator, which is most commonly the largest. The vascular pedicle for this flap is quite short and it is rarely used for free tissue transfer due to the abundance of other donor sites which are available.

David (7) introduced the concept of an innervated deltopectoral flap for intraoral reconstruction with sensory restoration reestablished through the supraclavicular nerves of the cervical plexus (Figure 6-4). Although he noted excellent sensation when

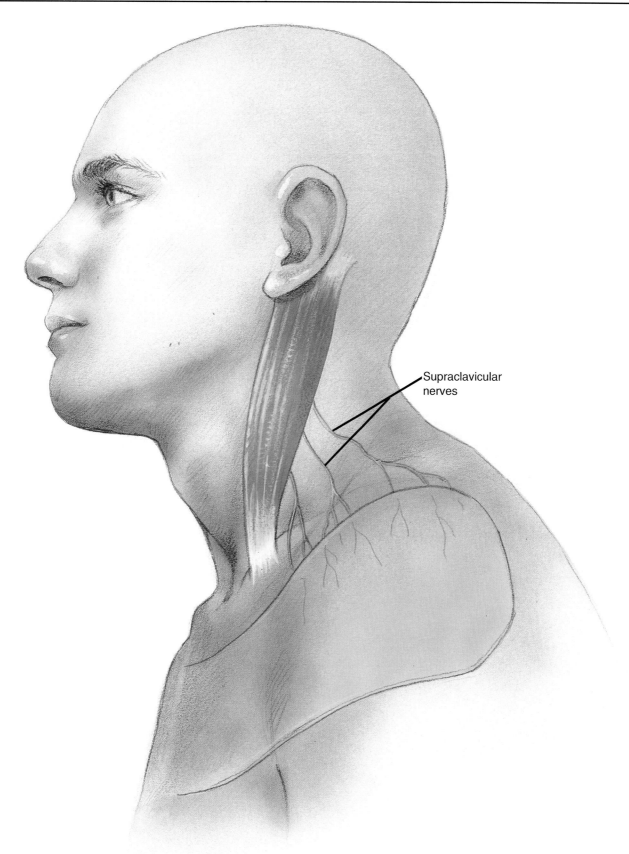

Supraclavicular
nerves

Figure 6-4. The supraclavicular sensory nerves arise from C-3 and C-4 and can easily be traced through the posterior triangle fat pad to be mobilized or transsected and then anastomosed to an appropriate recipient nerve.

the nerves were mobilized and not transsected, he did not report sensory recovery when the nerves were transsected and then reanastomosed to recipient sensory nerves in the neck. The potential for transfer of a sensate deltopectoral free flap is readily apparent. The concept of transferring sensate skin to the oral cavity and pharynx to assist in postoperative rehabilitation was not pursued until Urken et al. (26) reported the first sensate radial forearm flap in pharyngeal reconstruction.

The deltopectoral flap has been applied to a wide variety of reconstructive problems in the head and neck. As noted previously, Bakamjian (2) first described this flap as a solution to the problem of restoring continuity to the gullet following laryngopharyngectomy. In a landmark publication in 1965, he reported a two-stage technique that involved the transfer of a tubed deltopectoral flap. Following the initial procedure, a control salivary fistula was created at the lower end of the tube that was positioned lateral and inferior to the tracheostoma, permitting a safer and more manageable salivary egress. The stump of the esophagus was sutured in end-to-side fashion to the skin tube. After a 3- to 5-week interval, the base of the deltopectoral flap was transsected and closed to complete the pharyngoesophageal reconstruction. Bakamjian and Holbrook (4) later described the use of a staged secondary reconstruction of the pharyngoesophagus by tubing the deltopectoral flap on the chest wall prior to transfer.

Additional experience with the deltopectoral flap led to its application to intraoral reconstruction of the tongue, floor of the mouth, tonsil, and pharynx. It has also been widely used for external defects of the neck, cheek, ear, and mentum (19). Ingenious techniques, albeit through staged procedures, of reconstructing extensive mid and upper facial defects have been reported by "waltzing" the pedicle to more cephalad regions. Resurfacing hemifacial and orbitomaxillary defects have been described (6,23). A favorable body habitus and, more often, the institution of a prior delay are critical to the use of this flap for more cephalad defects of the face. McGregor and Reid (21) described the combined use of the forehead flap to achieve internal lining and the deltopectoral flap for external lining when reconstructing through-and-through defects of the cheek. Bakamjian and Poole (6) described the use of the deltopectoral flap for reconstructing the palate following ablative surgery. In most cases, except where an island flap is created, the use of the deltopectoral flap for relining any part of the gullet required the creation of a control salivary fistula that was subsequently closed at the time of returning the pedicle to the chest wall.

NEUROVASCULAR ANATOMY

The blood supply to the deltopectoral flap is derived from parasternal perforators of the internal mammary artery and vein, which traverse the intercostal interspaces. The 2-cm zone lateral to the border of the sternum should not be violated when raising this flap to avoid injury to these vessels. The second and third perforators are usually the largest in size with external diameters in the range of 1.2 mm. The venae comitantes are usually equal or greater in diameter (Figure 6-5).

The vessels of the deltopectoral flap run in a plane superficial to the fascia overlying the pectoralis major and deltoid muscles. Although this flap is most commonly harvested with this fascial layer to protect the circulation, it is not an absolute requirement to do so (16).

A number of articles have been written on the nature of the vascular supply to the deltopectoral flap and the implications for safely harvesting skin overlying the deltoid muscle. A review of the vascular territories of the upper chest provides a better understanding of the potential problems that may arise when using skin from distal portions of this flap. The angiosome concept may be applied to this discussion by defining the source vessels that supply the anterior thoracic skin. The primary region of the internal mammary perforators extends from the lateral border of the sternum to the deltopectoral groove. This territory is also supplied by musculocutaneous per-

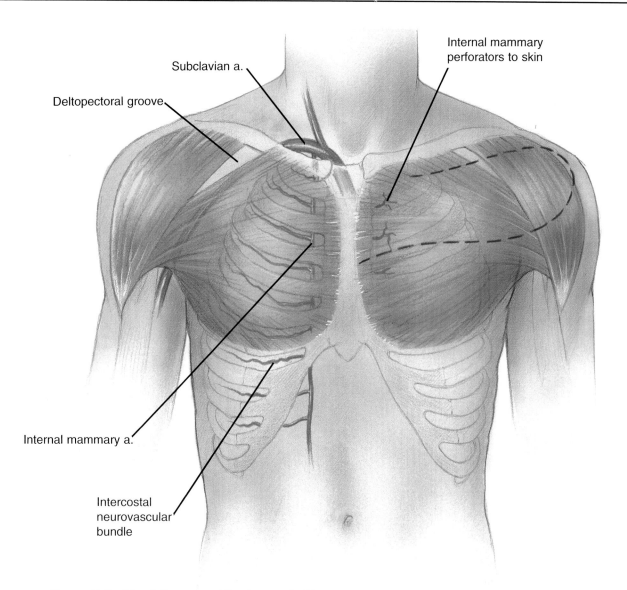

Figure 6-5. The deltopectoral flap is supplied by internal mammary perforators, which emerge from the second and third intercostal space in the parasternal region.

forators arising from the pectoralis major. In the region of the deltopectoral groove, there is a direct cutaneous artery arising from the thoracoacromial system, which supplies a small area of skin below the clavicle. The skin of the deltoid territory, lying lateral to the deltopectoral groove, is supplied by musculocutaneous branches arising from the deltoid branch of the thoracoacromial system and the anterior circumflex humeral artery. It is therefore evident that, in raising a deltopectoral flap, the skin overlying the deltoid muscle and the deltopectoral groove, which were previously supplied by musculocutaneous vessels and direct cutaneous vessels, respectively, must now be captured and made exclusively dependent on the internal mammary perforators. In the angiosome model described by Taylor et al. (25), the blood supply to skin in immediately adjacent angiosomes is usually quite reliable. However, the pressure gradient of the nutrient flow diminishes as one moves to the angiosome next in line, or "once removed," from the primary source vessel. The skin overlying the deltoid muscle is an angiosome once removed from the internal mammary angiosome, and therefore, that skin is at risk for partial or total necrosis. It is possible that the variable pattern of reliability of the tip of the deltopectoral flap is a function of the

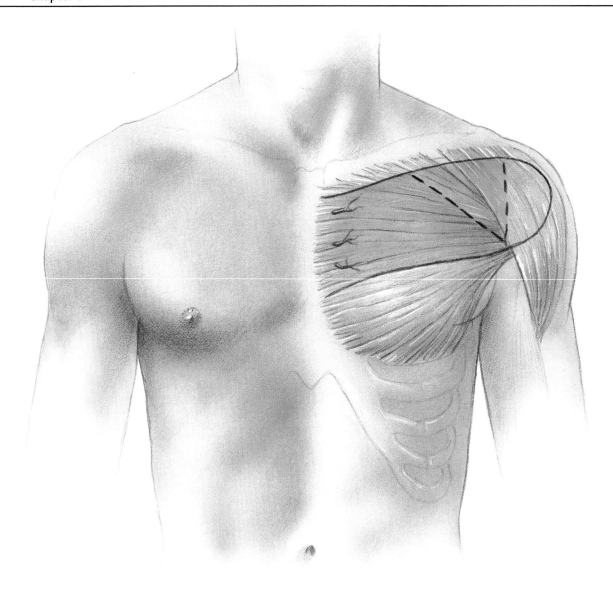

Figure 6-6. The three major angiosomes of the upper chest and shoulder, moving from medial to lateral, are the internal mammary, acromiothoracic, and the deltoid angiosomes. The regions that are marked represent the approximate territories of these source vessels. To capture the skin in the deltoid angiosome, or the angiosome once removed, flow from the internal mammary perforators must traverse the acromiothoracic angiosome which causes a pressure gradient prior to reaching the deltoid region.

size of the acromiothoracic angiosome that is the middle territory in this series. With a larger and more dominant cutaneous branch from the acromiothoracic axis, the deltoid skin may be rendered less reliable (Figure 6-6).

The angiosome concept provides a framework for describing delay procedures that are used to increase the reliability of the deltoid skin (Figure 6-7). To capture the blood supply of that territory, it is essential to reverse the direction of flow in the adjacent thoracoacromial angiosome and the third angiosome in line overlying the deltoid region. It is critical that the direction of flow across the choke arteries that connect adjacent angiosomes be uniformly oriented from the sternum to the tip of the shoulder. The most promising delay procedures are those that interrupt the source arteries and veins in the intermediate and distal angiosomes to allow reversal of flow and more favorable pressure gradients. This was demonstrated by the fluorescein injection studies of McGregor and Morgan (20). A successful delay procedure for the deltopectoral flap must interrupt the direct cutaneous branch of the thoracoacromial

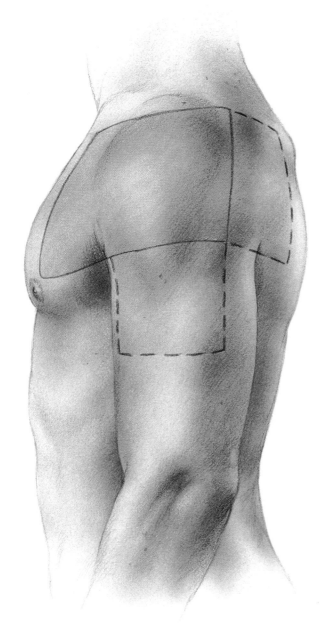

Figure 6-7. A delay procedure is required to enhance the chances of successfully transferring distal portions of the deltopectoral flap, which extend down the arm and around the shoulder.

system and the distal musculocutaneous branches of the deltoid achieved by raising the tip of the flap lateral to the deltopectoral groove and undermining in the infraclavicular fossa.

The sensory nerve supply to the deltopectoral skin is derived from the supraclavicular nerves of C-3 and C-4 and the anterolateral intercostal nerves of T-2, T-3, and T-4. The ability to maintain the sensory supply intact largely depends on whether a radical neck dissection is performed. As noted previously, the report by David (7) of a sensate deltopectoral flap was the first successful restoration of sensation to the reconstructed oral lining (Figure 6-4).

POTENTIAL PITFALLS

The technique of deltopectoral flap harvest is so straightforward that it is rare to encounter problems leading to total flap necrosis. The problem of partial tip necrosis has varied in different series, depending on the length of the flap and the use of a delay procedure. Park et al. (24) warned that factors contributing to flap loss included diabetes, wound infection, and a radiated recipient bed. In a series of 51 deltopectoral flaps placed in irradiated beds, Krizek and Robson (16) reported only five major complications. Kirkby et al. (15) noted an overall total flap failure rate of 26%, which required secondary reconstructive procedures. Higher rates of flap failure were noted in flaps placed for internal lining and for flaps used in an irradiated field. The total flap failure rate of 26% was considerably greater than that reported in other large series, *e.g.*, 9% (5), 12% (17), 16% (24), and 14% (22). Minor complications that did not require additional surgery ranged from 14% (5) to 26% (17).

Although extension of the flap over the deltoid leading to distal ischemia is the most common cause of partial necrosis, there are a variety of other etiologic factors that have been implicated, *e.g.*, placement of the flap over a mandibular K wire, folding of the flap for inner and outer lining, head movement causing flap tension or kinking, and inadequate oro- or pharyngostomal aperture through which to pass the deltopectoral flap for mucosal replacement (11). The wide array of flaps that are available for oral and pharyngeal defects have limited the current role of the deltopectoral flap to reconstruction of cervical cutaneous defects. For this purpose, the deltopectoral flap should be considered a highly reliable technique.

Flap Harvesting Technique

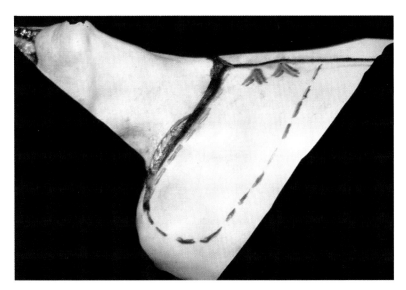

Figure 6-8. A deltopectoral flap is shown outlined over the right upper chest. The upper incision runs just inferior to the clavicle; the inferior incision extends from the fourth or fifth interspace, parallel to the upper incision. The distal extent of the flap is determined by the defect. The dominant pedicle to this flap arises in the second or third interspace, and therefore to ensure viability, the base should overlie these two interspaces.

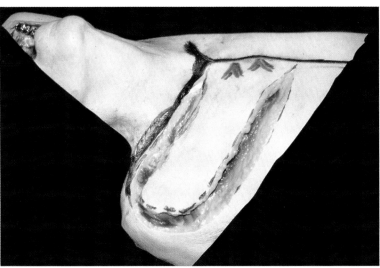

Figure 6-9. Incisions are made along the upper, lower, and distal margins. The incision is made through the skin, subcutaneous tissue, and deltopectoral fascia.

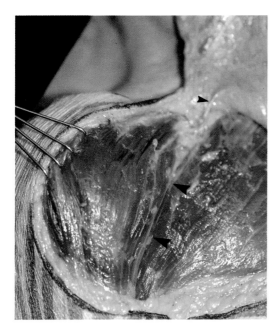

Figure 6-10. As the flap is elevated laterally to medially in a subfascial plane, the deltopectoral groove (*large arrows*) is encountered. The direct cutaneous branch arising from either the deltoid or acromial branches (*small arrow*) has been isolated in the cephalad aspect of the groove.

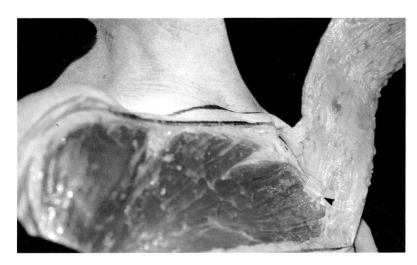

Figure 6-11. The medial extent of the dissection is usually to a point approximately 2 cm lateral to the sternal border. Although an internal mammary perforator (*arrow*) has been isolated to demonstrate its position, these vessels are not identified in the dissection for fear of injuring the blood supply to the flap.

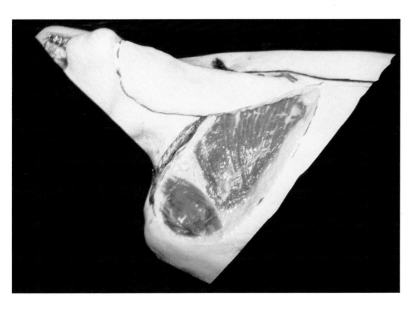

Figure 6-12. The deltopectoral flap has been completely isolated and transposed over the clavicle onto the anterior neck. Closure of the donor site is accomplished by wide undermining and the use of retention sutures. Although primary closure may be achieved, the use of a skin graft is the norm.

REFERENCES

1. Aymard JL: Nasal reconstruction with a note on nature's plastic surgery. *Lancet* 1917;2:888.
2. Bakamjian VY: A two-stage method for pharyngoesophageal reconstruction with a primary pectoral skin flap. *Plast Reconstr Surg* 1965;36:173.
3. Bakamjian VY: Total reconstruction of pharynx with medially based deltopectoral skin flap. *N Y State J Med* 1968;1:2771.
4. Bakamjian VY, Holbrook L: Prefabrication techniques in cervical pharyngoesophageal reconstruction. *Br J Plast Surg* 1973;26:214
5. Bakamjian VY, Long M, Rigg B: Experience with the medially based deltopectoral flap in reconstructive surgery of the head and neck. *Br J Plast Surg* 1971;24:174.
6. Bakamjian VY, Poole M: Maxillofacial and palatal reconstructions with the deltopectoral flap. *Br J Plast Surg* 1977;30:17.
7. David JD: Use of an innervated deltopectoral flap for intraoral reconstruction. *Plast Reconstr Surg* 1977;60:377.
8. East C, Flemming A, Brough M: Tracheostomal reconstruction using a fenestrated deltopectoral skin flap. *J Laryngol Otol* 1988;102:282.
9. Fujino T, Tanino R, Sugimoto C: Microvascular transfer of free deltopectoral dermal-fat flap. *Plast Reconstr Surg* 1975;55:428.
10. Gibson T, Robinson D: The mammary artery pectoral flaps of Jacques Joseph. *Br J Plast Surg* 1976;29:370.
11. Gingrass R, Culf N, Garrett W, Mladick R: Complications with the deltopectoral flap. *Plast Reconstr Surg* 1972;49:501.
12. Harii K, Ohmori K, Ohmori S: Free deltopectoral skin flaps. *Br J Plast Surg* 1974;27:231.
13. Jackson I, Lang W: Secondary esophagoplasty after pharyngolaryngectomy using a modified deltopectoral flap. *Plast Reconstr Surg* 1971;48:155.
14. Joseph J: *Nasenplastik und sonstige Gesichtsplastik nebs teinem Anhang uber Mammaplastik und einige weitere Operationen aus dem gebiek der ausseren Korperplastik.* Leipzig: Verlag von Curt Kabitzchl; 1931:673–677, 811–819.
15. Kirkby B, Krag C, Siemssen O: Experience with the deltopectoral flap. *Scand J Plast Reconstr Surg* 1980;14:151.
16. Krizek T, Robson M: The deltopectoral flap for reconstruction of irradiated cancer of the head and neck. *Surg Gynecol Obstet* 1972;135:787.
17. Krizek T, Robson M: Split flap in head and neck reconstruction. *Am J Surg* 1973;126:488.
18. McGregor I: The temporal flap in intraoral cancer; its use in repairing the post-excisional defects. *Br J Plast Surg* 1963;16:318.
19. McGregor I, Jackson I: The extended role of the deltopectoral flap. *Br J Plast Surg* 1970;23:173–185.
20. McGregor I, Morgan G: Axial and random pattern flaps. *Br J Plast Surg* 1973;26:202.
21. McGregor I, Reid W: The use of the temporal flap in the primary repair of full-thickness defects of the cheek. *Plast Reconstr Surg* 1966;38:1.
22. Mendelson B, Woods J, Masson J: Experience with the deltopectoral flap. *Plast Reconstr Surg* 1977;59:360.
23. Nickell W, Salyer K, Vargas M: Practical variations in the use of the deltopectoral flap. *South Med J* 1974;67:697.
24. Park J, Sako K, Marchette F: Reconstructive experience with the medially based deltopectoral flap. *Am J Surg* 1974;128:548.
25. Taylor GI, Palmer J: The vascular territories (angiosomes) of the body: experimental study and clinical applications. *Br J Plast Surg* 1987;40:113.
26. Urken ML, Vickery C, Weinberg H, Biller HF: The neurofasciocutaneous radial forearm flap in head and neck reconstruction—a preliminary report. *Laryngoscope* 1990;100:161.

REGIONAL FLAPS
Cutaneous and Fasciocutaneous Flaps

Anterior and Posterior Scalp

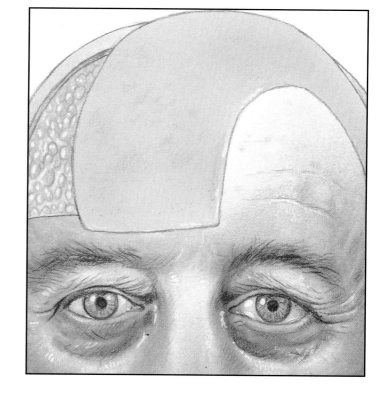

Mack L. Cheney, M.D., and
Mark L. Urken, M.D.

The myriad of regional and free flaps that are presently available has made it possible to transfer skin of virtually any size and shape to the facial region. However, the requirement of using skin of similar color and texture to that of the native facial skin greatly limits the available donor sites (2,5,14,18,20). The skin of the forehead and the posterior neck perhaps come closest to mimicking the facial skin. Tissue from both of these regions can be transferred to the midface for cheek and nasal reconstruction by using the scalp as a carrier. In the 1930s, Gillies (14,15) developed the principles of transferring forehead skin for nasal reconstruction.

MacGregor (21) is credited with introducing the forehead flap for intraoral reconstruction in 1963 (17). Along with the deltopectoral flap, this flap was the primary source of tissue for head and neck reconstruction until the development of the extensive range of regional musculocutaneous and free flaps that began in the 1970s and continued to the present. Although MacGregor's (21) transverse forehead flap is rarely used today because of the morbidity of the skin grafted donor site, the forehead continues to be widely utilized for resurfacing cutaneous and soft tissue defects of the nose and cheek (3). A variety of forehead flap designs have been reported during the last six decades, including the median, the paramedian, the sickle, and the oblique patterns of forehead skin transfers.

During World War II, Converse (7,9,10) introduced the anterior scalping flap, which transferred the skin of one half of the forehead. The flap is based on the contralateral vascular supply of the scalp. It was originally developed as a variation of Gillies "up-and-down flap" and includes the forehead skin, the scalp, and galea with its vascular supply derived from the vessels of the forehead and anterior portion of the scalp. Despite the necessity of a two-stage procedure, this technique continues to have specific applications for the reconstruction of large nasal, upper lip, and cheek cutaneous defects for which color match and tissue pliability are priorities.

Arena (1) recognized that the posterior neck skin has similar qualities to that of the facial skin and reported a two-stage technique for transferring skin from this region to the face. Using surgical principles similar to those developed by Gillies (14) and Converse (7) for transferring forehead skin to the nose, he used the rich vascularity of the scalp as a vehicle for transporting favorable skin from the nape of the neck to the midface. Closure of this donor site was accomplished with a skin graft or a scalp-advancement flap. As a result of its posterior location, the donor-site defect is more easily camouflaged than the deformity caused by an anterior scalp flap. This technique may be considered an extension of the flap developed by Washio (28,29) in which postauricular skin is transferred for reconstructing limited facial and nasal defects (22).

FLAP DESIGN AND UTILIZATION

The anterior scalp flap is most useful in the reconstruction of large nasal and paranasal defects. The pliability of the distal aspect of the flap allows it to be contoured to recreate the anatomic details that are required to satisfactorily reconstruct the nose (4). The anterior scalping flap offers some distinct advantages compared with other forehead flaps. The design of the flap provides an adequate pedicle length because of the extensive undermining that can be safely performed. Because of the limited tension in the forehead skin that is transferred, lower nasal and columella reconstruction can be safely performed when required. When columella reconstruction is needed, an adequate vertical length is essential to allow the tip of the reconstructed nose to be sufficiently projected (Figure 7-1) (11). The area of flap harvest is limited to one half of the forehead, which facilitates concealment of the donor site. This flap should be considered in patients whose foreheads are narrow or who have a low hairline. In such patients, a median or paramedian forehead flap would transfer hair-bearing skin when resurfacing caudal nasal defects. One of the unique features of the anterior scalp flap is that there is sufficient length to fold the flap on itself to create an inner lining for both the ala and the columella.

It is often helpful to fashion a template of the nasofacial defect that can be used to design the area of skin to be transferred from the forehead. The pattern that is created should be as accurate as possible to minimize the amount of skin transferred and the necessity for secondary flap debulking (2,3,16).

Secondary flap division is customarily performed at 21 days unless the recipient bed has been compromised by prior radiation or scar. At the time of the initial flap transfer, the donor site is covered with a full-thickness skin graft harvested from the postauricular or supraclavicular areas (23).

The anterior scalping flap's biggest drawback is the donor-site defect. The aesthetic deformity can be minimized by preserving innervated frontalis muscle. Placement of the skin graft over this muscle improves the contour of the forehead and preserves expressive movement in this region (23). As a secondary procedure, the donor site can be reduced by serial excisions or resurfaced with a temporofasciocervical flap (19,25). This technique may be particularly necessary in male patients and in cases in which hyperpigmentation of the graft develops. Additional options for donor-site camouflage include changes in the patient's hair style and the use of a tissue expander to allow advancement of the contralateral forehead for full-thickness skin coverage of the defect.

When contemplating the use of a posterior scalp flap it is important to examine the texture and color of the posterior neck skin to determine its suitability for replacing skin in the midface region. In women who have longer hair styles, the skin of this region tends to be well protected from the effects of the sun. In addition, longer hair

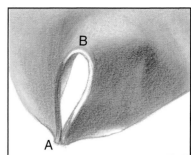

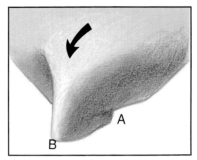

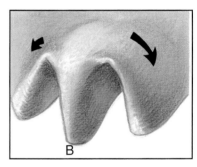

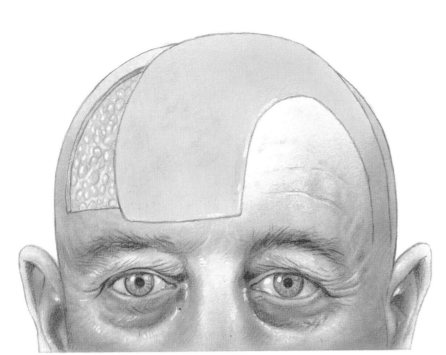

Figure 7-1. The anterior scalp flap transfers up to one half of the forehead skin, using the scalp as a carrier. Its primary advantages are that it provides skin of the closest color and texture to the skin of the cheek and nose. In addition, it has the viability and the length to achieve a detailed reconstruction of the caudal portion of the nose. Inner lining of the caudal portion of the nose may be achieved by folding this flap on itself. When significant defects of the nose require reconstruction, then local or distant flaps may be required to achieve an adequate lining. This factor is of paramount importance when replacing the architectural support of the nose by the use of free bone grafts. A reliable inner lining, under these circumstances, is critical for the protection and revascularization of these nonvascularized structural grafts.

makes the camouflage of this defect much easier. The posterior neck skin in patients who have spent considerable time in the sun may be unsuitable for resurfacing cutaneous defects of the face. In most individuals, however, the process of photoaging tends to affect the skin in the posterior neck in a similar manner to that of the skin of the face (27).

The scalp is the thickest skin in the human body. The dermis and epidermis of the scalp region vary in thickness from 3 to 8 mm. However, the skin in the postauricular area and the posterior neck is much thinner and more pliable. It is therefore suitable for the reconstruction of large defects of the nose, cheek, and orbital cavity. Its use in the reconstruction of the upper and lower lips has also been described (28,29). In addition to its use in oncological surgery, the posterior scalp flap may be extended onto the posterior shoulder to provide a large area of skin that may be utilized to replace areas of scar contracture caused by trauma, irradiation, or burns.

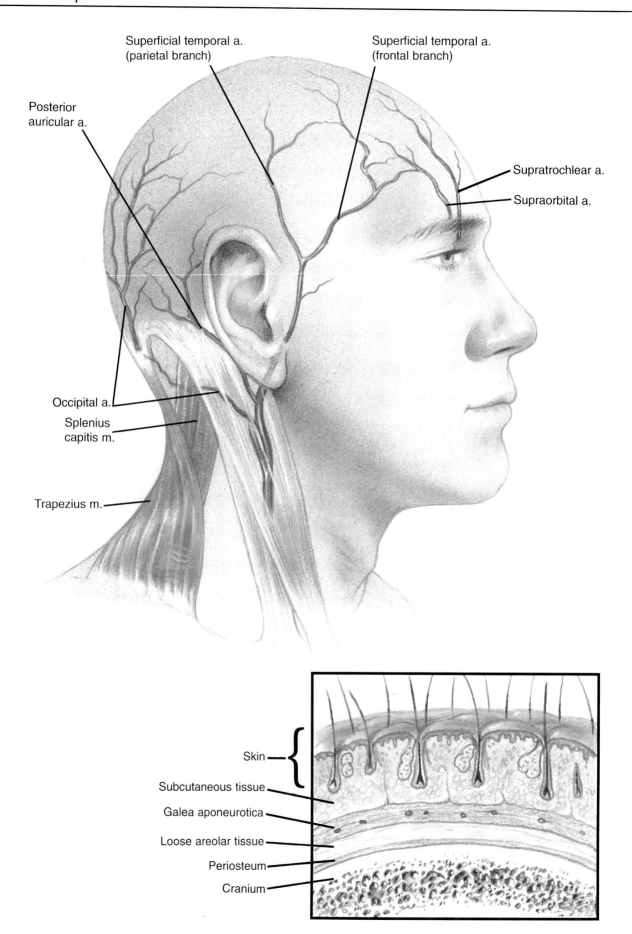

Superficial temporal a.
(parietal branch)

Superficial temporal a.
(frontal branch)

Posterior
auricular a.

Supratrochlear a.

Supraorbital a.

Occipital a.

Splenius
capitis m.

Trapezius m.

Skin

Subcutaneous tissue

Galea aponeurotica

Loose areolar tissue

Periosteum

Cranium

NEUROVASCULAR ANATOMY

The scalp is supplied by a rich array of arteries, including the superficial temporal, supraorbital, supratrochlear, occipital, and postauricular (Figure 7-2). There are significant anastomotic channels between the different primary scalp vessels that make it possible to transfer large areas of the scalp on a single arterial pedicle.

The anterior scalp flap is supplied by the supratrochlear, supraorbital, and superficial temporal vessels of the side opposite to that in which the forehead skin is harvested. The frontal branch of the superficial temporal artery should be identified prior to surgery by palpation or Doppler sonography. This branch should be incorporated by designing the flap so that the transverse limb of the incision that crosses over the scalp is placed behind this vessel.

The venous drainage to this area is reliable. The supraorbital veins run superficial to the frontalis and communicate with the frontal branch of the superficial temporal vein and the supraorbital vein. All these veins contribute to the vascular egress in the anterior scalping flap.

The vascular supply of the posterior scalping flap is similar to that of the anterior flap. The contributions from the occipital artery are transsected in the process of raising this flap, and therefore, it is entirely dependent on the blood flow from the anterior system. The parietal branch of the superficial temporal artery is preserved when harvesting the posterior scalp flap, and this branch plays a significant role in ensuring an adequate circulation to the posterior neck skin. The venous supply to the posterior scalp flap parallels that of the arteries. The full extent of the skin territory that can be harvested with this flap is unknown. We have safely harvested skin to the level of the scapular spine, which increases both the surface area and the arc of rotation.

The sensory supply to the anterior scalp is primarily derived from the supraorbital nerve, which is a branch of the ophthalmic branch of the trigeminal nerve. The auriculotemporal branch of the trigeminal nerve supplies sensation to the temporoparietal scalp. Contributions from the cervical plexus supply sensation to the posterior scalp through the greater auricular and the greater and lesser occipital nerves.

POTENTIAL PITFALLS

The rich vascularity of the scalp makes it uncommon for ischemic complications to occur in either the posterior or anterior flaps. These two flaps are unique in the head and neck because of the fact that the pedicle is located either cephalad or on an even plane to the defect and, therefore, the effects of gravity are not problematic in causing flap separation from a poor recipient bed. The latter problem is often encountered in heavily irradiated wounds when the flap pedicle is located in a dependent position.

Figure 7-2. The scalp has a rich vascular supply that arises from the supratrochlear, the supraorbital, the two major branches of the superficial temporal, the occipital, and the posterior auricular arteries. There are significant anastomoses between all of these systems that allow long narrow flaps to be transferred if at least one of these major arteries is incorporated in the base of the flap. The posterior scalp flap involves the transfer of skin from the nape of the neck region overlying the splenius capitis and trapezius. The major layers of the scalp are shown. The vascular channels are located in the galea and subcutaneous tissue layers. The loose areolar layer that separates the galea from the periosteum is a relatively avascular plane that is responsible for the mobility of the scalp over the bone.

POSTOPERATIVE WOUND CARE

Both the anterior and posterior scalp flaps have the disadvantage of requiring a two-stage procedure. The nutrient vascular flow through the scalp must be maintained for 2 to 3 weeks until neovascularization at the recipient site has occurred. The interval between the first and second procedures is uncomfortable for the patient because of the cosmetic deformity of the displaced scalp and the necessity for biologic dressings over the denuded portion of the skull. The patient must be advised preoperatively of these factors to be psychologically prepared.

Flap Harvesting Technique
Anterior Scalping Flap Dissection

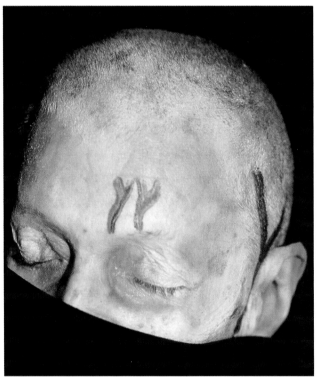

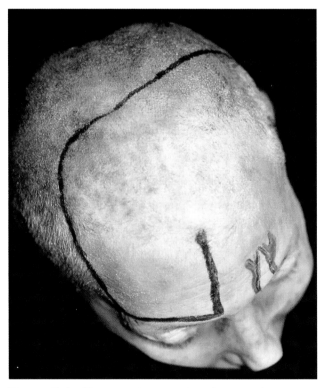

Figure 7-3. The primary vascular supply to the anterior scalp flap is from the supratrochlear and supraorbital vessels in conjunction with the frontal branch of the superficial temporal artery and vein.

Figure 7-4. The anterior scalping flap has been outlined to transfer skin from one side of the forehead. It is often fabricated from a template of the defect to transfer only that portion of the forehead that is needed. However, the aesthetic result is improved by skin grafting a defect that extends from the eyebrow to the hairline. The extension of the incision across the vertex of the scalp to the contralateral ear ensures vascularity through the three dominant pedicles of this flap.

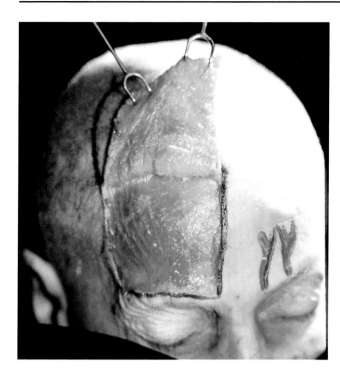

Figure 7-5. The skin of the forehead is elevated over the frontalis on which a split- or full-thickness skin graft is subsequently applied.

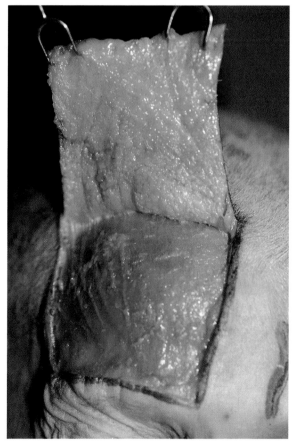

Figure 7-6. It is important when making the lateral incision to preserve the innervation to the frontalis. After the upper limit of the frontalis has been reached, the level of dissection is changed to the supraperiosteal plane, which is carried over the remainder of the skull.

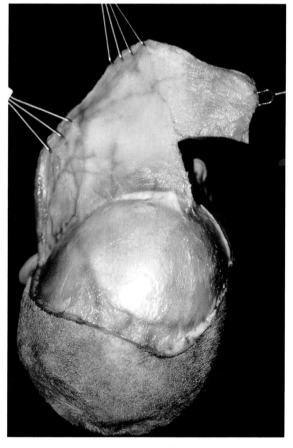

Figure 7-7. The anterior scalp flap has been elevated. The large area of denuded skull is noted. The transitional zone can be easily seen on the undersurface of the flap. Undermining over the contralateral forehead is performed to provide adequate mobility to achieve caudal transposition of the forehead skin.

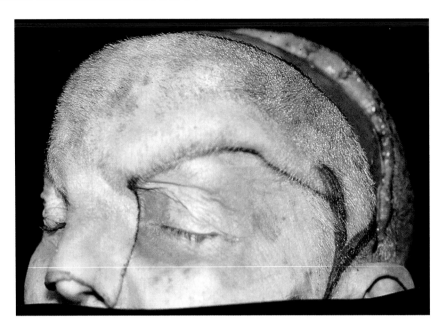

Figure 7-8. A large quantity of thin pliable skin can be transferred to reconstruct total or near-total nasal defects. Further undermining of the contralateral scalp allows the forehead skin to be placed onto the upper lip or cheek as needed. Following this stage of the procedure, the denuded scalp must be carefully covered with a biologic dressing for the 2- to 3-week period prior to the second stage.

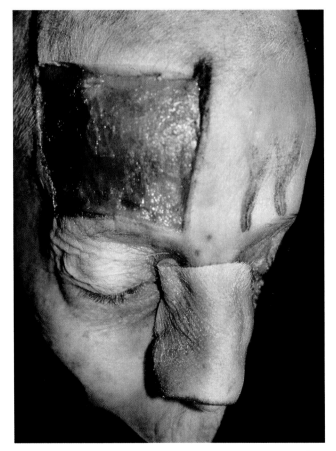

Figure 7-9. The scalp is transferred back to the donor site, leaving the forehead defect, which was previously covered at the time of the first procedure with a split- or full-thickness graft. Smaller defects may be covered with a skin graft harvested from the postauricular region. Advancement of the contralateral forehead may be achieved by either serial excision or use of a tissue expander.

Posterior Scalping Flap Dissection

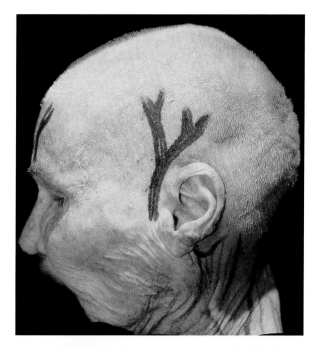

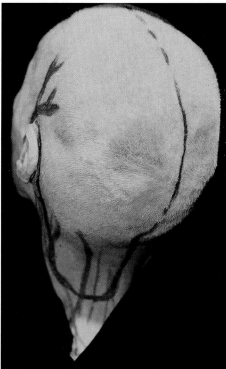

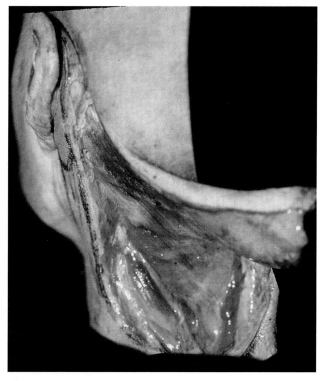

Figure 7-10. The dominant blood supply to the posterior scalping flap is derived from the anterior blood supply to the scalp through the supraorbital, the supratrochlear, and both branches of the superficial temporal artery and vein. The occipital branches that supply the posterior scalp are transsected in the process of elevating this flap.

Figure 7-11. The incisions for raising the posterior scalp flap are shown. The extension in the postauricular sulcus is required to achieve adequate mobilization of this flap. It is imperative that the postauricular incision stop at the superior attachment of the helix to avoid violating the vascular supply from the superficial temporal vessels. The *dotted line* in the midline of the scalp demonstrates a possible extension of the incision, depending on the degree to which the flap must be mobilized to achieve tension-free closure of the defect.

Figure 7-12. The skin of the posterior neck is elevated superficial to the trapezius, splenius capitis, and levator scapulae. At the superior nuchal line, the plane of dissection changes to a supraperiosteal level, which is continued over the remainder of the skull.

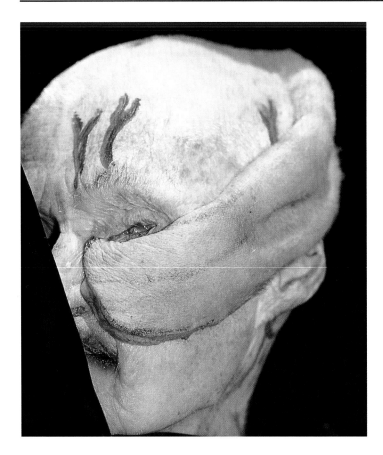

Figure 7-13. Elevation of the scalp is continued until the posterior neck skin can be placed in the desired recipient defect. The midface can be easily reached and a tension-free closure performed without doing extensive undermining.

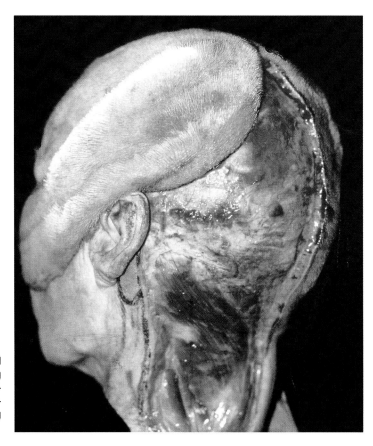

Figure 7-14. The arc of rotation can be increased to reconstruct the nose or upper lip by extending the incision in the midline of the scalp. Extensive undermining does not in any way hinder the blood supply to the posterior neck skin, which is running through the galea and subcutaneous tissue layers.

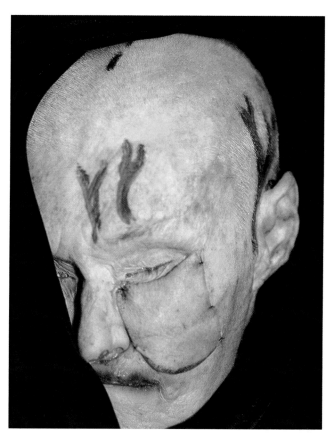

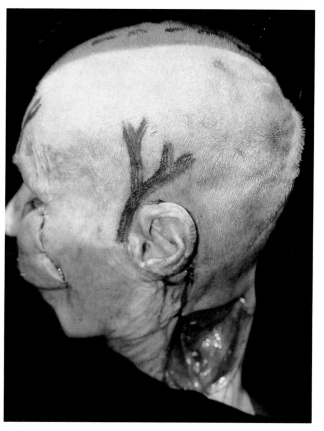

Figure 7-15. The skin of the posterior neck has been detached from the scalp pedicle. During the time interval prior to the second surgical procedure, the denuded posterior scalp must be covered with a biologic dressing. A skin graft is placed over the donor defect in the neck that overlies the posterior neck muscles.

Figure 7-16. The posterior neck defect can often be well camouflaged in individuals with longer hair styles and by the use of high-collared shirts. Over time, the aesthetic appearance of this defect improves. The size of the defect may be diminished by serial excision or the use of a tissue expander.

REFERENCES

1. Arena S: The posterior scalping flap. *Laryngoscope* 1977;137:98–104.
2. Blair VP: Reconstructive surgery of the face. *Surg Gynecol Obstet* 1922;34:701.
3. Burget GC, Menick FJ: *Aesthetic Reconstruction of the Nose.* St. Louis: CV Mosby; 1994:57–91.
4. Coiffman F: Total reconstruction of the nose.In: Stark RB: *Plastic Surgery of the Head and Neck, vol. 1.* New York: Churchill, 1986;704–705.
5. Coleman CC: Scalp flap reconstruction in head and neck cancer patients. *Plast Reconstr Surg* 1959;24:45.
6. Conley J: *Regional Flaps of the Head and Neck.* Stuttgart: Georg Thieme Verlag; 1976.
7. Converse JM: A new forehead flap for nasal reconstruction. *Proc R Soc Med* 1942;35:811.
8. Converse JM: Reconstruction of the nose by scalping flap technique. *Surg Clin North Am* 1959;39:335.
9. Converse JM: Clinical application of the scalping flap in the reconstruction of the nose. *Plast Reconstr Surg* 1969;43:247.
10. Converse JM: Full-thickness loss of nasal tissue. In: Converse JM: *Reconstructive Plastic Surgery. vol. 2.* Philadelphia: WB Saunders; 1977:1236.
11. Converse JM, McCarthy JG: The scalping forehead flap revisited. *Clin Plast Surg* 1981;8:413.
12. Denneny EC, Denneny J III: Forehead and scalp reconstruction. In: Papel ID, Nachlias NE, eds. *Facial Plastic and Reconstructive Surgery.* St. Louis: Mosby-Year Book; 1992:392–398.
13. Friedman M: Parietal occipital nape of neck flap. *Arch Otolaryngol Head Neck Surg* 1986;112:309.
14. Gillies HD: *Plastic Surgery of the Face.* London: Oxford University Press; 1920.
15. Gillies HD: The development and scope of plastic surgery. *Northwest Univ Bull* 1935;35:1.
16. Gonzalez-Ulloa M: Restoration of the facial covering by means of selected skin in regional aesthetic units. *Br J Plast Surg* 1956;46:265.
17. Hamaker RC, Singer MI: Regional flaps in head and neck reconstruction. *Otolaryngol Clin North Am* 1982;15:99.
18. Joseph J: Nasenplastik und sonstige Geisichtoplastik nebst einem Anhang uber Mammaplastik und

einige weitere Operationen aus dem Gebiete der ausserreu Korperplastik. In: *Bin Atlas und Lehrbuch.* Leipzig: Kabitzsh; 1931.

19. Juri J, Juri C, Cerisola J: Contribution to Converse's flap for nasal reconstruction. *Plast Reconstr Surg* 1982;69:697.

20. Kazanjian VH: The repair of nasal defects with the median forehead flap. Primary closure of the forehead wound. *Surg Gynecol Obstet* 1946;83:37.

21. MacGregor IA: The temporal flap in the intraoral defects: its use in repairing postexcisional defects. *Br J Plast Surg* 1965:16:318–335.

22. Maillard GF, Montandon D: The Washio tempororetroauricular flap: its use in 20 patients. *Plast Reconstr Surg* 1982;70:550.

23. McCarthy JG, Converse JM: Nasal reconstruction with scalping flap. In: Brent B, ed. *The Artistry of Reconstructive Surgery.* St. Louis: CV Mosby; 1987.

24. Millard DR: Total reconstructive rhinoplasty and a missing link. *Plast Reconstr Surg* 1966;37:167.

25. Schimmelbusch C: Bin neues Verfahren der Rhinoplastik und Operation der Sattelnase. *Verh Dtsch Ges Chir* 1895;24:342.

26. Smet HT: *Tissue Transfers in Reconstructive Surgery.* New York: Raven Press; 1980:6–7.

27. Stark RB, Khoury F: Anatomy of the skull, scalp, and brow. In: Stark RB, ed. *Plastic Surgery of the Head and Neck.* vol. 1. New York: Churchill Livingstone; 1987:3–6.

28. Washio H: Retroauricular-temporal flap. *Plast Reconstr Surg* 1969;43:162–166.

29. Washio H: Further experiences with the retroauricular temporal flap. *Plast Reconstr Surg* 1972;50:160.

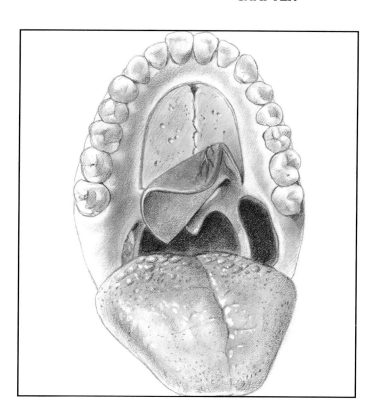

Palatal
Island

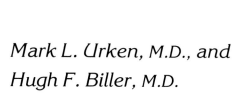

Mark L. Urken, M.D., and
Hugh F. Biller, M.D.

The reconstruction of mucosal defects of the oral cavity following trauma or ablative surgery can be a challenging problem. Primary closure, healing by secondary intention, or the application of skin grafts are effective techniques in most situations. It is tempting to borrow mucosa from adjacent areas of the oral cavity, and a wide variety of "oral flaps" have been described (3). In particular, the tongue has been subjected to assault as the source of well-vascularized mucosa to resurface defects from the palate to the hypopharynx. However, when the surgeon borrows tissue from the region that is being reconstructed, it is imperative that a critical appraisal be made of the potential deficits associated with borrowing that tissue. The availability of a wide range of alternative flaps from regional or distant sites makes it generally unnecessary to use tissue from the tongue to resurface the oral cavity or pharynx. The tongue is the most critical structure in the oral cavity for postoperative oral function. To interfere with its activity, in any way, should be condemned.

However, this philosophy does not take away from the desirability of using "like tissue" to accomplish the reconstruction. The transfer of well-vascularized, sensate mucosa is particularly appealing. The palatal island mucoperiosteal flap is an attractive reconstructive option for those reasons. Originally introduced by Millard (5) in 1962, it was popularized for use in ablative defects of the posterior oral cavity by Gullane and Arena (1). The latter authors expanded the utility of this flap by reporting the safe transfer of virtually the entire hard palate mucoperiosteum on a single neurovascular pedicle (2). Although the loss of mucosa from the palate creates a secondary defect of exposed bone, the healing of that defect by secondary intention causes no functional morbidity. The fact that the secondary defect overlies bone ensures that it will heal without contraction.

The vascular pedicle of the palatal island mucoperiosteal flap is unique because it traverses a bony canal, and also because of its nondependent position in the oral cavity, which eliminates the detrimental effects of gravitational pull.

FLAP DESIGN AND UTILIZATION

Because of the small area of mucosa of the palate, there is a limited range of flap designs. The island flap that was reported by Millard (5) was harvested from one side of the palate. Gullane and Arena (2) expanded the area of transfer to include virtually the entire palatal mucoperiosteum, providing approximately 8 to 10 cm² of tissue. The flap island is created by incising the palate 1 cm medial to the teeth and 1.5 cm anterior to the junction of the hard and soft palate. The flap can be rotated 180 degrees for inserting it into defects of the retromolar trigone and tonsillar fossa. To improve the arc of rotation, the hook of the hamulus can be removed, thereby providing an additional 1 cm of length.

The island palatal flap is ideal for resurfacing defects of the retromolar trigone, tonsil, and lateral pharyngeal wall. It has been used to restore velopharyngeal competence in combination with a mucosal flap from the posterior pharyngeal wall (6). This flap is also useful in cleft palate repair and for closure of oroantral fistulas (2).

NEUROVASCULAR ANATOMY

A thorough understanding of the osteology of the palate is crucial to raising the mucoperiosteal flap. The hard palate is formed by the palatine processes of the max-

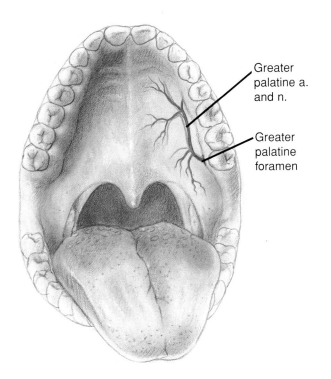

Greater
palatine a.
and n.

Greater
palatine
foramen

Figure 8-1. The greater palatine artery and nerve emerge from the greater palatine canal through the greater palatine foramen. The neurovascular pedicle runs forward on the palate, and the artery then ascends through the incisive canal to supply the nasal mucosa.

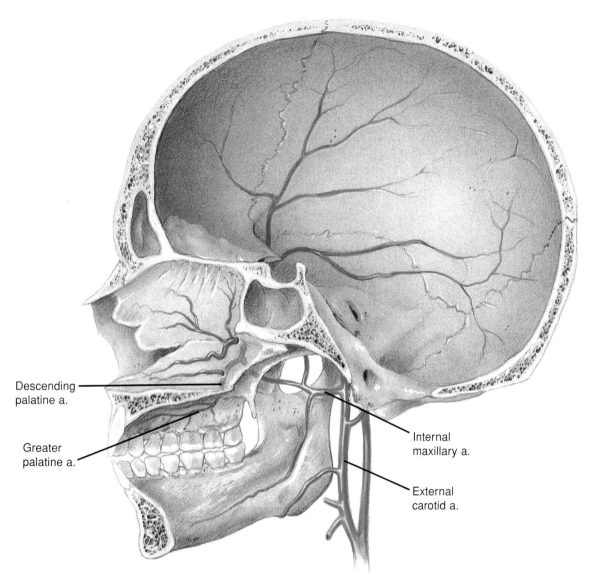

Descending palatine a.

Greater palatine a.

Internal maxillary a.

External carotid a.

Figure 8-2. The greater palatine artery is a branch of the descending palatine artery, which in turn, arises from the internal maxillary artery.

illae and the horizontal laminas of the palatine bones. There is a longitudinal suture that separates the palate in the midline and a transverse suture that separates the maxillary shelf from the palatine shelf posteriorly. The greater palatine foramen is located in the lateral aspect of the transverse suture just opposite the second molar (Figure 8-1). Posterolateral to the greater palatine foramen are the lesser palatine foramina, of which there are usually two. The latter foramina are located in the palatine bone and transmit the lesser palatine artery and nerves. The hard palate is covered by a mucosal layer, which is firmly adherent to the periosteum. The periosteum is firmly attached to the palatal bone through the fibrous pegs of Sharpey.

The blood supply to the palate is derived from the descending palatine artery, which is a branch of the internal maxillary artery (Figure 8-2). The descending palatine artery gives off the greater palatine branch, which emerges through the greater palatine foramen with the greater palatine nerve. The greater palatine artery runs forward on the lateral aspect of the palate to supply the mucoperiosteum. The descending palatine artery traverses the greater palatine canal, which connects the pterygomaxillary fossa with the hard palate. The lesser palatine artery, a branch of the descending palatine artery, emerges through the lesser palatine foramina to supply the soft palate. Additional blood supply to the palate comes through branches of the ascending pharyngeal, facial, and lingual arteries. This collateral supply is primarily to the soft palate.

The vascular supply to the palatal island mucoperiosteal flap is the greater palatine artery and vein. After running their posteroanterior course on the hard palate, these vessels ascend in the incisive canals to supply the nasal mucosa. The greater palatine vein drains into the pterygoid plexus of veins. Despite the presence of a midline longitudinal raphe that divides the palatal mucosa in half, Gullane and Arena (1,2) demonstrated that the entire palate could be supplied by one greater palatine pedicle. They referred to the work reported by Maher (4) in 1977, which showed an extensive arborization of the greater palatine vessels, which was termed the "macronet." By arteriographic studies, Maher found evidence of three vascular layers: mucosal, submucosal, and periosteal. The arterial network crossed the midline raphe to provide nutrient flow through one pedicle when the contralateral one was sacrificed.

POTENTIAL PITFALLS

Gullane and Arena (2) reported a 5% failure rate in a series of 53 palatal flaps. They warned against the use of this technique when any of the following three conditions were present: (a) ligation of the external carotid or internal maxillary artery, (b) prior palatal surgery with possible disruption of the greater palatine vessels, or (c) prior radiation to the palate. The surgeon should also be cautious about placing excess tension on the palatal blood supply, which may be less forgiving than most island flaps because of the course of the vessels through a bony canal.

POSTOPERATIVE CARE

The exposed palatal bone is cleansed on a regular basis with frequent oral irrigations. The ingrowth of mucosa from the edges of the defect occurs fairly rapidly. It has been our experience that the mucosal ingrowth brings sensory nerve fibers, which reduces the donor-site morbidity. The fact that the defect overlies bone ensures that there is no scar contracture, which would otherwise occur.

Flap Harvesting Technique

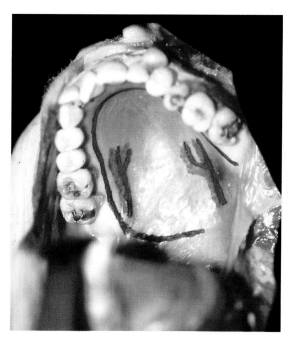

Figure 8-3. The palatal island mucoperiosteal flap is outlined with the approximate position of the greater palatine neurovascular pedicles on either side.

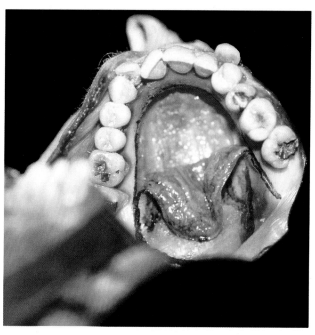

Figure 8-4. The mucoperiosteal flap is elevated by sharp and blunt dissection, moving in an anterior to posterior direction. The mucosal layer is intimately associated with the palatal periosteum.

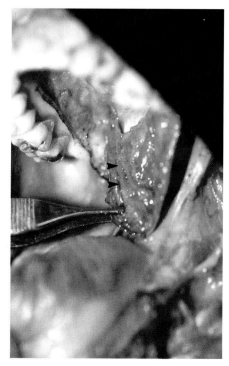

Figure 8-5. The neurovascular arcade (*arrows*) is visualized on the undersurface of the periosteum. It is best to begin the dissection on the side opposite the pedicle that is to be preserved.

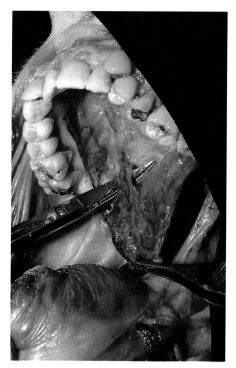

Figure 8-6. The contralateral neurovascular pedicle has been isolated and is now ready to be transsected.

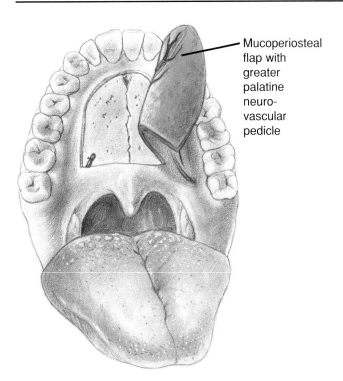

Mucoperiosteal flap with greater palatine neuro-vascular pedicle

Figure 8-7. The mucoperiosteal flap is carefully elevated toward the nutrient neurovascular pedicle. The fixed position of the vessels exiting through the greater palatine foramen provides little leeway in mobilizing the flap. The contralateral pedicle has been ligated and transsected.

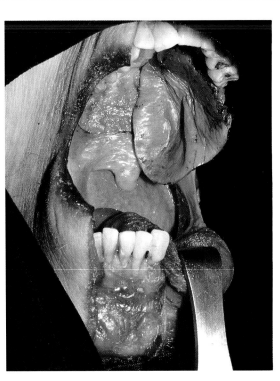

Figure 8-8. The palatal flap is completely isolated on its pedicle and can now be rotated to resurface the mucosal defect.

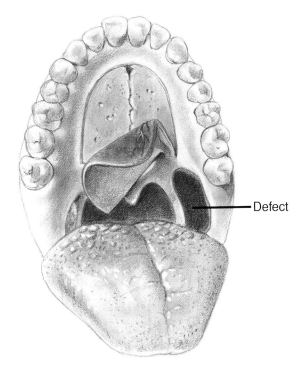

Defect

Figure 8-9. The most frequent use of the palatal flap is to close defects of the tonsillar fossa and the retromolar trigone.

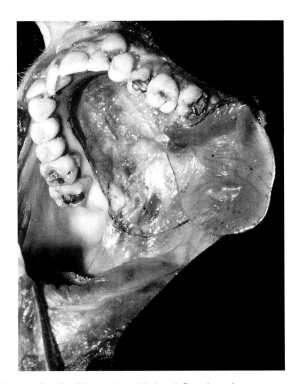

Figure 8-10. The palatal island flap has been rotated 180 degrees. Further mobilization can be achieved by cutting the hook of the hamulus and decompressing the posterior wall of the greater palatine foramen.

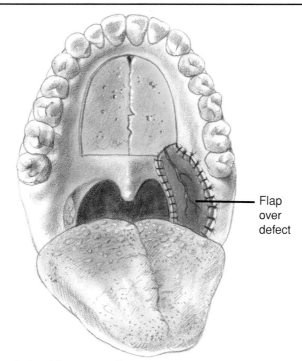

Flap over defect

Figure 8-11. The palatal flap is sutured into the defect. It is important that undue tension is not placed on the flap because the pedicle's course through the greater palatine canal is unforgiving.

REFERENCES

1. Gullane P, Arena S: Palatal island flap for reconstruction of oral defects. *Arch Otolaryngol Head Neck Surg* 1977;103:598.
2. Gullane P, Arena S: Extended palatal island mucoperiosteal flap. *Arch Otolaryngol Head Neck Surg* 1985;111:330.
3. Komisar A, Lawson W: A compendium of intraoral flaps. *Head Neck* 1985;8:91.
4. Maher W: Distribution of palatal and other arteries in cleft and non-cleft human palates. *Cleft Palate Craniofac J* 1977;14:1.
5. Millard DR: Wide and/or short cleft palate. *Plast Reconstr Surg* 1962;29:40.
6. Millard DR, Seider H: The versatile palatal island flap: its use in soft palate reconstruction and naso-pharyngeal and choanal atresia. *Br J Plast Surg* 1977;30:300.

II
PART

Free Flaps

9

Rectus Abdominis

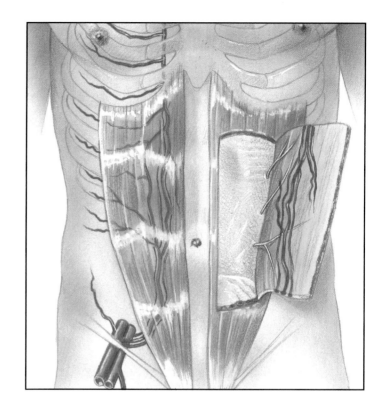

Mark L. Urken, M.D.

Brown et al. (3) are credited with being the first to use abdominal cutaneous flaps based on the perforators of the rectus abdominis muscle. However, Drever's (7) report of the "epigastric island flap" was the first to recognize the potential of transferring an island of skin supplied by a segment of the underlying muscle. He described a vertically oriented musculocutaneous flap that was transferred to a defect of the chest wall based on the deep superior epigastric vascular supply. Pennington and Pelly (27) are credited with the first report of transferring a free rectus abdominis musculocutaneous flap based on the deep inferior epigastric artery (DIEA) and vein (DIEV). These authors described the results of ink-injection studies that demonstrated the rich vascularity of the abdominal skin through the DIEA.

The rectus abdominis musculocutaneous flap has assumed an important role in head and neck reconstruction because of its ease of harvest, long vascular pedicle, and tremendous reliability. Pedicle flaps based on the deep superior epigastric vascular supply to the rectus abdominis have been used extensively in reconstruction of the breast. Pedicled transposition flaps can also be based on the deep inferior epigastric system for use in reconstructing defects in the groin and upper thigh (20). The DIEA and DIEV are much more useful for free tissue transfers because of their greater diameter and length and the larger skin territory that can be captured.

The rectus abdominis muscles occupy the paramedian position of the anterior abdominal wall. Each muscle spans the entire length of the abdomen, arising from the pubis and inserting into the anteroinferior part of the thorax (Figure 9-1). The primary action of the rectus abdominis is to flex the trunk. The rectus abdominis donor

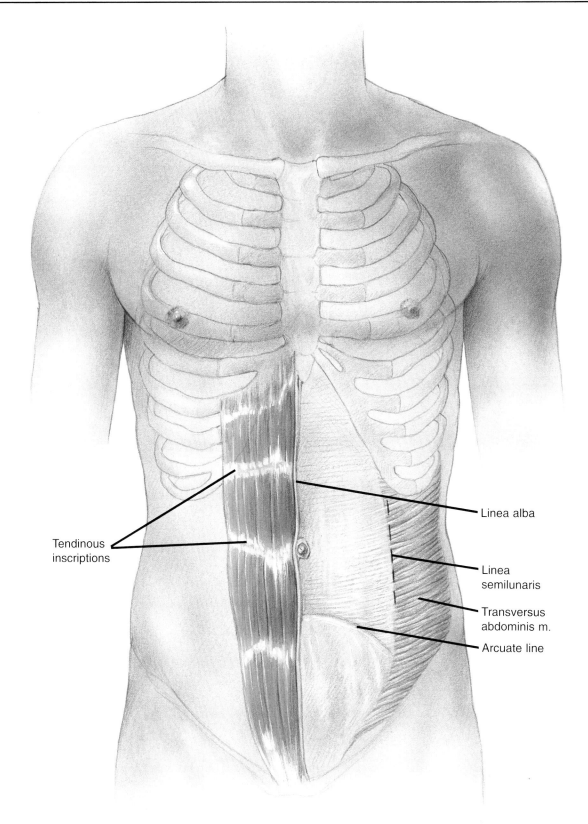

Figure 9-1. The rectus abdominis arises from the pubis and runs the entire length of the abdomen to insert on the fifth, sixth, and seventh costal cartilages and the xiphoid process. The muscle is wider in its cephalad portion. Two to five tendinous inscriptions divide the muscle transversely. These inscriptions are firmly adherent to the anterior, but not the posterior, rectus sheath.

site is a useful source of vascularized muscle and skin for a variety of ablative defects of the head and neck (23). It offers several unique features compared with the regional musculocutaneous flaps based on the pectoralis major, trapezius, and latissimus dorsi. The area of skin that can be reliably harvested with a single rectus muscle encompasses a substantial portion of the abdomen and lower chest. The size of the muscle component ranges from the entire muscle to only a small portion in the paraumbilical region where the dominant perforators are located. The caudal portion of the muscle may be trimmed to add length to the vascular pedicle. The thickness of the subcutaneous tissue varies from being very thick in the lower abdomen to rather thin in the region above the costal margin. The rich vascularity of the skin territory permits a greater flexibility in the flap design, leading to more accurate contouring to the surgical defects. Finally, the ability to harvest this flap with the patient in the supine position greatly facilitates the use of a two-team approach.

FLAP DESIGN AND UTILIZATION

The rectus abdominis may be transferred alone, with overlying fascia and subcutaneous tissue, or as a composite flap consisting of muscle, fascia, skin, and subcutaneous tissue. Dye-injection studies by Boyd et al. (2) showed vascularity to the sixth rib and, therefore, introduced the possibility of incorporating bone in this flap. The segmental nerve supply to the muscle provides the potential for a dynamic reconstruction, and we have successfully used this flap for facial reanimation (36). Although there are no reported cases of sensate rectus abdominis flaps, this potential exists through the mixed motor-sensory nerves.

There are a multitude of flap designs that have been reported that permit the contouring of this flap to virtually any defect in the head and neck. The patient's body habitus may be a limiting factor with regard to excess thickness of the subcutaneous tissue component. However, the muscle alone may be transferred and then resurfaced with a split-thickness skin graft. The skin of a significant portion of the abdomen may be reliably transferred because of the network of subcutaneous vessels emanating from the musculocutaneous perforators in the paraumbilical region. These perforators are located in a zone that extends from 2 cm above to 3 cm below the umbilicus. Boyd et al. (2) speculated that the deep inferior epigastric flap may provide the largest potential territory of vascularized skin of any donor site in the body (Figure 9-2).

There are many factors that enter into the decision in regard to flap design. The defect's size and volume play a significant role, along with its proximity to the recipient vessels. Lengthening of the donor vascular pedicle may be achieved by placing the skin paddle in a more cephalad position on the abdominal wall. The entire rectus abdominis may be transferred if needed. Preservation of a portion of that muscle at the donor site adds little to maintain the integrity of the abdominal wall to prevent ventral herniation. As with any musculocutaneous flap, the muscle component provides little long-term bulk as a result of denervation atrophy. The degree of atrophy may be diminished by reestablishing a motor input through repair of the flap motor nerves to suitable recipient motor nerves in the neck. A more accurate method to provide bulk for contour is to transfer vascularized subcutaneous tissue.

The most commonly used design for this donor site is the transverse rectus abdominis musculocutaneous flap (TRAM) (29). Popularized for use in breast reconstruction, this design incorporates skin from the entire lower abdomen. Four different skin zones have been identified. Zone 1 refers to the skin overlying the ipsilateral rectus muscle. Zone 2 denotes the skin of the contralateral lower abdomen overlying the opposite rectus muscle. The skin territory on the ipsilateral side of the abdomen, lateral to the linea semilunaris is referred to as zone 3, and the skin lateral to the opposite linea semilunaris is zone 4. The blood supply to zone 4 is the most tenuous. Investigations of the vascular supply to the TRAM flap reveal vessels that arise from one rectus abdominis and cross the midline to supply the skin of zone 3. The exami-

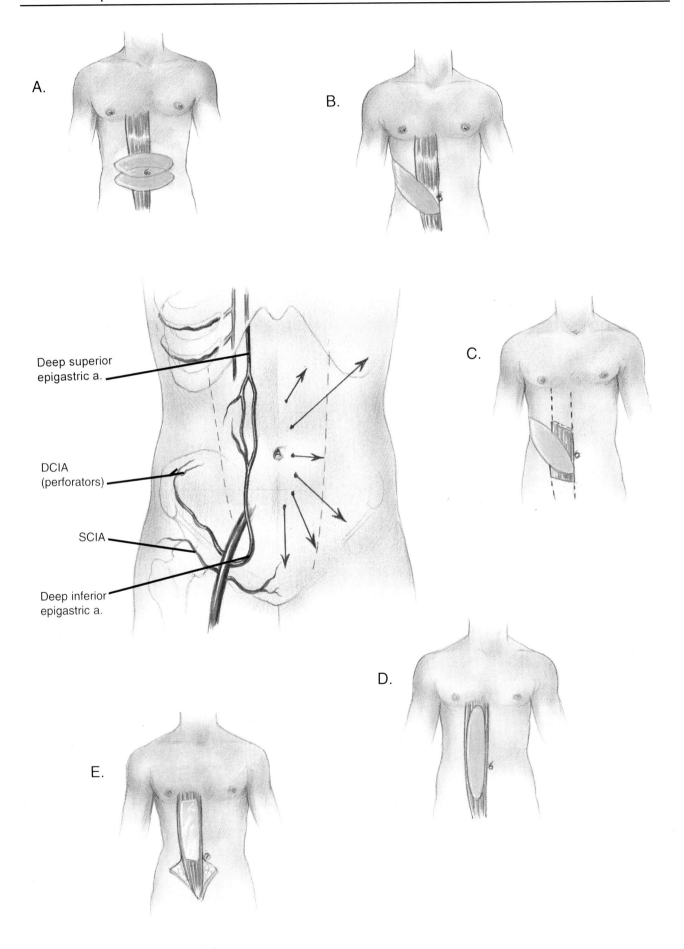

Deep superior epigastric a.

DCIA (perforators)

SCIA

Deep inferior epigastric a.

nation of these crossing vessels and contrast-injection studies have confirmed the poor blood supply to zone 4 (17). However, Takayanagi and Ohtsuka (30) reported a technique that augmented the vascular supply in the zone 4 skin when its viability was deemed critical to the success of the reconstruction. They anastomosed the superficial epigastric or the superficial circumflex iliac pedicle to enhance the vascular supply to that region.

A vertically oriented skin paddle that overlies the entire length of the rectus muscle may be harvested from the pubis to the xiphoid. This design is reliable but has the disadvantage of the additional bulk of the muscle. An alternative flap design (referred to as the thoracoumbilical flap or the extended deep inferior epigastric flap) crosses the abdomen in an oblique fashion, extending from the infraumbilical region to above the ipsilateral costal margin (Figure 9-2). The advantage of this skin design is that it introduces a range of tissue thickness that is at its greatest in the portion overlying the muscle and least in the region that extends above the costal margin. More accurate flap contouring may be achieved by trimming the muscle component to only that portion in the periumbilical region with the greatest concentration of dominant musculocutaneous perforators (32).

In patients with excessive amounts of subcutaneous tissue in the anterior abdominal wall, a thinner flap may be harvested by skin grafting the muscle or just using the anterior rectus sheath above the arcuate line. We have used the latter technique in reconstructing through-and-through defects of the cheek. In such cases, the external skin is restored with a skin paddle from the periumbilical region, and the inner lining is resurfaced with the anterior sheath overlying the cephalad portion of the muscle. The muscle is folded upon itself to achieve inner and outer epithelial surfaces. As noted previously, the anterior sheath from the region above the arcuate line can be harvested without fear of ventral herniation. The anterior sheath provides a thin tough layer to achieve a watertight seal. We have also used this technique in palatal reconstruction in which the rectus sheath provides a suitable lining for the oral cavity following ablative procedures of the sinuses, nasopharynx, or skull base. Chicarilli and Davey (6) used the rectus abdominis flap to reconstruct a cranio-orbitomaxillary defect. The anterior rectus sheath was sutured to the bony margins of the cranial defect above the orbit to serve as a hammock to support the intracranial contents.

An alternative technique to harvest a thinner flap from this donor site was described by Koshima et al. (18). They reported the transfer of "thinned, paraumbilical" flaps based solely on the musculocutaneous perforators. The dominant perforators were dissected through the muscle to the DIEA and DIEV. Branches to the muscle were ligated, and no muscle was transferred with the skin. The advantages of this flap included not only its thinness, but also the fact that the integrity of the abdominal wall musculature was not disturbed. The authors warned, however, that the dissection through the muscle may be technically difficult . Along similar lines, Akizuki et al. (1) described harvesting the "extremely thinned" rectus abdominis free

Figure 9-2. The versatility of the deep inferior epigastric system of flaps is largely the result of the periumbilical perforators, which send branches in all directions on the anterior abdominal wall like the spokes on a wheel. The deep superior epigastric artery (DSEA) and the DIEA communicate through a system of choke vessels. Other vascular systems that contribute to the blood supply of the abdominal wall are the deep circumflex iliac artery (DCIA) and superficial circumflex iliac artery (SCIA). Not shown in this illustration are the superficial inferior epigastric pedicle and the superficial epigastric artery. An array of different flap designs are shown that may be combined to meet the needs of the particular defect. A: Transverse skin paddle placed below or above the umbilicus. It is imperative to capture the dominant periumbilical perforators. B: The extended DIEA flap may be transferred with the entire rectus muscle. C: The extended DIEA flap may be transferred with only a small cuff of muscle in the region of the umbilicus. D: A longitudinal skin paddle oriented over the entire length of the muscle provides a rich vascularity to the skin but a thicker flap due to the large muscle component. E: A thinner flap can be achieved by harvesting the rectus abdominis with the anterior rectus sheath above the arcuate line.

flaps. The basic design was an extended deep inferior epigastric flap based on a small segment of muscle in the periumbilical region. The portion of the flap that extended lateral to the muscle was thinned by removing all fatty tissue deep to Scarpa's fascia, thereby preserving the vascularity through the subdermal plexus. This technique is an important contribution because it provides a method to utilize the rectus abdominis donor site in individuals who might otherwise not be considered candidates because of an unfavorable body habitus.

Virtually any combination of these flap designs may be used. Two separate skin paddles may be oriented over the longitudinal axis of the muscle to reconstruct composite defects requiring inner and outer lining. Although primary closure of the abdominal wall skin is highly desirable, the application of a skin graft may be performed and, certainly, represents a better option when wound tension and respiratory compromise become an issue.

We have used this donor site for a variety of head and neck defects. It serves as an alternative source of skin for external coverage when regional flaps are not available or are unsuitable because of the defect's size or distance from the donor site. Although the radial forearm flap remains the workhorse flap for oral cavity reconstruction, the rectus abdominis is useful to supply bulk following total glossectomy. The goal in total tongue reconstruction is to supply sufficient soft tissue height for an approximation of the neotongue to the palate without the use of a palatal augmentation prosthesis. The rectus abdominis flap is an excellent choice as a result of the tendinous inscriptions of the anterior rectus sheath, which can be sutured to the mandible to form a platform for the overlying skin paddle. The tissue above this platform does not atrophy, and therefore, the shape and volume of the neotongue can be precisely contoured (36).

Perhaps the greatest use of this flap has been in skull base reconstruction; it has become the flap of choice for many skull base defects requiring free tissue transfer (35). Jones et al. (16) reported the use of this flap for defects involving the middle and posterior cranial fossa; Yamada et al. (37) described its application to defects of the anterior cranial fossa. In the latter report, the free rectus abdominis flap was used in patients who had undergone prior surgery or radiation to help prevent a cerebrospinal fluid leak, to prevent ascending infection, and to provide vascularity to free bone grafts used in the periorbital region. I have used the rectus abdominis free flap in the anterior cranial fossa in a patient who had a postoperative collection of pus following resection of a recurrent frontal meningioma. The free rectus muscle successfully achieved a functional separation of the nasal and anterior cranial cavities, with complete resolution of the infectious process (35). I normally do not like to place a microvascular free flap in a grossly infected field because of the extremely detrimental effect that infection has on the microvascular pedicle. However, this was a unique circumstance, and the ability of the rectus flap to survive in this environment is a testimony to its hardiness.

The versatility of flap design of the rectus abdominis flap is extremely useful when trying to achieve a watertight seal of the various cavities that are opened following many skull base procedures (10). This is particularly challenging in the "three-cavity defect," which involves the nasal, oral, and intracranial cavities in which multiple epithelial surfaces are required for a successful outcome. De-epithelialized portions of the flap can be used to enhance the contour of regions such as the infratemporal fossa or the orbit following exenteration. Finally, the extremely reliable nature of this flap is a critical factor in ensuring protective coverage to exposed portions of the brain (35).

Many different free flaps have been used to reconstruct defects of the scalp. Miyamoto et al. (25) reported four cases of extensive scalp reconstructions using the rectus abdominis free flap. Aside from the large surface area, the length of the vascular pedicle was noted to be a particular advantage for this donor site. The vascular pedicle can be lengthened by judicious skin paddle placement and careful removal of the caudal portion of the rectus muscle. These techniques help to avoid the use of vein grafts.

NEUROVASCULAR ANATOMY

According to the classification system of Mathes and Nahai (22), the rectus abdominis is a type III muscle with two dominant vascular pedicles, the deep superior epigastric artery (DSEA) and vein (DSEV) and the DIEA and DIEV. The DSEA is a continuation of the internal mammary artery; the DIEA is a branch of the external iliac artery arising directly opposite the deep circumflex iliac artery (Figure 9-3). The DSEA and DIEA pedicles arborize as they approach each other in a longitudinal direction on the undersurface of the muscle. The two systems connect above the umbilicus through a system of small-caliber vessels that Taylor and Palmer (34) referred to as "choke" vessels.

Through cadaveric studies, the degree of arborization of the DIEA and the DSEA has been classified into three different types. In the type 1 pattern, the DIEA does not divide, remaining a single vessel as it runs its course on the undersurface of the muscle (29%). The type 2 pattern refers to a DIEA that divides into two dominant branches (57%). The type 3 pattern is a trifurcation of the DIEA (14%). The extent of branching of the inferior system is mirrored by the DSEA (25). The division of the vascular pedicle into two or three branches is the basis for the "split muscle" transfer that was reported by Sadove and Merrell (28).

The DIEA, measuring an average of 3 to 4 mm, is roughly twice the diameter of the DSEA. The venous supply of the inferior muscle is composed of paired venae comitantes, which usually join to form a single venous pedicle prior to their junction with the external iliac vein. The DIEV is approximately 3.5 mm in diameter. Extensive studies of the venous circulation of the TRAM flap revealed a superficial and deep system. The veins of the superficial system were above Scarpa's fascia and communicated extensively across the midline. The superficial veins drained into the deep inferior epigastric system by way of the veins accompanying the musculocutaneous arterial perforators. Valves located in the connecting veins regulated the direction of flow from the superficial toward the deep system. The findings from this study confirmed the safety of thinning the rectus abdominis musculocutaneous flaps by removing fat from below Scarpa's fascia as long as the musculocutaneous perforators were preserved (5).

In addition to the size of the vascular pedicle, there are a variety of compelling reasons why the inferior pedicle is a better supply for free tissue transfer than is the superior pedicle. The musculocutaneous perforators are direct branches of the DIEA and DIEV and are therefore capable of supplying a much larger territory of skin. Although the deep superior epigastric system is capable of capturing these perforators, it does so through a reversal of flow in the DIEA and DIEV, across the choke system of vessels that connect the two systems. Boyd et al. (2) studied the distribution of musculocutaneous perforators exiting through the anterior rectus sheath. By dividing the length of the muscle into horizontal segments, they found that the dominant perforators were located in a zone close to the umbilicus, with very few perforators arising in the most caudal or cephalad portions of the muscle. These perforators were also mapped according to a longitudinal division of the muscle into thirds. The greatest concentration of large perforators traversing the anterior sheath was located in the middle and medial zones, with few exiting laterally.

The inferior pedicle runs an extraperitoneal course in close proximity to the deep inguinal ring. It crosses the lateral border of the rectus muscle and pierces the transversalis fascia approximately 3 to 4 cm caudal to the arcuate line. The DIEA gives off a number of smaller branches to the pubis and the caudal aspect of the rectus muscle prior to entering the rectus sheath.

Additional cadaveric studies by Taylor et al. (31) demonstrated the rich connections between different arterial supplies to the anterior abdominal wall skin. The periumbilical musculocutaneous perforators of the DIEA give off a series of radiating branches that anastomose with the cutaneous branches of the following arteries: superficial superior epigastric, intercostal, deep and superficial circumflex iliac, the superficial inferior epigastric (SIEA), and the pudendal arteries. The dominant connec-

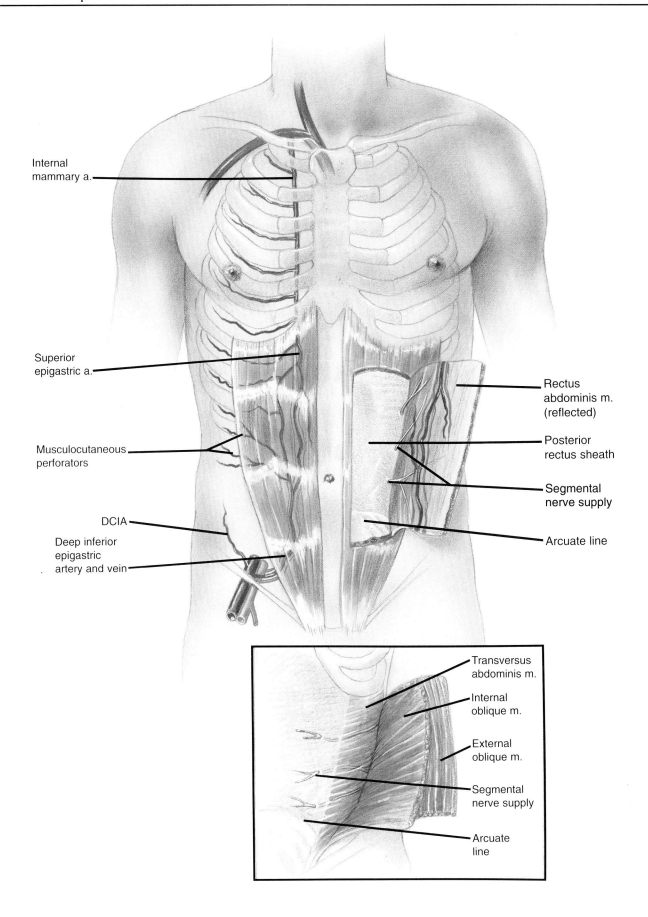

Internal
mammary a.

Superior
epigastric a.

Musculocutaneous
perforators

DCIA

Deep inferior
epigastric
artery and vein

Rectus
abdominis m.
(reflected)

Posterior
rectus sheath

Segmental
nerve supply

Arcuate line

Transversus
abdominis m.

Internal
oblique m.

External
oblique m.

Segmental
nerve supply

Arcuate
line

tions between these systems were found to occur within the subdermal plexus (Figure 9-2). There are also anastomotic connections in the intermuscular layer running between the transversus abdominis and internal oblique muscles. The primary connections occurring in this layer are between the branches of the epigastric system and the lower six intercostal vessels.

Taylor et al. (33) used the angiosome concept of defining the vascular territories of the abdominal wall to describe a technique of surgical delay to enlarge the territory of skin that can be safely transferred on the DIEA and DIEV. The angiosome theory proposes that the region of skin that is most reliably harvested on the deep inferior epigastric vascular system is defined by a line that marks the interface between the DIEA and the other source arteries of the abdominal wall. This line of demarcation denotes the system of choke vessels that connect two adjacent angiosomes. Thus, the system of choke vessels between the DIEA and the DSEA is consistently located above the umbilicus. The interface zone with the contralateral DIEA is along the linea alba. In a two-stage procedure, surgical delay can be achieved by ligating the source artery in the adjacent territory, which varies depending on the orientation of the desired skin flap. This delay procedure causes a dilation of the choke vessels connecting the two adjacent territories leading to a more favorable hemodynamic gradient across the two systems. Although the surgeon can usually capture the skin in an adjacent angiosome without surgical delay, it becomes progressively more difficult when more than one system of choke vessels is traversed in series. If a longer vertically oriented flap is desired, then the appropriate delay procedure would involve interruption of the deep superior epigastric pedicle. Enhancement of the vascularity to the skin of the transverse rectus abdominis musculocutaneous flap can be achieved by interruption of the vascular supply to the skin of the lower abdomen. On the ipsilateral side, the delay procedure would involve ligation of the SIEA. Improving the vascular supply to the skin of zones 2 and 4 can be achieved by interrupting the contralateral DIEA and SIEA. Although the area of skin that can be reliably harvested on a single DIEA is so great that a delay phenomenon is rarely needed in head and neck reconstruction, there are certain complex defects in which this technique may be helpful.

The system of branches of the periumbilical perforators has the appearance of the radiating spokes of a wheel with the hub located at the umbilicus, thus giving credence to the clinical observation that incorporation of the periumbilical perforators permits a skin flap to be harvested with virtually any orientation from the midline. However, the dominant orientation of these branches is 45 degrees from the horizontal toward the inferior scapular border (32). This explains the extremely reliable oblique flap design that was previously referred to as the extended deep inferior epigastric or the thoracoumbilical flap. Taylor reported that this design may safely incorporate skin above the costal margin as far lateral as the midaxillary line (32).

The nerve supply to the rectus abdominis is derived from the lower six intercostal nerves, which traverse the plane between the transversus abdominis and the internal oblique muscles. These nerves are mixed motor and sensory nerves, providing a segmental innervation to the rectus muscle and sensory supply to the overlying skin. The intercostal nerves enter the midportion of the muscle on its posterior surface (9). By stimulating one of the segmental nerves, it is possible to select a portion of the rectus muscle for use in facial reanimation. We have done this successfully in one

Figure 9-3. The rectus abdominis has a type III vascular supply with two dominant pedicles, the DSEA and DSEV and the DIEA and DIEV. These two systems communicate through a rich system of anastomoses located approximately halfway between the xiphoid and the umbilicus. Musculocutaneous perforators arise in the paraumbilical region and send an array of dominant branches which are oriented toward the inferior border of the scapula. The segmental nerve supply to the rectus abdominis arises from the terminal branches of the lower six intercostal nerves, which run across the abdominal wall from lateral to medial in the layer between the transversus abdominis and the internal oblique muscles. These nerves penetrate the posterior rectus sheath approximately 3 cm medial to the linea semilunaris.

patient who underwent a composite reconstruction of the cheek following radical parotidectomy. Good dynamic activity was obtained by anastomosing two segmental nerves to the main trunk of the ipsilateral facial nerve (36). Hata et al. (15) reported successful facial reanimation in two patients with chronic facial paralysis. A cross facial nerve graft was initially placed and then followed at 1 year with a free rectus abdominis transfer in which several of the segmental nerves were anastomosed to the cross facial graft. The rectus abdominis was considered a good muscle for facial reanimation because of the ease of harvest and the length of the neurovascular pedicle. A particular advantage that is unique to the rectus abdominis is the tendinous inscriptions, which allow placement of anchoring sutures. To my knowledge, restoration of sensation to the skin of the rectus abdominis musculocutaneous flap has not been reported.

ANATOMY OF THE RECTUS SHEATH

An understanding of the anatomy of the fascial envelope of the rectus abdominis is perhaps more critical than with any other flap. The prevention of herniation depends on restoring the integrity of the abdominal wall by effectively closing the fascial layers.

The aponeurotic extensions of the three muscles of the anterior abdominal wall merge to form the anterior and posterior sheaths of the rectus fascia (Figure 9-4). The compositions of these sheaths vary in different locations between the pubis and the xiphoid. Above the costal margin, there is no posterior sheath, and the anterior sheath is formed by an extension of the external oblique aponeurosis. In the upper two thirds of the muscle, the anterior sheath is formed by the external oblique plus a contribution from the internal oblique aponeurosis. The internal oblique aponeurosis also contributes to the posterior sheath where it joins with the aponeurosis of the transversus abdominis. An important transition occurs in the posterior sheath at the arcuate line (semicircular line or arch of Douglas), which is approximately at the level of the anterosuperior iliac spine. From this point to the pubis, the posterior sheath is composed only of the transversalis fascia. The strength of the posterior rectus sheath above the arcuate line is sufficient to prevent an abdominal bulge or herniation. Below the arcuate line, these sequelae undoubtedly occur if the transversalis fascia is not augmented. It is rarely necessary to design a flap that requires harvest of the anterior rectus sheath below the arcuate line. Maintaining the integrity of the blood supply to the skin requires only that the anterior rectus sheath is harvested in the paraumbilical region where the dominant perforators are located. Although it is probably not essential to do so above the arcuate line, we routinely augment the posterior sheath by closing cuffs of the anterior sheath that are preserved both medially and laterally. Taylor et al. (31) described a fascial sparing technique whereby cuts in the anterior rectus sheath are made based on direct visualization of the dominant perforators. The amount of anterior sheath that is harvested may be minimized by this technique.

Three other terms related to the fascia must be defined (Figure 9-1). The linea alba is the midline fascial condensation that divides the two rectus muscles. The linea semilunaris refers to the fascial condensation that marks the lateral extent of each rectus muscle. The rectus abdominis is subdivided by two to five tendinous inscriptions. The anterior sheath but not the posterior sheath is firmly adherent to each inscription. These fascial condensations do not extend to the posterior sheath. Moon and Taylor (26) reported that 93.5% of a series of 108 muscles had three tendinous inscriptions with the most caudal one at the level of the umbilicus.

ANATOMIC VARIATIONS

In a series of 25 cadaver dissections reported by Boyd et al. (2), the average diameter of the DIEA was 3.4 mm. The vessel was slightly larger in instances in which the DIEA was the source of an abnormal obturator artery. The authors reported that the

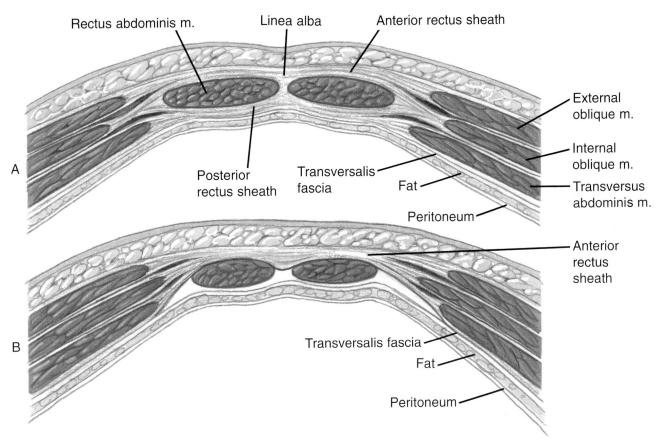

Figure 9-4. Transverse sections through the anterior abdominal wall reveal the fascial anatomy of the anterior and posterior rectus sheaths at two different levels in the abdomen. **A:** Above the arcuate line, the posterior sheath is composed of contributions from the aponeuroses of the transversus abdominis and the internal oblique muscles. The aponeurosis of the internal oblique muscle splits to form part of the anterior rectus sheath with the external oblique aponeurosis. **B:** Below the arcuate line, at about the level of the anterior superior iliac spine, the aponeurotic extensions of all three muscle layers contribute to the anterior rectus sheath. The posterior sheath is composed only of the transversalis fascia.

DIEV entered the external iliac vein as a single trunk in 68% of cases and as a double trunk in 32%. In a series of 115 cadaver dissections, Milloy et al. (24) reported no cases of absent DIEA and DIEV and only three cases in which the DSEA and DSEV could not be identified. In the vast majority of cases, the DIEA–DIEV pedicle runs its usual course along the deep surface of the rectus abdominis. We have encountered two cases in which the pedicle tracked for an unusual distance along the lateral aspect of the muscle before taking a medial intramuscular route. Another anomalous course of the deep inferior epigastric pedicle has been described in which it winds around the medial aspect of the muscle and does not give feeders to the muscle until assuming a position along its superficial surface. In this particular instance, the perforators to the skin run directly through the anterior rectus fascia without traversing the muscle (11).

POTENTIAL PITFALLS

The reliability of the rectus abdominis free flap is reflected by the success rate of 93% in a large series of cases in which this flap was used throughout the body (23). In a review of all reported cases used for head and neck reconstruction, we found only one failure in 73 free flaps transferred to the head and neck (36).

The preoperative assessment must include a careful history and examination of the abdomen to be certain that prior surgery will not interfere with flap harvest. Most intraperitoneal procedures involve a longitudinal incision through the linea alba, even though the skin incision is transverse. A right subcostal incision for an open cholecystectomy does not preclude the use of the rectus muscle. This procedure almost invariably interrupts the nerve supply to the cephalad portion of the muscle. The surgeon should be aware of the potential for denervation atrophy in the post-cholecystectomy patient. However, this does not interfere with the vascularity of the atrophic muscle or its suitability for transfer.

On more than one occasion, we have found that the DIEA and DIEV run a longitudinal course along the lateral aspect of the muscle prior to arborizing on the undersurface of the muscle. Extreme care must be taken when making the cuts in the anterior rectus sheath medial to the linea semilunaris.

Although the requirements of the recipient defect usually dictate the size and design of the abdominal skin paddle, there are situations in which the surgeon has options for planning the incisions and the approach to the rectus muscle. Taylor et al. (31) and Hallock (12) advocated a transverse suprapubic incision for the exposure of the vascular pedicle. The resulting scar is well camouflaged. Alternatively, Hallock described the use of an abdominoplasty approach but warned that proper case selection was imperative.

Removal of one rectus abdominis along with a portion of the overlying fascia creates a potential weakness in the anterior abdominal wall that may predispose the patient to ventral herniation or a midline bulge. A pre-existing hernia or diastasis recti may complicate donor-site closure and mitigate against the use of this flap. Taylor et al. (31) warned that divarication of the recti must be recognized preoperatively to account for the more lateralized position of the rectus muscles in designing the flap.

The rectus abdominis muscles assist in flexion of the torso and also provide static support to the anterior abdominal wall. There is a tremendous amount of controversy regarding the optimum method for closure of the abdominal wall defect following rectus abdominis flap harvest. Much of the data on donor-site complications are derived from large series of pedicled flaps that were used for breast reconstruction. For the purposes of this discussion, we will not cover the issues regarding closure of the abdominal wall following harvest of rectus abdominis muscles. There are two major camps that are divided over the necessity of introducing a synthetic mesh for closure of the anterior rectus sheath. Drever and Hodson-Walker (8) described the technique of placing a mesh of the exact dimensions to the area of the anterior rectus sheath that was removed with the flap. Using this method in 87 cases, they reported no cases of ventral hernias and only 2 cases of abdominal wall bulging. In a comparable group of 31 patients who were closed primarily without a mesh, there was a 43% incidence of bulging or hernias. These authors argued that the mesh maintained the position of the remaining abdominal wall musculature and did not cause an increased resting tone resulting from direct approximation of the linea alba to the linea semilunaris. Lejour and Dome (19) reported using a 4-cm wide double-layered synthetic mesh between the posterior sheath and the direct closure of the anterior sheath. They reported no hernias or bulging in their series of unilateral flaps. Hartrampf (13) espoused a different view of this controversy. He argued for direct approximation of the residual anterior fascial margins to achieve a centralization of the remaining muscles. By so doing, he believes that the mechanical advantage of the residual abdominal muscles is restored. In 300 patients who underwent either unilateral or bilateral rectus muscle transfers, there was a 0.3% incidence of abdominal hernia and a 0.8% incidence of abdominal wall laxity (14). In my experience of more than 50 unilateral rectus abdominis free flap transfers in which the abdominal wall was closed in this manner, there have been no patients who have had abdominal wall hernias or abdominal wall bulges. An additional technique of anterior sheath closure using autologous tissue should be mentioned. A "turnover," contralateral, anterior rectus sheath flap based at the midline has been reported for donor site closure (23).

The postoperative function of the abdominal wall is generally believed to be unaffected by transfer of a single rectus abdominis. Bunkis et al. (4) warned that, in patients who are active in sports or who engage in other physical activities, there may be an impact on their lifestyle. However, there are few reports that quantify the actual effects of removing a rectus abdominis. Hartrampf and Bennett (14) conducted the most extensive study of abdominal wall function in 300 patients, of whom the majority returned to their preoperative level of function, based on the parameters used in their investigation. Lejour and Dome (19) reported that follow-up studies in 57 patients revealed a significant discrepancy between a patient's responses to a questionnaire and objective findings that were recorded by a physiotherapist. Although the majority of patients reported either no disturbance or improvements in abdominal strength and sports activities following surgery, the physiotherapist reported a marked decrement in the functions of the recti and the external oblique muscles.

POSTOPERATIVE CARE

Because of retraction of the peritoneal cavity for dissection of the vascular pedicle, it is not uncommon for patients to have an ileus in the early postoperative period. Interim feedings must be delayed for a short period until this resolves. Early postoperative ambulation is encouraged. Exercises that involve the abdomen may be resumed in approximately 6 weeks following surgery.

Flap Harvesting Technique

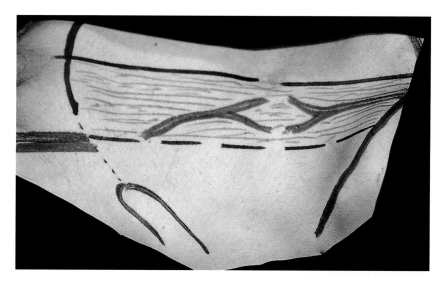

Figure 9-5. The topographical anatomy of the rectus abdominis flap is outlined on the abdomen. The position of the palpable pulse of the femoral vessel is shown. In addition, the iliac crest and costal margins are outlined. In the midline, the linea alba has been drawn from the pubis to the xiphoid. The approximate position of the linea semilunaris is outlined by a *dashed line* at the midpoint between the pubis and the anterior superior iliac spine. The DIEA and DIEV and the DSEA and DSEV are shown in their approximate course on the undersurface of the rectus abdominis.

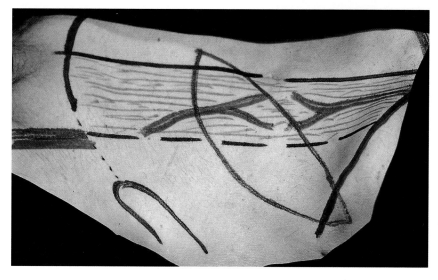

Figure 9-6. An extended deep inferior epigastric flap has been outlined on the left side of the abdomen. This flap extends over the costal margin and provides an abundance of thin well-vascularized pliable skin. The vascularity to this flap depends on capture of the dominant periumbilical perforators. This flap may extend across the midline, capturing well-vascularized tissue to approximately the level of the contralateral linea semilunaris. The arcuate line is approximately at the level of the anterior superior iliac spine. The anterior rectus sheath should not be harvested below this level.

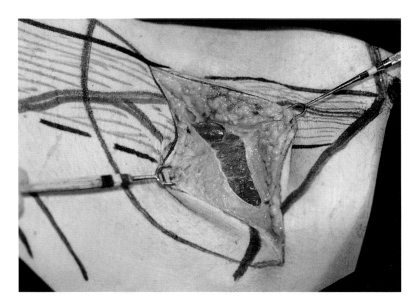

Figure 9-7. The dissection begins in the cephalad portion of the flap by incising the skin and subcutaneous tissue to the level of the fascia. The full breadth of the rectus abdominis is identified by incising the anterior rectus sheath to expose the rectus abdominis from the linea alba to the linea semilunaris.

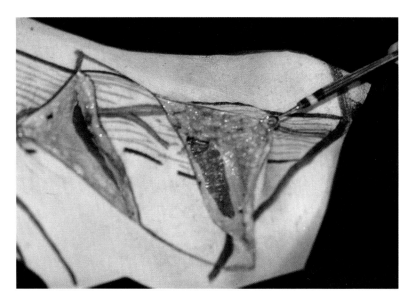

Figure 9-8. The dissection is continued inferiorly in a similar plane through the skin and subcutaneous tissue to expose the full width of the caudal portion of the rectus abdominis. This is achieved by incising the anterior rectus sheath and exposing the rectus abdominis from the linea alba to the linea semilunaris.

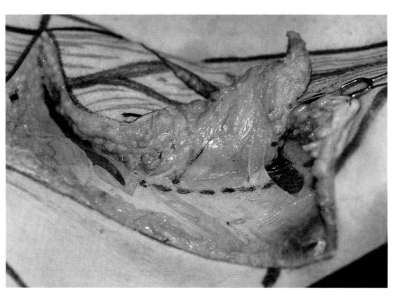

Figure 9-9. Having identified the linea semilunaris in its cephalad portion and in its caudal portion, the skin paddle can now be elevated off the external oblique muscle and aponeurosis to the linea semilunaris, which is identified by the *dashed line*. Defatting of the portion of this flap which has been elevated may be safely performed deep to Scarpa's fascia.

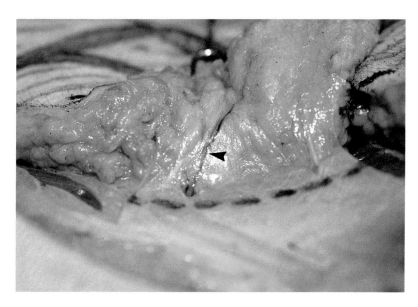

Figure 9-10. Meticulous dissection in this plane superficial to the external oblique fascia is performed to identify the first set of musculocutaneous perforators (*arrow*). The anterior sheath is then incised laterally, preserving these dominant perforators.

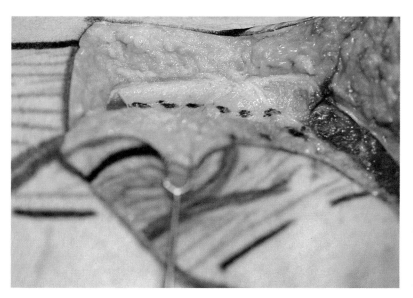

Figure 9-11. The medial dissection is performed by elevating the skin and subcutaneous tissue in a prefascial plane above the contralateral anterior rectus sheath. The exact position of the linea alba is marked by a *dotted line,* having been identified in both the cephalad and caudad exposure. A cuff of anterior rectus sheath is preserved by making a longitudinal incision lateral to the linea alba, as indicated by the *dashed line.*

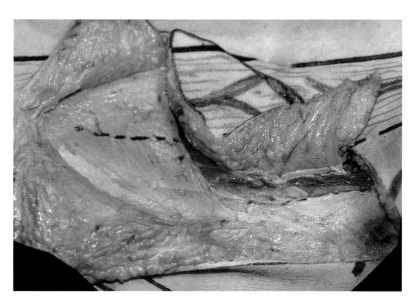

Figure 9-12. The lateral aspect of the dissection is completed by incising the anterior rectus sheath medial to the linea semilunaris, preserving a small cuff of fascia to facilitate closure of the anterior sheath. Exposure of the caudal aspect of the rectus fascia has been obtained through a vertical incision. A corresponding vertical incision in the anterior rectus sheath is then made (*dashed line*) in order to expose the caudal portion of the muscle for harvest.

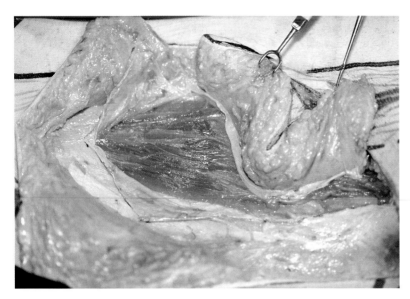

Figure 9-13. Full exposure of the rectus abdominis has been achieved by longitudinally incising the anterior rectus sheath inferiorly in the midportion between the linea alba and the linea semilunaris. Flaps of rectus fascia are elevated both medially and laterally to obtain full exposure of the muscle. The skin paddle is completely isolated, except for its attachments to the anterior rectus sheath in the midportion of the muscle. Only that portion of the anterior rectus sheath that is immediately subjacent to the skin paddle needs to be harvested. The cephalad portion of the rectus abdominis may be incorporated in this flap by gaining exposure through elevation of the anterior rectus sheath to the costal margin. The attachments of the anterior sheath to the muscle at the level of the tendinous inscriptions require that sharp dissection be utilized.

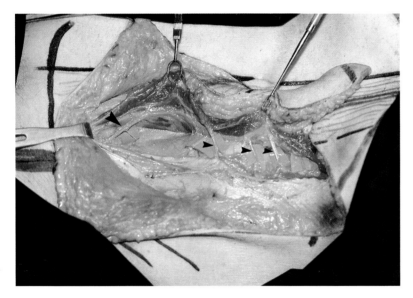

Figure 9-14. The dissection progresses from cephalad to caudad by elevating the rectus abdominis off the posterior rectus sheath. This is achieved by transecting the rectus abdominis above and bluntly dissecting between the muscle and the posterior sheath. Blunt dissection along the linea semilunaris reveals the segmental nerve supply (*small arrows*). In the caudal aspect of this exposure, the deep inferior epigastric pedicle (*large arrow*) is identified.

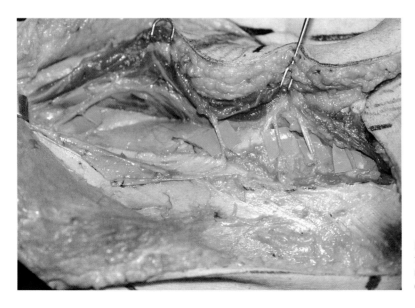

Figure 9-15. A closer view of the undersurface of the rectus abdominis reveals the segmental nerve supply and the deep inferior epigastric pedicle.

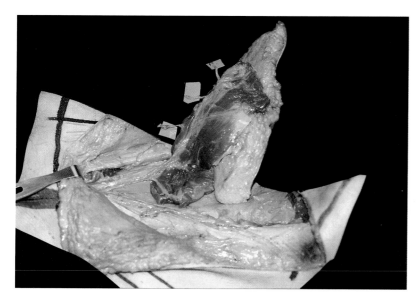

Figure 9-16. The extended deep inferior epigastric flap has been completely isolated on its vascular supply, and the segmental nerves are shown against the blue background. Proximal dissection of the vascular pedicle is achieved by the use of deep abdominal retractors. Despite the large caliber and length of the DIEA, it is helpful to extend the dissection to the takeoff from the external iliac artery and vein because the venae comitantes join in most cases to create a single DIEV at a variable distance from the external iliac vein.

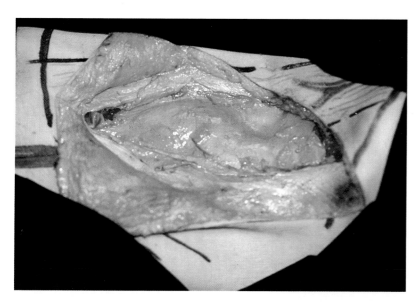

Figure 9-17. Meticulous closure of the donor defect is required to prevent weakening or herniation of the anterior abdominal wall. It is imperative to close the anterior rectus sheath below the arcuate line. This can be readily achieved by designing the skin paddle so that only that portion of the anterior rectus sheath above the arcuate line is harvested.

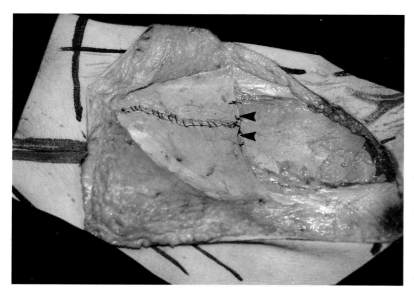

Figure 9-18. Closure of the anterior rectus sheath below the arcuate line has been accomplished. The integrity of the anterior abdominal wall is fortified by suturing the anterior rectus sheath to the posterior rectus sheath at the level of the arcuate line (*arrows*). Although the posterior rectus sheath cephalad to the arcuate line is probably of sufficient strength, it can be augmented by closing the preserved cuff of anterior fascia attached to the linea semilunaris and the linea alba. A ribbon retractor is usually placed along the posterior rectus sheath to prevent the errant placement of a suture into the peritoneal cavity.

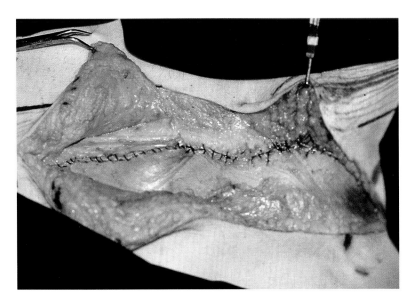

Figure 9-19. The anterior rectus sheath has been closed.

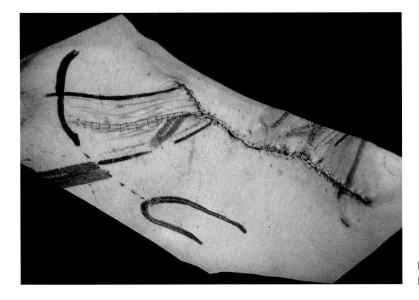

Figure 9-20. Closure of the skin is accomplished by wide undermining.

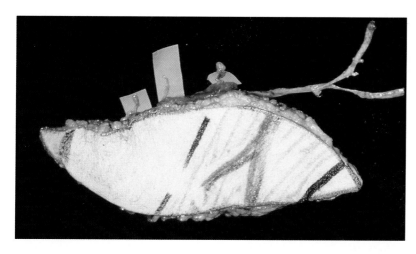

Figure 9-21. The rectus abdominis musculocutaneous flap provides a large area of skin, a long vascular pedicle, and a segmental nerve supply.

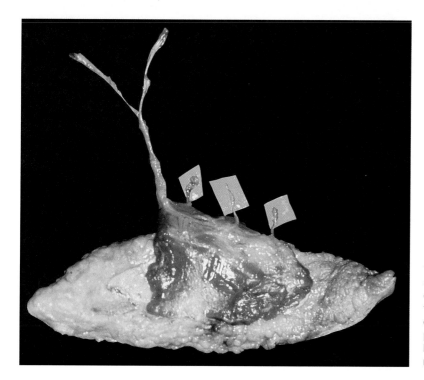

Figure 9-22. If desirable, because of excess bulk or the necessity for a longer vascular pedicle, the amount of muscle that is incorporated in this flap may be significantly reduced by separating the loose attachments of the DIEA and DIEV on the undersurface of the muscle in its proximal portion. In so doing, the caudal aspect of the rectus abdominis may be removed. This provides further length to the vascular pedicle and reduces the amount of muscle to only that portion in the paraumbilical region that harbors the dominant musculocutaneous perforators.

REFERENCES

1. Akizuki T, Harii K, Yamada A: Extremely thinned inferior rectus abdominis free flap. *Plast Reconstr Surg* 1993;91:936–941.
2. Boyd JB, Taylor GI, Corlett R: The vascular territories of the superior epigastric and the deep inferior epigastric systems. *Plast Reconstr Surg* 1984;73:1–14.
3. Brown R, Vasconez L, Jurkiewicz M: Transverse abdominal flaps and the deep epigastric arcade. *Plast Reconstr Surg* 1975;55:416–419.
4. Bunkis J, Walton R, Mathes S, Krizek J, Vascomez L: Experience with the transverse lower rectus abdominis operation for breast reconstruction. *Plast Reconstr Surg* 1983;72:819–827.
5. Carramenha e Costa M, Carriquiry C, Vasconez L, Grotting I, Herrera R, Windle B: An anatomic study of the venous drainage of the transverse rectus abdominis musculocutaneous flap. *Plast Reconstr Surg* 1987;79:208.
6. Chicarilli ZN, Davey LM: Rectus abdominis myocutaneous free-flap reconstruction following a cranio-orbital-maxillary resection for neurofibrosarcoma. *Plast Reconstr Surg* 1987;80:726–731.
7. Drever J: The epigastric island flap. *Plast Reconstr Surg* 1977;59:343–346.

8. Drever J, Hodson-Walker N: Closure of the donor defect for breast reconstruction with rectus abdominis myocutaneous flaps. *Plast Reconstr Surg* 1985;76:558–567.

9. Duchateau J, Declety A and Lejour M: Innervation of the rectus abdominis muscle: implications for rectus flaps. *Plast Reconstr Surg* 1988;82:223–227.

10. Ebihara H, Maruyama YU: Free abdominal flaps: variations in design and application to soft tissue defects of the head. *J Reconstr Microsurg* 1989;5:193–201.

11. Godfrey P, Godfrey N, Romita M: The "circummuscular" free TRAM pedicle: a trap. *Plast Reconstr Surg* 1994;93:178–180.

12. Hallock G: Aesthetic approach to the rectus abdominis free tissue transfer. *J Reconstr Microsurg* 1989;5:69–73.

13. Hartrampf CR: Discussion of article by Drever JM, Hodson-Walker N: Closure of the donor defect for breast reconstruction with rectus abdominis myocutaneous flaps. *Plast Reconstr Surg* 1985;76:563–565.

14. Hartrampf CR, Bennett GK: Autogenous tissue reconstruction in the mastectomy patient. *Ann Plast Surg* 1987;205:508–519.

15. Hata Y, Yano K, Matsuka K, Ito O, Matsuda H, Hosokawa KI: Treatment of chronic facial palsy by transplantation of the neurovascularized free rectus abdominis muscle. *Plast Reconstr Surg* 1990;86:1178.

16. Jones N, Sekhar L, Schramm V: Free rectus abdominis muscle flap reconstruction of the middle and posterior cranial fossa. *Plast Reconstr Surg* 1986;78:471–473.

17. Kaufman T, Hurwitz D, Boehnke M, Futrell J: The microcirculatory pattern of the transverse-abdominal flap: a cross-sectional xerographic and CAT scanning study. *Ann Plast Surg* 1985;14:340.

18. Koshima I, Moriguchi T, Fukuda H, Yoshikawa YS-S: Free thinned paraumbilical perforator-based flaps. *J Reconstr Microsurg* 1991;7:313–316.

19. Lejour M, Dome M: Abdominal wall function after rectus abdominis transfer. *Plast Reconstr Surg* 1991;87:1054.

20. Logan S, Mathes S: The use of a rectus abdominis myocutaneous flap to reconstruct a groin defect. *Br J Plast Surg* 1984;37:351.

21. Markowitz BL, Satterberg T, Calcaterra T, Orringer J, Cohen S, Burstein F, Shaw W: The deep inferior epigastric rectus abdominis muscle and myocutaneous free tissue transfer: further applications for head and neck reconstruction. *Ann Plast Surg* 1991;27:577.

22. Mathes S, Nahai F: *Clinical Applications for Muscle and Musculocutaneous Flaps.* St. Louis: CV Mosby; 1982:44–45.

23. Meland N, Fisher J, Irons G, Wood M, Cooney W: Experience with 80 rectus abdominis free-tissue transfers. *Plast Reconstr Surg* 1989;83:481.

24. Milloy F, Anson B, McAfee D: The rectus abdominis muscle and the epigastric arteries. *Surg Gynecol Obstet* 1960;110:293–302.

25. Miyamoto Y, Harada K, Kodama Y, Takahashi H, Okano S: Cranial coverage involving scalp, bone and dura using free inferior epigastric flap. *Br J Plast Surg* 1986;39:483.

26. Moon H, Taylor GI: The vascular anatomy of rectus abdominis musculocutaneous flaps based on the deep superior epigastric system. *Plast Reconstr Surg* 1988;82:815–829.

27. Pennington D'Lai M, Pelly A: The rectus abdominis myocutaneous free flap. *Br J Plast Surg* 1980;33:277.

28. Sadove R, Merrell J: The split rectus abdominis free muscle transfer. *Ann Plast Surg* 1987;18:179–181.

29. Scheflan M, Dinner M: The transverse abdominal island flap. Part II. Surgical technique. *Ann Plast Surg* 1983;10:120–129.

30. Takayanagi S, Ohtsuka M: Extended transverse rectus abdominis musculocutaneous flap. *Plast Reconstr Surg* 1989;83:1057.

31. Taylor G, Corlett RJ, Boyd B: The versatile deep inferior epigastric (inferior rectus abdominis) flap. *Br J Plast Surg* 1984;37:330–350.

32. Taylor G, Corlett R, Boyd J: The extended deep inferior epigastric flap: a clinical technique. *Plast Reconstr Surg* 1983;72:751.

33. Taylor I, Corlett R, Caddy C, Zelt Z: An anatomic review of the delay phenomenon II. Clinical applications. *Plast Reconstr Surg* 1992;89:408.

34. Taylor G, Palmer J: The vascular territories (angiosomes) of the body: experimental and clinical applications. *Br J Plast Surg* 1987;40:113–131.

35. Urken ML, Catalano PJ, Sen C, Post K, Futran N, Biller HF: Free tissue transfer for skull base reconstruction. Analysis of complications and a classification scheme for defining skull base defects. *Arch Otolaryngol Head Neck Surg* 1993;119:1318.

36. Urken ML, Turk J, Weinberg H, Vickery C, Biller HF: The rectus abdominis free flap in head and neck reconstruction. *Arch Otolaryngol Head Neck Surg* 1991;117:857–866.

37. Yamada A, Harii K, Ueda K, Asato H: Free rectus abdominis muscle reconstruction of the anterior skull base. *Br J Plast Surg* 1992;45:302–306.

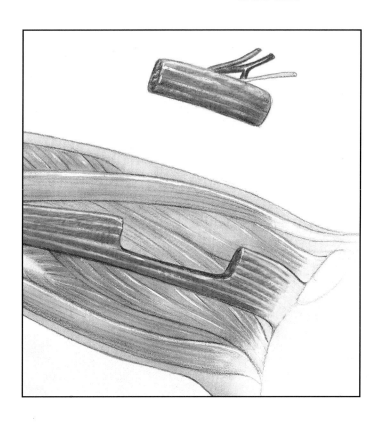

Gracilis

Michael J. Sullivan, M.D., and
Mark L. Urken, M.D.

The gracilis muscle was one of the first musculocutaneous flaps to be transferred by microvascular techniques. Harii et al. (3) introduced this free flap in 1976 and subsequently popularized the use of this muscle alone for dynamic facial reanimation. The gracilis flap has also been used extensively as a pedicle flap for defects of the perineum, including the vagina, rectum, and even pressure ulcers underlying the ischium. The gracilis muscle has an easily identifiable vascular pedicle with a large motor nerve that makes it suitable for transfer and reinnervation.

The gracilis muscle is an adductor and a medial rotator of the thigh. It is a long straplike muscle that arises from the pubic symphysis and ramus and inserts below the knee into the tibia. The powerful adductor longus and adductor magnus muscles compensate for the functional loss of the gracilis muscle (Figures 10-1 and 10-2).

FLAP DESIGN AND UTILIZATION

The gracilis muscle is a long thin muscle that measures 4 to 6 cm in width. The neurovascular pedicle enters the proximal portion of the muscle, approximately 8 to 10 cm caudal to the pubic tubercle (Figure 10-3). The dominant musculocutaneous perforator is also located in the same vicinity.

The primary use of the gracilis muscle in the head and neck has been for facial reanimation in which the muscle is both revascularized and reinnervated to restore its contractile activity. In Harii et al.'s (3) original description of this technique, a segment of the gracilis muscle was transferred to the paralyzed side of the face, and

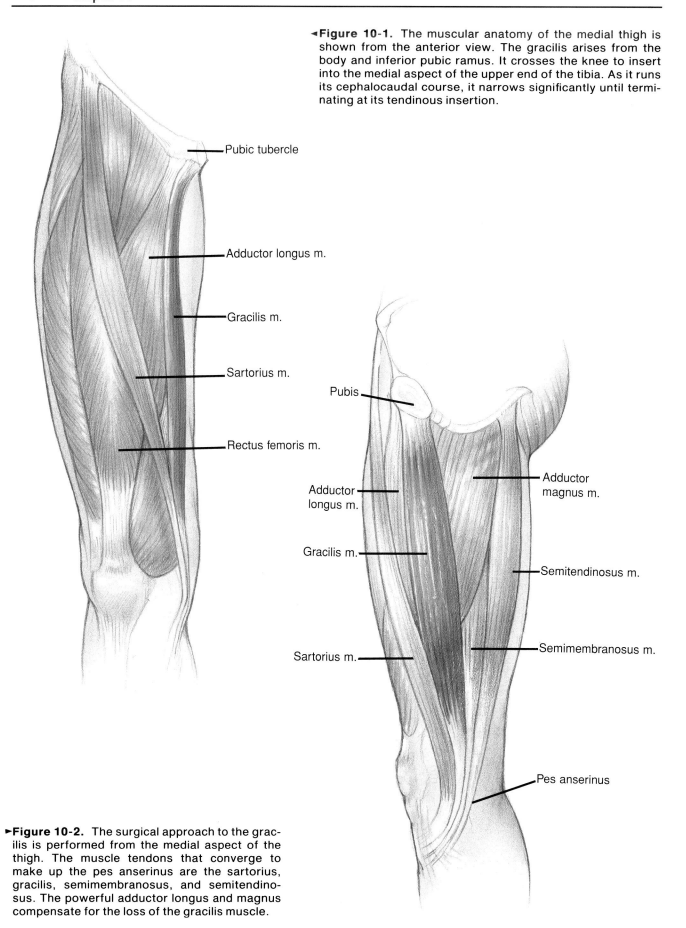

◄**Figure 10-1.** The muscular anatomy of the medial thigh is shown from the anterior view. The gracilis arises from the body and inferior pubic ramus. It crosses the knee to insert into the medial aspect of the upper end of the tibia. As it runs its cephalocaudal course, it narrows significantly until terminating at its tendinous insertion.

Pubic tubercle

Adductor longus m.

Gracilis m.

Sartorius m.

Rectus femoris m.

Pubis

Adductor longus m.

Adductor magnus m.

Gracilis m.

Semitendinosus m.

Semimembranosus m.

Sartorius m.

Pes anserinus

►**Figure 10-2.** The surgical approach to the gracilis is performed from the medial aspect of the thigh. The muscle tendons that converge to make up the pes anserinus are the sartorius, gracilis, semimembranosus, and semitendinosus. The powerful adductor longus and magnus compensate for the loss of the gracilis muscle.

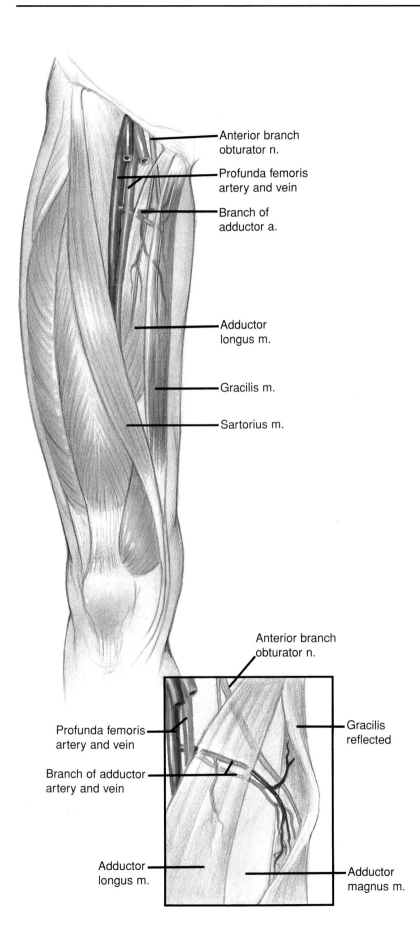

Anterior branch
obturator n.

Profunda femoris
artery and vein

Branch of
adductor a.

Adductor
longus m.

Gracilis m.

Sartorius m.

Anterior branch
obturator n.

Profunda femoris
artery and vein

Branch of adductor
artery and vein

Adductor
longus m.

Gracilis
reflected

Adductor
magnus m.

Figure 10-3. The vascular supply to the gracilis muscle is from a terminal branch of the adductor artery and vein, which arise from the profunda femoris artery and vein. The adductor artery usually arises from the profunda femoris artery, but it may also arise from the medial circumflex femoral artery. The gracilis branch of the adductor artery, accompanied by paired venae comitantes, passes between adductor longus and adductor magnus. The anterior division of the obturator nerve supplies the motor innervation to the gracilis muscle. It enters the muscle in a more cephalad location with a more oblique course than the main vascular pedicle.

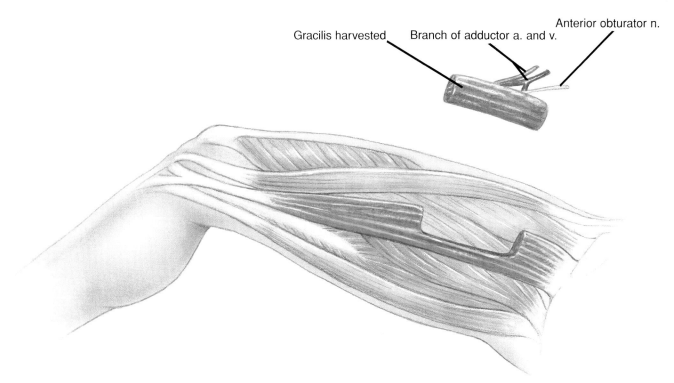

Gracilis harvested   Branch of adductor a. and v.   Anterior obturator n.

Figure 10-4. The branching pattern of the anterior division of the obturator nerve allows the gracilis muscle to be separated into at least two functional muscular units. A single fascicle usually supplies the anterior 25% of the muscle; the remaining nerve fascicles supply the rest of the muscle. A small portion of the muscle can be harvested with the main vascular pedicle and the fascicle from the anterior branch of the obturator nerve.

then its motor branch, the anterior branch of the obturator nerve, was anastomosed to the deep temporal nerve. One end of the muscle was sutured to the orbicularis oris at the lateral commissure, and the other end was sutured under tension to the temporal fascia.

Over time, there have been several refinements to Harii's original technique. To restore synchronous mimetic movement when the proximal stump of the facial nerve was not available, a two-stage procedure was described utilizing a cross face sural nerve graft in the initial stage. There is a considerable amount of cross innervation of the muscles in the midface, which are supplied by the buccal division of the facial nerve. The selection of an appropriate recipient branch can be made by intraoperative electrical stimulation. The Tinel's sign is used to monitor the progression of axonal growth across the face, which usually requires 9 to 12 months after the initial transfer. When the patient's examination reveals that the distal end of the sural graft has viable axons, then the free muscle is transferred, revascularized, and reinnervated to the stump of the cross facial graft (1).

In addition to introducing cross facial nerve grafts to achieve mimetic activity, an effort was made to reduce the bulk of the muscle in the face. Harii (1) described transfer of a gracilis muscle segment 10 cm in length and 3 cm in width, which is approximately one half the breadth of the muscle belly. Manktelow (4) investigated the fascicular pattern of the motor branch of the obturator nerve, which supplies the gracilis. Of the three fascicles usually present in that nerve, one was usually responsible for the innervation of the anterior 25% to 50% of the muscle. Interfascicular dissection and intraoperative stimulation allow selective harvest of only a small portion of the muscle innervated by a single- or double-nerve fascicle. Through this technique, Manktelow has transferred a smaller portion of the muscle

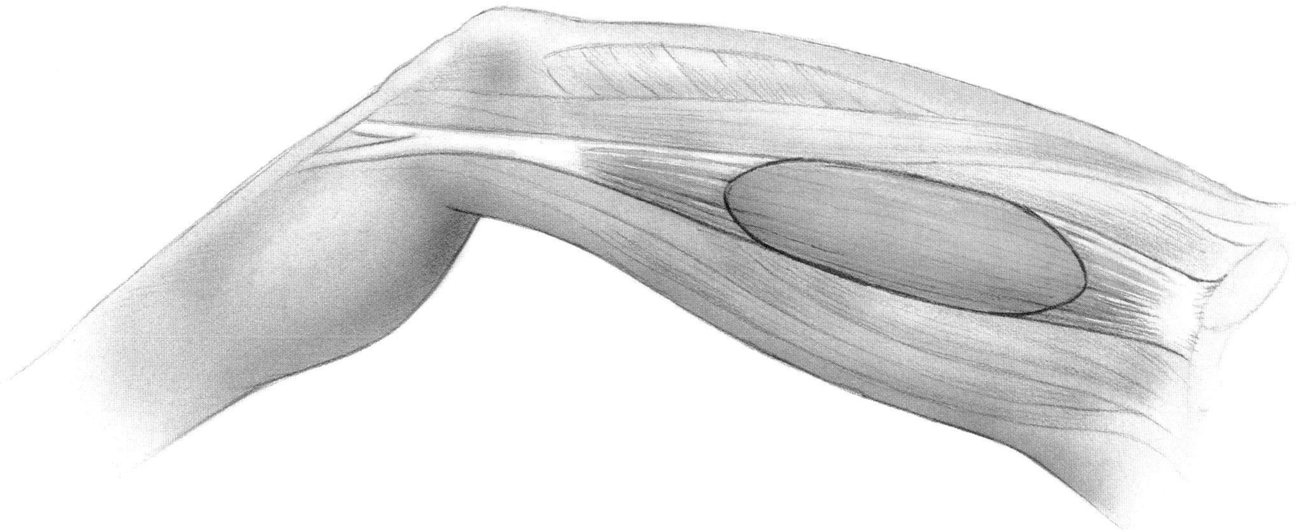

Figure 10-5. The skin paddle of the gracilis musculocutaneous flap was originally oriented longitudinally over the lengthwise direction of the muscle. An alternative transverse orientation has also been shown to be reliable. Either flap design must be centered over the dominant musculocutaneous perforator, which is located from 8–10 cm distal to the pubic tubercle.

while maintaining a neurovascular pedicle suitable for microvascular anastomosis (Figure 10-4).

Harii (1) reported a wide range of results in the quality of facial reanimation using the free gracilis muscle transfer in 122 patients. The selection of the recipient nerve that was used to drive the transplanted muscle seemed to have the greatest impact on the results of reanimation. The most consistently good results were achieved with anastomosis of the motor nerve of the gracilis to the stump of the ipsilateral facial nerve. However, good to satisfactory results were achieved with the two-stage cross facial nerve graft method when the ipsilateral facial nerve was not usable.

The gracilis musculocutaneous flap was originally described by Harii et al. (3) with a skin island designed over the proximal muscle. A longitudinally oriented skin paddle overlying the proximal muscle was transferred for a variety of defects (Figure 10-5). An alternative transverse skin paddle design was described by Yousif et al. (9) and is believed to offer several advantages. Three to six major musculocutaneous perforators are in the upper portion of the muscle. The dominant perforator measured approximately 1.5 mm in diameter and was located almost directly over the point where the main pedicle entered the gracilis. Yousif et al. reported that the perforators took either an anterior or posterior course after exiting the muscle. This superficial course of the perforators stimulated the authors to introduce a transverse skin flap that extended anteriorly over the adductor longus and sartorius and posteriorly over the adductor magnus and semitendinosus. The pattern of skin staining following dye-injection studies confirmed the validity of this skin flap design. Primary closure of the cutaneous defect limits the width of the flap in the vertical dimension. Yousif et al. reported the successful transfer of a flap measuring 10 × 25 cm. Donor-site closure was better disguised with the transverse design.

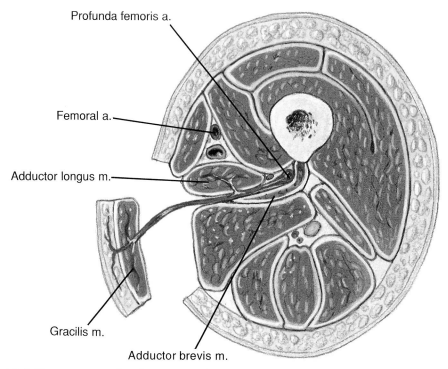

Profunda femoris a.

Femoral a.

Adductor longus m.

Gracilis m.

Adductor brevis m.

Figure 10-6. The cross-sectional anatomy of the medial thigh shows the course of the adductor artery arising from the profunda femoris and running between the adductor muscles with brevis and magnus posterior and longus anterior. The musculocutaneous perforator enters the skin opposite the point where the main pedicle enters the muscle.

NEUROVASCULAR ANATOMY

The gracilis muscle has a type II pattern of vascularity, according to the classification system of Mathes and Nahai (5). The dominant pedicle is the terminal branch of the adductor artery, which arises from the profunda femoris and runs a circuitous course between the adductor longus anteriorly and the adductor brevis and magnus posteriorly before entering the gracilis at the junction of the upper third and lower two thirds (Figure 10-6). This point of entry is consistently located between 8 and 10 cm inferior to the pubic tubercle. The adductor artery arises from the profunda femoris in the vicinity of the first perforator or from the medial femoral circumflex artery. It gives off branches to adductor longus and brevis, which must be ligated to obtain adequate pedicle length, which is usually 6 cm; the average arterial diameter is 2 mm. It is important to point out that, although the adductor artery may take its origin from the medial circumflex femoral artery, the main vascular supply to the gracilis muscle is not the medial circumflex femoral artery itself.

The minor vascular pedicle arises from the superficial femoral artery and enters the lower third of the muscle. An additional minor vascular supply arises from the medial circumflex femoral artery.

The major artery to the gracilis is accompanied by two venae comitantes. These veins may either join or drain separately into the profunda femoris vein. The average diameter of the veins is about 1.5 to 2.5 mm.

The blood supply to the skin through the system of musculocutaneous perforators was described earlier. The dominant perforators exit the muscle in the upper third, with few noted in the middle and lower portions. Yousif et al. (9) described an additional skin supply through septocutaneous vessels that exited through the intermuscular septum between the gracilis and the adductor longus. The orientation of the terminal branches of the septocutaneous vessels was also in a transverse direction.

The septocutaneous vessels in the distal thigh are branches of the superficial femoral artery, rather than the profunda system.

The motor supply to the gracilis muscle is the anterior branch of the obturator nerve, which enters the muscle in a more oblique course approximately 2 to 3 cm cephalad to the entry point of the vascular pedicle. The nerve may be traced proximally between adductor longus and brevis to gain additional length. The sensory supply to the medial thigh skin is from branches of the obturator nerve, which may be dissected in the subcutaneous tissues cephalad to the skin paddle. There are no published reports of sensory reinnervation with the gracilis musculocutaneous flap. However, the sensory nerves have been identified in the upper medial thigh in cadaver dissections. By tracing these nerves toward the obturator canal, a suitable length can be obtained.

ANATOMIC VARIATIONS

The vascular and nerve supply to the muscle is consistent. The major variability is noted in the blood supply to the overlying skin, both in the number and the size of musculocutaneous perforators. Yousif et al. (9) described several dissections in which there were no musculocutaneous perforators exiting the gracilis, and the major skin supply was derived from septocutaneous vessels or from the inferior branch of the superior external pudendal artery, which extended into the territory of the gracilis.

POTENTIAL PITFALLS

The potential pitfalls in harvesting the gracilis muscle flap are few because of the consistency of the neurovascular pedicle. The major problem may arise when harvesting a musculocutaneous flap because of the occasional variations in the vascular supply to the skin of the medial thigh. In addition, an attempt to harvest a long cutaneous paddle often results in necrosis of the skin overlying the distal third of the muscle. The morbidity of removing this muscle is limited as a result of the strength of the remaining adductor muscles.

Flap Harvesting Technique follows on page 146.

Flap Harvesting Technique

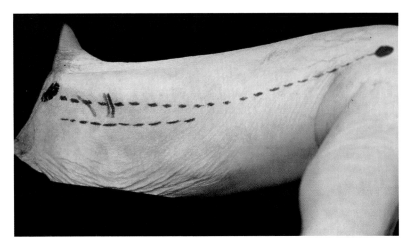

Figure 10-7. This dissection demonstrates the harvest of the gracilis muscle flap. With the leg flexed and abducted, a *dotted line* is drawn between the pubic tubercle and the medial condyle of the tibia. The superior edge of the gracilis muscle lies approximately 1–1.5 cm posterior to this line. The neurovascular pedicle enters the muscle on its undersurface approximately 8 to 10 cm below the publc tubercle. If a musculocutaneous flap was harvested, the skin paddle would be centered over this point, oriented either in a transverse or longitudinal direction.

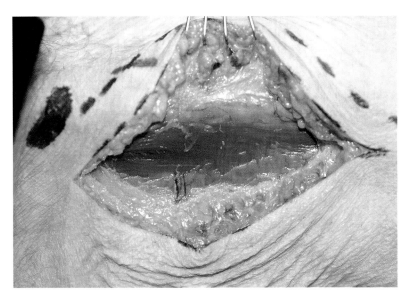

Figure 10-8. The initial incision is carried through the skin and subcutaneous tissue to identify the midbelly of the gracilis muscle. The sartorius is a good landmark to help identify the gracilis in the midthigh. From the surgical position, the sartorius is located immediately above the gracilis. In the proximal thigh, the adductor longus is immediately above the gracilis, which is shown at this point in this dissection.

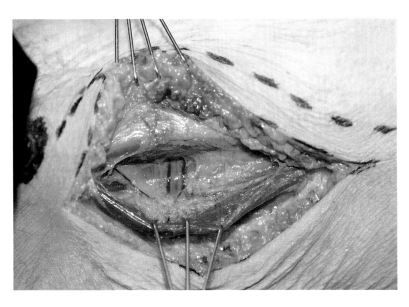

Figure 10-9. With the superior edge of the gracilis muscle reflected inferiorly, the neurovascular pedicle is easily identified as it enters the muscle on its deep surface. The neurovascular pedicle exits between the adductor longus above and adductor magnus below before entering the gracilis.

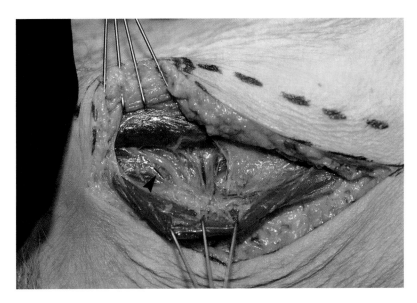

Figure 10-10. After the artery and vein are identified, the anterior obturator nerve (*arrow*) is found entering the muscle in a more oblique course and 2–3 cm proximal to the vascular pedicle.

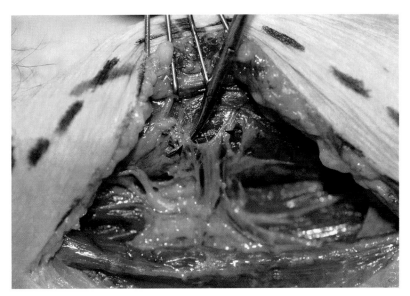

Figure 10-11. Branches (*arrows*) from the vascular pedicle to the adductor longus muscle must be ligated to maximize the length.

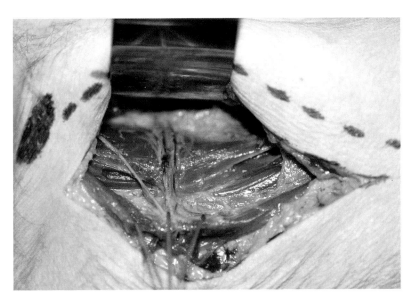

Figure 10-12. The vascular pedicle can be dissected medially to obtain approximately 6 cm of length. The maximum diameter of the artery is about 2 mm, and the vein may reach a diameter of 2.5 mm.

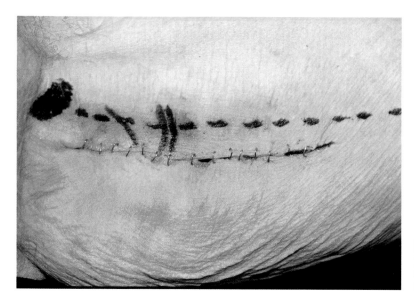

Figure 10-13. The wound is closed by reapproximating the fascia of adductor longus and magnus and then closing the skin in layers.

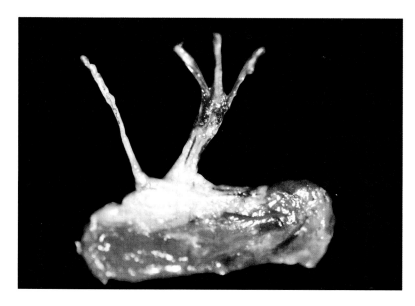

Figure 10-14. A segment of the gracilis muscle has been harvested with the nutrient artery and its paired venae comitantes. The anterior obturator nerve is shown entering the muscle in a more proximal location. The muscle may be divided longitudinally to reduce the bulk while preserving the neurovascular pedicle.

REFERENCES

1. Harii K: Microneurovascular free muscle transplantation. In: Rubin L, ed. *The Paralyzed Face.* Philadelphia: Mosby Yearbook; 1991:178–200.
2. Harii K, Ohmori K, Sekiguchi J: The free musculocutaneous flap. *Plast Reconstr Surg* 1976;57:294–303.
3. Harii K, Ohmori K, Torii S: Free gracilis muscle transplantation with microvascular anastomosis for the treatment of facial paralysis. *Plast Reconstr Surg* 1976;57:133–135.
4. Manktelow R: *Microvascular Reconstruction; Anatomy, Applications and Surgical Technique.* New York: Springer-Verlag; 1986.
5. Mathes S, Nahai F: *Clinical Application for Muscle and Musculocutaneous Flaps.* London: CV Mosby; 1982.
6. McGraw J, Massey F, Shanklin K, Horton C: Vaginal reconstruction with gracilis myocutaneous flaps. *Plast Reconstr Surg* 1976;58:176.
7. Pickrill K, Georgiade N, Maquire C, Crawford H: Gracilis muscle transplants for rectal incontinence. *Surgery* 1956;40:349.
8. Wingate G: Report of ischial pressure ulcers with gracilis myocutaneous island flaps. *Plast Reconstr Surg* 1978;62:245.
9. Yousif N, Matloub H, Kabachalam R, Grunert B, Sanger J: The transverse gracilis musculocutaneous flap. *Ann Plast Surg* 1992;29:482–490.

FREE FLAPS
Fascial and Fasciocutaneous Flaps

Radial
Forearm

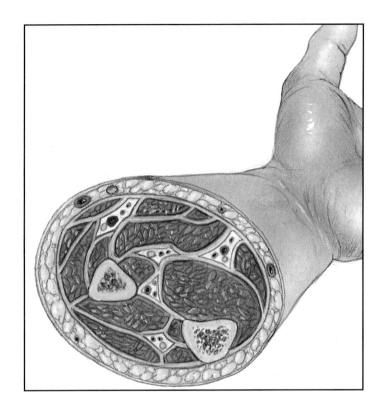

Mark L. Urken, M.D.

The first free flap to be transferred on the radial artery was a segment of the superficial branch of the radial nerve and was performed by Taylor in 1976 (46). However, the radial forearm flap as a fasciocutaneous flap was first introduced by Yang et al. (55) in the Chinese literature in 1981. This initial report of 60 radial forearm flaps with only 1 failure was soon followed by additional publications from China (38), and hence, this flap became known as the "Chinese flap." Soutar's group (40–42) popularized the radial forearm flap for intraoral reconstruction through a number of publications, the first of which appeared in 1983.

Based on the radial artery and either the cephalic vein or the venae comitantes, this flap may be transferred as a composite flap containing vascularized bone (39), vascularized tendon (34), the brachioradialis muscle (36), vascularized nerve (19), or sensory nerves (20). However, its thin pliable skin with its rich vascularity, permitting a flexibility in design and a high degree of reliability, is the key reason why the forearm flap has assumed such an important place in head and neck reconstruction.

FLAP DESIGN AND UTILIZATION

The skin of virtually the entire forearm, extending from the antecubital fossa to the flexor crease of the wrist, may be harvested (Figure 11-1). The thickness of this flap varies among individuals but tends to be thinner in its distal portion. The flap is also usually thinner in male than in female patients. The degree and pattern of hair-bearing skin also varies between individuals.

The radial forearm fasciocutaneous flap has been used more extensively and for

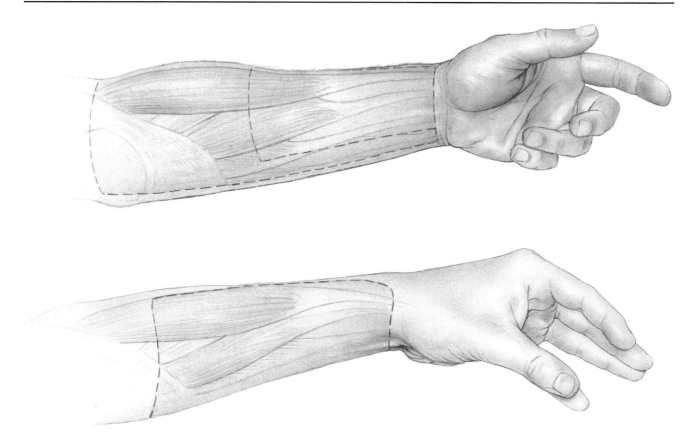

Figure 11-1. The size and shape of the radial forearm flap vary with the defect. The axis of the flap should be centered over the course of the radial artery and the cephalic vein. The flap may extend from the flexor crease of the wrist to above the antecubital fossa. There are regional differences in the thickness of the subcutaneous tissue with the thinnest flaps harvested from the distal forearm. The donor site is more easily camouflaged when the majority of it is located on the volar surface.

more diverse reconstructive problems that any other free flap. Unquestionably, its greatest application is in the restoration of oral mucosal defects following ablative surgery. It has been used in virtually every portion of the oral cavity (23,27,28,40,41,53). In 1994, Urken et al. (50) described a bilobed design for the radial forearm flap to help preserve the mobility of the residual tongue following significant glossectomy. Toward that end, this flap provides thin and redundant tissue. The bilobed design allows one lobe to be used to resurface the tongue defect; the second lobe is placed in the floor of mouth. In so doing, the rest of the tongue remains separate from the inner table of the mandible. The deep fascia and subcutaneous tissue can be harvested without the overlying skin. Ismail (20) described this fascial-subcutaneous flap for extremity reconstruction and also reported the improved aesthetic result of a straight-line closure of the preserved forearm skin. This fascial flap may be covered with a skin graft to resurface epithelial defects. It is also highly effective in skull base surgery to assist in dural repair; this thin well-vascularized tissue is more easily inset in locations adjacent to the brain that will not accommodate thicker flaps. Martin and Brown (27) introduced the free radial forearm fascial flap for intraoral reconstruction. They described a rapid re-epithelialization of the fascial–subcutaneous tissue layer to achieve a mucosal surface. In addition, this technique produced a thinner and less mobile layer over the mandible that was more conducive to the placement of a dental prosthesis. The avoidance of a skin graft produced a more favorable donor-site appearance. Although this technique has merit in resurfacing the alveolus, it may lead to tethering in the floor of the mouth as a result of scar formation.

Another disadvantage of using a fascial free flap is that it removes the sensory receptors present in the skin and, therefore, leads to less predictable sensory restoration following anastomosis of the antebrachial cutaneous nerves to recipient nerves in the head and neck. We reported the first successful sensate radial forearm flap in head and neck reconstruction (52). A young woman with a pharyngeal defect underwent reconstruction with a forearm flap, and the sensory nerve was anastomosed to the greater auricular nerve. The patient experienced sensation when drinking hot and cold liquids that was referred to her ear. Arguably the greater auricular nerve was not the best recipient nerve for a pharyngeal defect, but it provided a valuable result. It showed that sensate flaps could be successfully used in the head and neck and that the mechanism for sensory recovery was through the nerve anastomosis. Our experience with sensate flaps has grown to include more than 60 cases, and our enthusiasm for this technique remains high, based on the predictable level of sensory recovery and the functional impact on patient rehabilitation (48). The primary defects in which we believe sensate flaps have their greatest applications are mobile and tongue base reconstruction, pharyngeal wall reconstruction, laryngeal reconstruction following partial laryngectomy, and restoration of the upper and lower lips.

In addition to defects of the lower half of the oral cavity, the radial forearm flap has been used for palatal reconstruction. Hatoko et al. (18) reported their favorable experience with reconstructing the hard palate with a folded double-layer forearm flap following maxillectomy. One layer was used for the oral side and the other layer, for the nasal and sinus floor. These patients were reportedly able to wear a maxillary denture. We have had considerable success in reconstructing partial and total soft palate defects with a folded radial forearm flap. The two layers of the flap are used for the oropharyngeal and nasopharyngeal sides of the defect. To achieve velopharyngeal competence, the folded edge of the flap is sutured to the posterior pharyngeal wall by de-epithelializing opposing surfaces. Bilateral mucosa-lined ports provide communication on either side of the midline attachment.

The desire to add to the versatility of the forearm donor site has led investigators to include additional components to this flap. The use of the brachioradialis is a product of that desire. It has been shown that, although the dominant muscular perforator to the brachioradialis may arise from the radial artery (40%), radial recurrent artery (33%), or the brachial artery (37%), it can be reliably transferred with the radial artery because of a series of secondary perforators. There are a large number of musculocutaneous perforators that exit the surface of the brachioradialis that allow a separate skin paddle to be harvested with the muscle as a carrier. Not only does this add bulk to the flap, but it also permits separate epithelial surfaces to be harvested for complex defects. The brachioradialis may also be transferred as a functional muscle unit if desired (36).

The brachioradialis has been used for total upper lip reconstruction by suturing the two ends of the muscle to the inferior orbicularis oris. Reinnervation of the muscle was accomplished by suturing the motor nerve of the brachioradialis to a buccal branch of the facial nerve. Takada et al. (45) reported excellent functional results and electromyographic evidence of electrical activity in the muscle. Total lower lip reconstruction with a radial forearm flap was reported by Sadove et al. (35). The palmaris longus tendon was transferred with the forearm skin to provide support to and to maintain the height of the lower lip. The combination of the palmaris longus tendon with the sensory nerve supply would provide an elegant total lower lip reconstruction.

There are occasions in head and neck reconstruction in which multiple skin paddles are required. The radial forearm flap has been divided into two epithelial surfaces separated by a de-epithelialized zone for providing inner and outer linings (5). The intervening zone has been divided down to the level of the fascia while still providing adequate vascularity to the distal skin paddle (3). Yousif and Ye (56) divided the perforators to the forearm skin into three clusters of vessels along the lateral intermuscular septum, each capable of supporting a segment of skin.

A segment of radius, limited proximally by the insertion of the pronator teres and

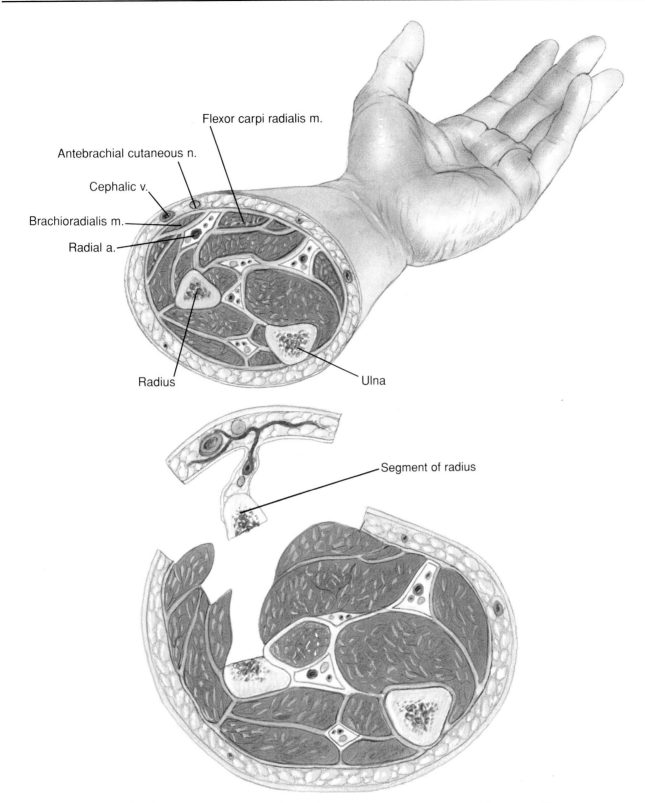

Figure 11-2. The cross-sectional anatomy of the forearm reveals the radial artery with its venae comitantes in the lateral intermuscular septum. The connection of the septum to the radius provides vascularity through perforators that supply the periosteum. The amount of radius that may be safely harvested is limited to 40% of the circumference.

distally by the insertion of the brachioradialis, may also be harvested (Figure 11-2). The length of bone is no greater than 10 to 12 cm, and the bone stock is restricted to 40% of the circumference of the radius. Soutar and Widdowson (42) reported the successful use of the osteocutaneous radial forearm flap in 12 of 14 patients who underwent oromandibular reconstruction. Osteotomies were created in nine patients to achieve a more favorable contour of the neomandible. Although the composite osteocutaneous flap is conceptually attractive for the reconstruction of oromandibular defects, there are two major factors that restrict its use. The dimensions of the bone that can be safely harvested are limited by the necessity to maintain the structural integrity of the remaining radius. Other donor sites for vascularized bone provide much better bone stock for functional mandibular reconstruction (31,49). The second major factor mitigating against the use of the radius is the potential morbidity resulting from pathologic fractures that have occurred in up to 23% of reported cases (49). Although specific techniques in creating the osteotomies, and prolonged postoperative immobilization, help to limit the incidence of fractures, the potential morbidity and the poor bone stock make this a less favored site for harvesting vascularized bone.

The superficial branches of the radial nerve may be transferred as vascularized nerve grafts. An isolated case report using this technique for the repair of the facial nerve revealed excellent results (20). However, the true value of vascularized nerve grafts over nonvascularized grafts remains controversial.

The radial forearm flap has been used successfully to cover large cutaneous defects of the head and neck, in particular, those involving the scalp where thin coverage is desirable (8). The radial forearm flap has also been applied to restoring complex defects of the nose and forehead (1,7).

Regional differences in the thickness of the skin of the forearm can be used to achieve a more aesthetic result, as dictated by the particular defect. More proximal skin paddles offer thicker tissue and the potential for wider flaps. Skin grafts placed over the proximal muscle bed are more reliable than are those placed over the distal tendons. The disadvantage of a skin flap harvested from a proximal location is that it significantly shortens the arterial pedicle. Baird et al. (1) described a proximal forearm flap for forehead reconstruction in which perfusion was maintained by retrograde flow through the distal radial artery, which was attached to the superficial temporal artery on one side of the head. The cephalic vein was dissected proximally in the arm for additional length and was anastamosed to the external jugular vein in the contralateral neck.

The radial forearm flap has also been applied to smaller defects in the head and neck. Tahara and Susuki (44) reported favorable results when introducing a radial forearm flap into the orbit to correct malignant contracture of an irradiated enophthalmic eye socket. The creation of an epithelium-lined socket permitted the patient to wear an orbital prosthesis.

Another application for the radial forearm flap is in circumferential pharyngoesophageal reconstruction. Harii et al. (17) introduced the concept of a tubed radial forearm flap to reconstruct a laryngopharyngectomy defect. The thin pliable tissue from this donor site is more readily tubed than is a thicker musculocutaneous flap. In addition, this method of reconstruction offers distinct advantages over free jejunal autografts because of the avoidance of a laparotomy.

The versatility of the forearm donor site is further reflected by its use in reconstructing defects of the larynx and pharynx. Chantrain et al. (6) described the application of the radial forearm flap to the reconstruction of a vertical hemipharyngolaryngectomy defect in three patients with a pyriform sinus cancer and one patient with a transglottic carcinoma. The tendon of the palmaris longus was included with the flap and fixed anteriorly to the thyroid cartilage and posteriorly to a hole drilled in the midline of the rostrum of the cricoid cartilage. This maneuver provided a fixed position for the neocord. The cutaneous portion of the flap was folded to line the hemilarynx and the medial wall of the pyriform sinus. All four patients were able to

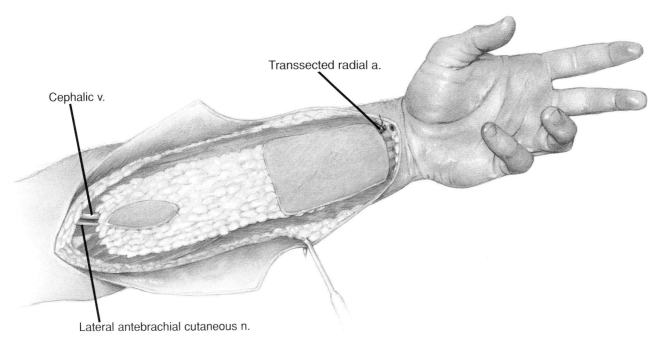

Figure 11-3. A modified design of the radial forearm flap has a distal skin paddle for resurfacing a mucosal defect and a proximal skin paddle that is exteriorized in the neck to serve as a monitor. The intervening subcutaneous tissue provides coverage of the great vessels and the microvascular pedicle and also leads to augmentation of the radial neck dissection deformity.

eat orally, and three of the patients were decannulated. The full extent to which this technique can be applied in partial laryngeal surgery has not yet been realized.

Hagen (14) presented a modified design of the radial forearm flap for postlaryngectomy voice rehabilitation. The forearm flap was tubed to create a skin-lined tube that was sutured to the cephalad end of the trachea. An epiglottis-like structure that was reinforced with autologous cartilage was sutured over the open end of the tube positioned at the base of tongue. The advantage of this form of alaryngectomy speech was that there was no prosthesis required, and the phonation pressure was less than that with a tracheoesophageal prosthesis. Most importantly, the seven patients in the series were able to swallow without aspiration.

The use of the radial forearm flap in the oro- or hypopharynx creates a problem for postoperative monitoring because of the limited access to these regions. I introduced a new design for the buried radial forearm flap in which there are two skin paddles, a distal one for resurfacing the mucosal defect and a smaller proximal one that is exteriorized in the neck (Figure 11-3) (51). The intervening fascial subcutaneous tissue is used to cover the carotid artery and provide augmentation to the radical neck dissection defect. Because the superficial veins and the radial artery are completely encompassed by this vascularized subcutaneous tissue, it provides an effective barrier for the pedicle in the event of a salivary fistula.

NEUROVASCULAR ANATOMY

The blood supply to the lower arm and the hand is derived from the brachial artery, which divides into the radial and ulnar arteries in the antecubital fossa. The radial

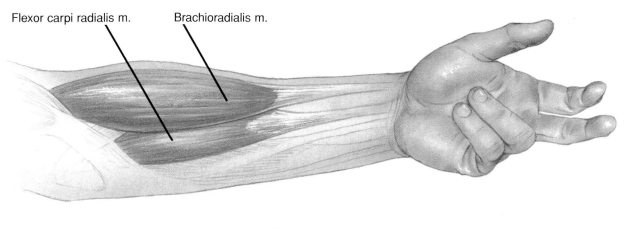

Flexor carpi radialis m.   Brachioradialis m.

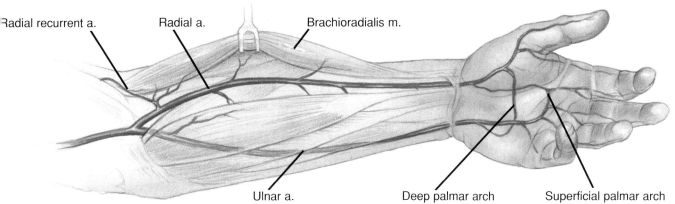

Radial recurrent a.   Radial a.   Brachioradialis m.

Ulnar a.   Deep palmar arch   Superficial palmar arch

Figure 11-4. The radial artery runs a course between the flexor carpi radialis and the brachio-radialis muscles before terminating in the deep palmar arch. The deep palmar arch supplies the principal circulation to the thumb and index finger. The ulnar artery terminates in the superficial palmar arch, which primarily supplies the third, fourth, and fifth digits and often also the index finger.

artery gives rise to the deep palmar arch; the ulnar artery terminates in the superficial palmar arch. Harvest of the radial forearm flap requires complete interruption of the radial artery and, therefore, total reliance on the ulnar system to maintain the vascular supply to the hand (Figure 11-4).

There are four vascular systems that supply the forearm skin through an array of septocutaneous and musculocutaneous perforators. These four vessels are the radial, ulnar, anterior, and posterior interosseous arteries (24).

The flexor and extensor muscles of the forearm are enclosed by a common fascial sheath. A condensation of this fascia, referred to as the lateral intermuscular septum, separates the brachioradialis and the flexor carpi radialis in the forearm (Figure 11-2). The radial artery, with its two venae comitantes, runs in the lateral intermuscular septum and gives off 9 to 17 fascial branches in the forearm. This fascial plexus supplies the skin of virtually the entire forearm. There are few fascial branches in the middle third of the forearm, and in fact, the connections between the radial artery and the deep fascia are attenuated because of the overlap between the flexor carpi radialis and the brachioradialis. The radial artery gives off a few fascial branches in the proximal third of the forearm. There is one dominant fasciocutaneous branch in the proximal forearm, the inferior cubital artery, which has been used to supply a proximally based fasciocutaneous flap. This vessel may arise from either the radial or the radial recurrent arteries (24). Ink-injection studies revealed that the vessels in the distal zone are capable of supplying a fasciocutaneous flap that extends proximally to the elbow (48). The maximum dimensions of the skin territory that can be based on the radial artery is undetermined. Yang et al. (55) reported a radial forearm flap that measured 35 × 15 cm. There is at least one case in the literature in which the entire skin of an amputated forearm was transferred as a free flap based on the radial artery (54).

In addition to supplying the forearm skin through the fascial plexus, the radial artery sends branches to the muscles of the flexor compartment, the palmaris longus tendon, and the radial nerve. The lateral intermuscular septum is attached to the distal radius, and it is through this connection that it supplies branches to the periosteum, allowing harvest of a segment of vascularized bone (10). A longitudinal vascular arcade has been described on the surface of the periosteum that originates in close proximity to the insertions of flexor pollicis longus and pronator quadratus (40).

The radial forearm flap has a deep venous supply through the two paired venae comitantes, which run in the intermuscular septum as well as the larger superficial veins, such as the cephalic vein. Both venous systems have valves that mandate unidirectional flow. The veins that supply the fascial plexus run with the branches of the radial artery and drain into the venae comitantes. The multiple connections between the venae comitantes and the superficial veins form the basis for using either of these two systems to drain the flap. The branching patterns of the deep and superficial venous systems have been classified into five different types (47). In the type 1 pattern (20%), there is a wide communication through an anastomotic vein between the superficial and deep systems. In addition, the median cubital vein splits into two large branches: the cephalic median vein and the basilic medial vein. The type 2 pattern (43%) is the most common and is identical to type 1 except that the median cubital vein does not bifurcate. The type 3 pattern (18%) includes a confluence of the two venae comitantes to a sizable common trunk, but there is no significant communication of this common trunk with the cephalic vein to form a median cubital vein. In the type 4 pattern (5%), the venae comitantes do not converge or join with the cephalic vein, but each is of suitable caliber for microvascular anastomosis. The type 5 pattern (15%) is similar to type 4 except that one of the venae comitantes is dominant relative to the other. I prefer to use the subcutaneous venous system because of the larger caliber vessels and the thicker wall, which permits an easier anastomosis. Often, there are multiple subcutaneous veins suitable for anastomosis, depending on the design of the radial forearm flap. When the types 1 and 2 patterns are identified, I prefer to use the median cubital vein for anastomosis based on the theoretical advantage that both the deep and superficial systems are being directly drained. However, I have never encountered a problem of venous insufficiency when using either the superficial or deep systems independently.

The length of the arterial pedicle to this flap is limited by the radial recurrent artery, which is the first major branch of the radial artery following its takeoff from the brachial artery. The radial recurrent artery is primarily a muscular branch. Alternatively, the cephalic vein may be traced throughout its entire course in the upper arm to its junction with the subclavian vein in the infraclavicular region. The additional length of vein that can be harvested by extending the dissection above the antecubital fossa may be helpful in skull base reconstruction in which vein grafts are frequently needed. This flap has been used in the head and neck in which the venous outflow is maintained without interruption of the cephalic vein while performing only an arterial anastomosis (32). Using this technique of an extensively mobilized but uninterrupted cephalic vein, Bhathena and Kavarana (3) described using a proximal forearm flap that was revascularized through retrograde arterial flow through the distal radial artery. The reliance on retrograde flow through the radial artery is routinely used when the "reversed radial forearm flap" is transferred as a pedicled flap to the hand (21).

The cutaneous innervation of the forearm is derived from the medial, lateral, and posterior antebrachial cutaneous nerves (Figure 11-5). The lateral antebrachial cutaneous nerve, the continuation of the musculocutaneous nerve, is the primary sensory nerve to the territory of forearm skin most commonly harvested. This nerve usually runs in close proximity to the cephalic vein in the upper forearm before ramifying in

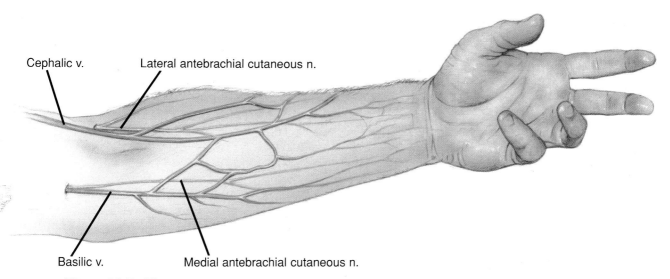

Cephalic v.   Lateral antebrachial cutaneous n.

Basilic v.   Medial antebrachial cutaneous n.

Figure 11-5. The sensory nerve supply to the forearm skin consistently follows a course that parallels the major subcutaneous veins. Depending on the size and orientation of the flap, either the medial, the lateral, or both antebrachial cutaneous nerves would be incorporated.

the distal forearm and continuing onto the hand in the region of the thenar eminence. The medial antebrachial cutaneous nerve arises from the medial cord of the brachial plexus, runs with the basilic vein, and supplies the skin of the medial aspect of the forearm. The skin of the dorsum of the forearm is supplied by posterior branches of the medial and lateral antebrachial cutaneous nerves and by the posterior antebrachial cutaneous nerve, a branch of the radial nerve. The medial and posterior antebrachial cutaneous nerves are rarely encountered in the dissection of a forearm flap, except when very large flaps are harvested.

The radial nerve is a mixed motor and sensory nerve. It supplies most of the muscles of the extensor compartment and the abductor pollicis longus and brevis. The sensory distribution of this nerve includes portions of the upper arm and the dorsum of the forearm through the posterior antebrachial cutaneous nerve. The superficial branch of the radial nerve courses in the forearm, deep to the brachioradialis, and passes laterally to the brachioradialis tendon where it divides into the dorsal digital nerves supplying sensation to the dorsum of the hand, thumb, and index and middle fingers. Although the distal branching pattern is highly variable, the major branches are always encountered in the wrist while elevating the radial forearm flap. This nerve and all its branches can be routinely preserved to maintain sensation to the hand.

ANATOMIC VARIATIONS

The anatomy of the superficial venous system in the forearm is highly variable. However, the pattern of veins can be easily mapped prior to surgery by placing a tourniquet on the upper arm and tracing the course of the engorged veins.

The greatest concern in harvesting the radial forearm flap is the integrity of the ulnar arterial supply to the hand through the superficial palmar arch. It is therefore the anomalies of the arterial blood supply to the hand that must be addressed. On the most basic level, the blood supply to the hand following radial artery transsection relies on the presence of an ulnar artery. In a cadaveric study of 750 upper extremities, McCormack et al. (30) found the ulnar and radial arteries to be present in all cases. The ulnar artery supplies the hand through the superficial palmar arch, which is either "complete," in the sense that it provides branches to four fingers and the thumb, or completed through communications with the deep palmar arch. Cadaveric studies by Coleman and Anson (9) revealed that the ulnar artery supply to the third, fourth, and fifth digits is rarely, if ever, compromised by anomalous patterns. When harvesting a radial forearm flap, it is the vascular supply to the thumb and the index finger that is most at risk by the combination of two concurrent arterial variations. The first is an incomplete superficial arch that does not send branches to the thumb and index finger. The second anomaly, which must also be present for there to be a problem of digital ischemia, is a complete lack of communication between the superficial and deep arches. In 265 cadaveric specimens, Coleman and Anson found a complete superficial arch in 77.3% of cases. The coexistence of the two anomalies, which would put the thumb at least at risk of ischemia in the event of radial artery occlusion, occurred in 12% of specimens.

A third source of blood supply to the hand may arise from a persistent median artery, which has been noted in up to 16% of cases (9). This vessel usually joins the superficial palmar arch. It is therefore possible that this vessel may supply protective circulation to the hand in those cases in which the thumb and index finger are otherwise at risk following sacrifice of the radial artery.

Heden and Gylbert (19) reported an aberrant radial artery that was encountered while raising a radial forearm flap. A small branch of the radial artery was found in the normal anatomic position, but the main vessel ran a divergent course in the distal forearm that was superficial to the extensor pollicis tendons and entered the hand several centimeters radial to its normal location. This anomaly has been reported to occur in 1% of the population, and its importance is evident when considering the implications for performing an accurate Allen test (19,26). Compression of the rudimentary branch may not demonstrate an abnormality in the palmar arch, putting the thumb at risk for ischemia. If encountered during a dissection of a forearm flap, it is imperative that the true aberrant radial artery is temporarily occluded and the tourniquet released to assess the impact on the vascularity of the hand.

Additional, although rare, anomalies of the radial artery have been reported. Otsuka and Terauchi (33) reported an aberrant dorsal course of the radial artery that passed around Lister's tubercle of the radius to enter the hand above the extensor tendons. Small and Millar (37) reported a radial artery that passed deep to the pronator teres.

Anomalies of the ulnar artery are equally rare. However, Fatah et al. (12) described an ulnar artery that ran a course superficial to the flexor muscles in the forearm. The importance of recognizing such an anomaly is essential to avoid catastrophic injury to the remaining blood supply to the hand following harvest of the radial forearm flap.

POTENTIAL PITFALLS

Although the radial forearm flap is a highly reliable method of reconstruction, there are a number of donor site problems that may be encountered. The performance of an accurate Allen test is the most important consideration in avoiding the catastrophic complication of an ischemic hand. There is one report in the literature by Jones and O'Brien (22) in which insufficient flow to the hand resulted from flap harvest despite a normal Allen test result. The hand was salvaged by intraoperative recognition of the problem and reconstruction of the radial artery by an interposition vein graft. Bardsley et al. (2) reported on a subset of 12 patients in their total series of 100 patients who underwent radial forearm flaps in whom reconstitution of the radial artery was performed. This group constituted the earliest patients in their series. Despite reestablishing flow in the operating room, only six vein grafts remained patent over time. None of the patients with occluded grafts suffered any complications. Vascular insufficiency may also result from too tight a closure of the forearm skin or compression from the forearm dressing. Careful observation of the hand both during and after surgery will help to avoid such problems.

Poor take of the skin graft may result from shearing forces of the underlying muscles as a result of inadequate immobilization of the hand. Failure to preserve the paratenon over the flexor tendons may also contribute to problems with the skin graft.

Infection of the forearm donor site is uncommon. However, the devastating effects of this complication were reported by Hallock (16) who described a patient with a frozen hand resulting from a descending suppurative tenosynovitis. Meticulous sterile technique and avoidance of cross contamination from the head and neck by using a separate set of instruments is absolutely imperative.

The aesthetic deformity of the skin-grafted donor site is recognized as one of the major disadvantages of the radial forearm free flap. A variety of different techniques have been reported to modify the appearance of the skin-grafted forearm defect. Direct closure of distal cutaneous defects has been reported by the use of an ulnar transposition flap. Long fascial attachments provide a reliable blood supply to these flaps, which can be used to close small to medium-sized defects. In muscular individuals, there is often a problem of closing the secondary defect in the proximal forearm which results from using an ulnar transposition flap. The usual technique of a V-to-Y closure will not work, and in such cases, a skin graft can be placed proximally while achieving full thickness skin coverage of the flexor tendons distally (2,11). Poor take of the skin graft over the distal flexor tendons can be problematic, despite care in preserving the paratenon. Coverage of the flexor carpi radialis tendon with turnover muscle flaps of the flexor pollicis longus and the flexor digitorum superficialis was described to improve the donor site bed to accept a skin graft (13).

The use of tissue expanders has been reported to achieve full-thickness coverage of the donor defect. Masser (28) placed a tissue expander several weeks prior to flap harvest to facilitate forearm coverage. The expanders were placed deep to the forearm fascia and deep to the radial artery. Careful monitoring of the Doppler signal during the expansion phase was critical to prevent occlusion of the radial artery. The preexpansion was believed to achieve a greater flap surface area and to delay marginal areas that may have been ischemic following transfer. In addition, Masser reported reduced thickness of the forearm flaps.

As an alternative to this approach, Hallock (15) placed tissue expanders under the residual forearm skin at the time of harvesting a radial forearm flap. He waited a minimum of 2 weeks to begin serial expansion. In ten patients so treated, five had linear scars; the remaining patients had a significant reduction in the size of the skin-grafted area.

The transfer of a fascial flap alone avoids the problem of a cutaneous donor-site defect. Such a fascial flap can be transferred and covered with a split-thickness skin graft. To eliminate the necessity of using a separate donor site for harvesting a skin graft, Kawashina et al. (23) described the de-epithelialized forearm flap for resurfacing the lining of the upper aerodigestive tract. The forearm flap was harvested and then de-epithelialized on a drum dermatone. The resulting split-thickness graft was returned to the forearm, avoiding the deformity of a second donor site for a skin graft. The de-epithelialized flaps healed uneventfully and were rapidly covered by an epithelial layer.

The most common neurologic problems in the forearm are related to sensory loss following injury to the superficial branches of the radial nerve and transsection of the antebrachial cutaneous nerves. Painful neuromas have not been a problem in my experience, but the potential is certainly present.

The function of the hand following routine harvest of a radial forearm flap is usually normal. The potential for morbidity in the hand mounts when an osteocutaneous flap is harvested. Fracture of the radius can have a significant detrimental effect on supination, wrist flexion, grip strength, and pinch strength (4). As noted previously, this potential morbidity and the poor bone stock greatly limit the advisability of routinely using the osteocutaneous flap. However, there are situations in which a very small composite flap may be needed. Under these circumstances, the method by which the osteotomy is created may be important in avoiding a significant donor-site problem. Bardsley et al. (2) recommended removal of as small a segment of bone as possible, and in the process, they advised creating smooth "boat-shaped" bone cuts rather than right-angled ones, which were prone to fracture. Prolonged immobilization and serial radiographs of the healing donor site were also advised to ensure adequate bone remodeling prior to stressing the forearm.

Swanson et al. (43) tested the hypothesis that the type of osteotomy influenced the mechanical strength of the residual radius. They did not find a statistically significant difference in the breaking force between a right-angled and beveled bone cut. There was a significant difference in breaking strength (24%) in the group of osteotomized radii compared with that in intact controls. However, the authors did advise the use of a beveled bone cut to reduce the concentration of stress at the corners of right-angled cuts and to minimize the amount of bone removed, which they believe should not exceed one third of the radial diameter. In addition, they advised an above-elbow splint for 8 weeks after surgery.

PREOPERATIVE MANAGEMENT

Factors, such as tissue thickness, hair-bearing skin, and the distribution of superficial veins, can be assessed preoperatively to plan the design of the forearm flap. The flap's dimensions and shape can usually be accurately determined by direct laryngoscopy and manual palpation. However, we usually wait to harvest this flap until frozen sections on tumor margins have been determined. The Allen test is the most important preoperative evaluation to assess the adequacy of the circulation to the hand through the ulnar artery. The Allen test must be performed properly. Simultaneous compression of the ulnar and radial arteries is applied by the examiner while the hand is alternately opened and closed. This pumping action causes the hand to become pale as a result of mechanical exsanguination. The hand is then opened to a relaxed position prior to the release of the ulnar artery. It is important that the fingers are not held in a hyperextended position, which can cause them to remain pale and, therefore, provide a false-positive result. Release of the ulnar artery should cause a blush of the hand within 15 to 20 seconds. If there is a delay beyond this time, then this raises concern about the ulnar circulation, and a radial forearm flap should not be performed. In dark-skinned individuals in whom capillary blush is not easily assessed, the perfusion of the hand can be confirmed by checking the capillary refill of the nail bed on compression and release of the fingernail. It is imperative that the examiner observe the vascularity to the thumb for the reasons outlined earlier. It is our preference to select the nondominant arm for flap harvest. The Allen test should be repeated to confirm the initial findings. A final check may be performed in the operating room where a pulse oximeter can be attached to the thumb to assess the wave-form changes when the radial artery is compressed. Little et al. (25) reported a 3% incidence of positive Allen test findings in the general population. The reliability of this test for screening individuals with poor ulnar circulation is attested by my experience with 100 patients and Soutar's (39) experience with 200 radial forearm flaps in which no cases of hand ischemia have occurred.

On admission to the hospital for a radial forearm flap, a bandage is placed over the donor forearm to prevent anyone from using that arm for arterial or venipunctures. The patient must also be instructed to warn all hospital personnel against violation of the forearm. Patients who have been hospitalized for prolonged periods may have few patent superficial veins in their arms. A forearm flap may be harvested in these patients based on the venae comitantes, or perhaps more prudently, an alternative donor site should be selected.

The patency of the radial artery is rarely an issue except in those patients who have had a previous indwelling radial artery catheter. Although flow in these vessels is usually restored over time, I have encountered a small number of cases in which this has not occurred. Although the length of the radial artery that remains occluded is uncertain, it is prudent to select another donor site.

POSTOPERATIVE CARE

After applying a split-thickness skin graft, a volar plaster splint is formed that extends from the fingers to the antecubital fossa. An elastic bandage is then placed over the splint, and the forearm is elevated. Immobilization of the forearm is important to prevent shearing of the muscles underneath the skin graft. It is imperative that the vascularity of the hand be confirmed after releasing the tourniquet. The circulation to the thumb must be assessed to ensure once again that the collateral circulation through the ulnar artery provides sufficient vascularity. The dressing and the volar splint are left in place for approximately 7 days following surgery. During this time, the forearm is elevated, and monitoring of the vascularity to the hand is continued to be certain that the bandage does not cause compression of the circulation as a result of postoperative edema. On the 7th day following surgery, the dressing is removed, and the skin graft is observed. A conforming elastic stocking is then used to assist in wound healing and reduce edema in the hand resulting from the interruption of the venous and lymphatic supply.

Flap Harvesting Technique follows on page 162.

Flap Harvesting Technique

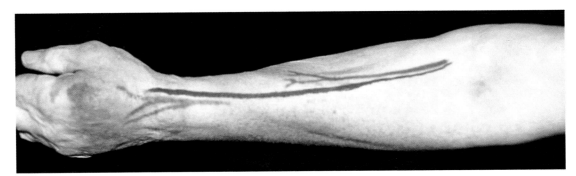

Figure 11-6. The design of the radial forearm flap begins by outlining the path of the dominant subcutaneous veins and the palpable pulse of the radial artery. The path of the cephalic vein and the radial artery have been drawn on the left forearm. In this dissection, the approximate topographical anatomy of the sensory nerves is outlined in orange. The lateral antebrachial cutaneous nerve runs adjacent to the cephalic vein, and the approximate course of the superficial branches of the radial nerve is shown as the branches terminate on the dorsum of the hand.

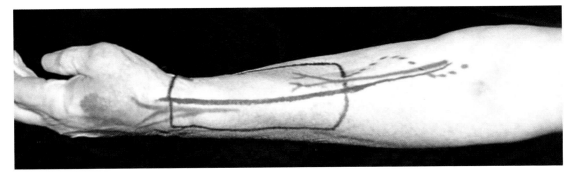

Figure 11-7. A rectangular radial forearm flap has been outlined on the distal forearm. The axis of this flap is centered on the radial artery and the cephalic vein. A *curvilinear dotted line* indicates the incision in the proximal forearm where skin flaps will be elevated to provide access to the proximal portion of the neurovascular pedicle. A larger skin paddle can be harvested that extends proximally to the antecubital fossa and encompasses virtually the entire circumference of the forearm, except for a bridge of skin along the ulnar aspect.

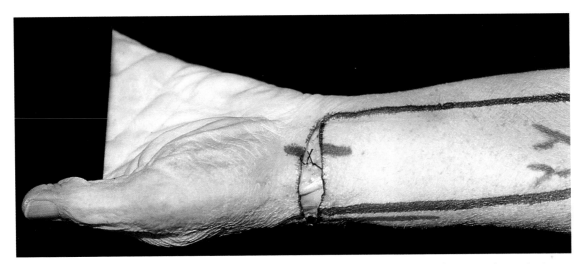

Figure 11-8. The dissection begins distally after exsanguination of the forearm through the use of an elastic bandage and raising the tourniquet to approximately 250 mmHg. The distal skin incision is made to gain exposure of the radial artery and its adjacent venae comitantes.

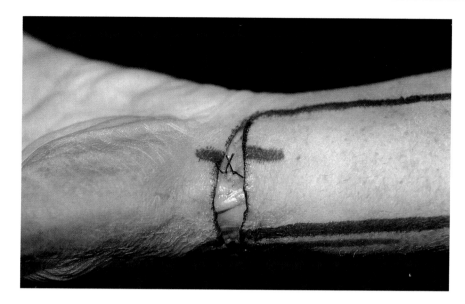

Figure 11-9. The radial artery is then ligated and divided.

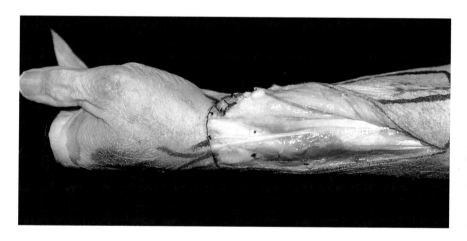

Figure 11-10. Dissection may begin either from the ulnar or from the radial direction. In this particular dissection, the skin flap has been elevated, starting from the radial aspect. The distal portion of the cephalic vein must be ligated and transsected.

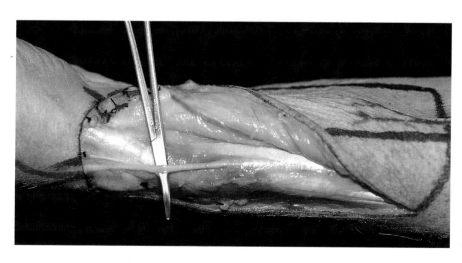

Figure 11-11. The skin flap has been elevated with the deep fascia to the level of the lateral intermuscular septum marked by the border of the brachioradialis. The superficial branches of the radial nerve are isolated and preserved to maintain sensation to the dorsum of the hand. The dissection of the radial nerve requires that the subfascial plane of dissection be broken.

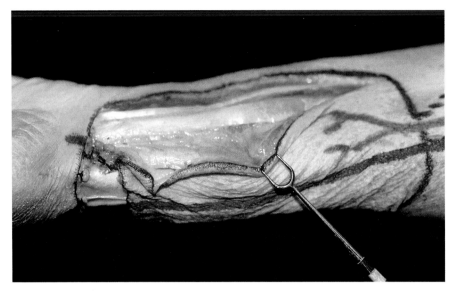

Figure 11-12. The ulnar dissection of the flap is carried out in a subfascial plane, elevating the flap off the tendons of the muscles in the flexor compartment. It is imperative to maintain the integrity of the paratenon when performing this dissection. The forearm flap has been elevated in an ulnar direction to the border of the flexor carpi radialis, which marks the position of the intermuscular septum.

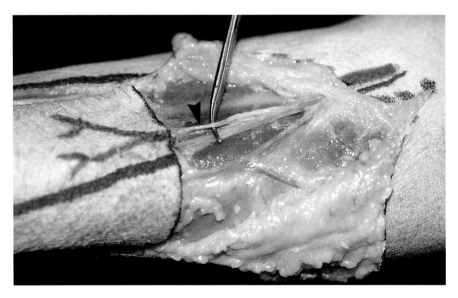

Figure 11-13. Skin flaps are elevated in the dissection proximal to the skin paddle by making an incision along the dotted line. The skin flaps are elevated in a subcutaneous plane to preserve the integrity of the subcutaneous veins and the adjacent sensory nerves. In this dissection, there are two subcutaneous veins, and the lateral antebrachial cutaneous nerve *(arrow)* is demonstrated lying adjacent to the cephalic vein.

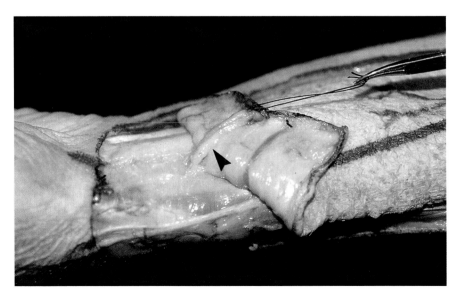

Figure 11-14. At this point in the procedure, the radial artery *(arrow)* is dissected distally to proximally by transsecting and cauterizing the deeper branches that supply the muscles of the forearm and the radius.

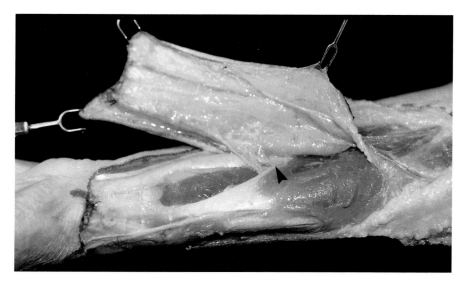

Figure 11-15. Dissection along the intermuscular septum is continued proximally until the point of overlap *(arrow)* of the brachioradialis and the flexor carpi radialis.

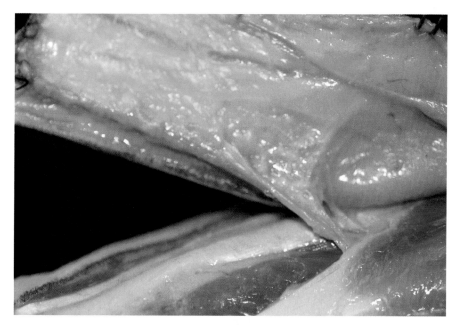

Figure 11-16. In the proximal forearm, the radial artery courses deep to the brachioradialis. Therefore, it is apparent that the primary arterial inflow to the skin component of the forearm flap arises through its fasciocutaneous perforators, which are given off in the distal third of the forearm.

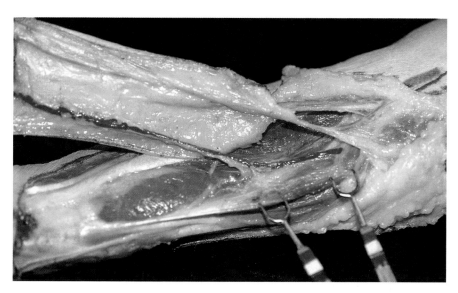

Figure 11-17. Exposure of the proximal radial artery and the venae comitantes is achieved by separating the brachioradialis from the flexor carpi radialis. The radial artery may be traced all the way to the brachial artery, but this is rarely necessary. The forearm flap is then reperfused by releasing the tourniquet. The vascularity is ensured through observation of the color and dermal bleeding. At this point, hemostasis is obtained, and the flap is prepared for harvest when the recipient site is ready.

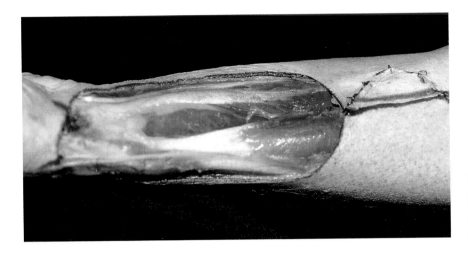

Figure 11-18. The donor site is closed by reapproximating the proximal skin flaps as shown. The remainder of the defect is closed with a split-thickness skin graft.

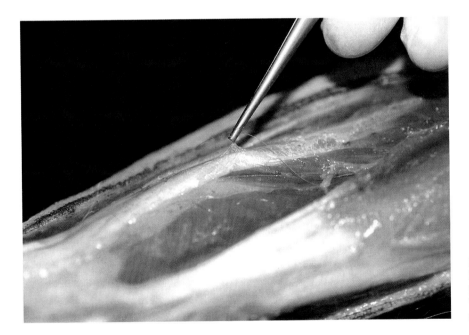

Figure 11-19. As noted previously, it is imperative to maintain the thin paratenon layer over the tendons in the distal forearm to facilitate skin grafting of this donor site.

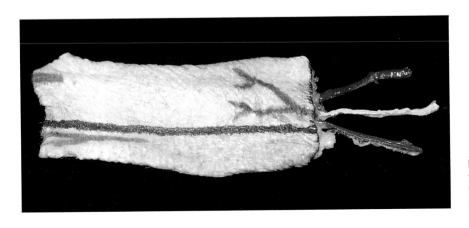

Figure 11-20. The radial forearm flap is shown with the radial artery, the cephalic vein, and the lateral antebrachial cutaneous nerve.

REFERENCES

1. Baird W, Wornom I, Culbertson J: Forehead reconstruction with a modified radial forearm flap: a case report. *J Reconstr Microsurg* 1988;4:363.
2. Bardsley A, Soutar D, Elliot D, Batchelor A: Reducing morbidity in the radial forearm flap donor site. *Plast Reconstr Surg* 1990;86:287.
3. Bhathena H, Kavarana N: Bipaddled retrograde radial extended forearm flap with microarterial anastomoses for reconstruction in oral cancer. *Br J Plast Surg* 1988;41:354.
4. Boorman J, Brown J, Sykes P: Morbidity in the forearm flap donor arm. *Br J Plast Surg* 1982;40:207.
5. Boorman JG, Green MF: A split Chinese forearm flap for simultaneous oral lining and skin cover. *Br J Plast Surg* 1986;39:179.
6. Chantrain G, Deraemaecker R, Andry G, Dor P: Wide vertical hemipharyngolaryngectomy with immediate glottic and pharyngeal reconstruction using a radial forearm free flap: preliminary results. *Laryngoscope* 1991;101:869.
7. Chicarelli Z, Ariyan S, Cuono C: Free radial forearm flap versatility for the head and neck and lower extremity. *J Reconstr Microsurg* 1986;2:221.
8. Chicarelli Z, Ariyan S, Cuono C: Single-stage repair of complex scalp and cranial defects with the free radial forearm flap. *Plast Reconstr Surg* 1986;77:577.
9. Coleman T, Anson B: Arterial patterns in the hand based upon a study of 650 specimens. *Surg Gynecol Obstet* 1961;113:409.
10. Cormack G, Duncan MJ, Lamberty B: The blood supply of the bone component of the compound osteocutaneous radial artery forearm flap—an anatomical study. *Br J Plast Surg* 1986;39:173.
11. Elliot D, Bardsley F, Batchelor A, Soutar D. Direct closure of the radial forearm flap donor site. *Br J Plast Surg* 1988;41:358.
12. Fatah M, Nancarrow J, Murray D: Raising the radial artery forearm flap: the superficial ulnar artery "trap." *Br J Plast Surg* 1985;38:394.
13. Fenton O, Roberts J: Improving the donor site of the radial forearm flap. *Br J Plast Surg* 1985;38:504.
14. Hagen R: Laryngoplasty with a radialis pedicle flap from the forearm: a surgical procedure for voice rehabilitation after total laryngectomy. *Am J Otolaryngol* 1990;11:85.
15. Hallock G: Refinement of the radial forearm flap donor site using skin expansion. *Plast Reconstr Surg* 1988;81:21.
16. Hallock G: Complication of the free flap donor site from a community hospital perspective. *J Reconstr Microsurg* 1991;7:331.
17. Harii K, Ebihara S, Ono I, Saito H, Terui S, Takato T: Pharyngoesophageal reconstruction using a fabricated forearm free flap. *Plast Reconstr Surg* 1985;75:463–476.
18. Hatoko M, Harashina T, Inoue T, Tanaka I, Imai K: Reconstruction of palate with radial forearm flap; a report of 3 cases. *Br J Plast Surg* 1990;43:350.
19. Heden P, Gylbert L: Anomaly of the radial artery encountered during elevation of the radial forearm flap. *J Microsurg* 1990;6:139.
20. Ismail TI: The free fascial forearm flap. *Microsurgery* 1989;10:155–160.
21. Jin Y, Guan W, Shi T, Quiwan Y, Xe L, Chang T: Reversed island forearm fascial flap in hand surgery. *Ann Plast Surg* 1985;15:340.
22. Jones B, O'Brien C: Acute ischemia of the hand resulting from elevation of a radial forearm flap. *Br J Plast Surg* 1985;38:396.
23. Kawashina T, Harii K, Ono I, Ebihara S, Joshizumi T: Intraoral and oropharyngeal reconstruction using a deepithelialized forearm flap. *Head Neck* 1989;11:358.
24. Lamberty B, Cormack G: The forearm angiosomes. *Br J Plast Surg* 1982;35:420.
25. Little J, Zylstra P, West J, May J: Circulatory patterns in the normal hand. *Br J Plast Surg* 1973;60:652.
26. Loetzke HH, Kleinau W: Gleichzeitiges Vorkommen der Aa. brachialis superficialis, radialis und antebrachialis dorsalis superficialis sowie deren Aufzweigungen. *Anat Anz* 1968;122:137–141.
27. Martin IC, Brown AE: Free vascularized fascial flap in oral cavity reconstruction. *Head Neck* 1994;16:45.
28. Masser M: The pre-expanded radial free flap. *Plast Reconstr Surg* 1990;86:295.
29. Matthews RN, Fatah F, DM Davies, Eyre J, Hodge RA, Walsh-Waring GP: Experience with the radial forearm flap in 14 cases. *Scand J Plast Reconstr Surg* 1984;18:303.
30. McCormack L, Cauldwell E, Anson B: Brachial and antebrachial arterial patterns, a study of 750 extremities. *Surg Gynecol Obstet* 1953;96:43.
31. Moscoso J, Keller J, Genden E, Weinberg H, Biller HF, Buchbinder D, Urken ML: Vascularized bone flaps in oromandibular reconstruction. A comparative study of bone stock from various donor sites to assess suitability for enosseous dental implants. *Arch Otolaryngol Head Neck Surg* 1994;120:36.
32. Nakayama Y, Soeda S, Iino T: A radial forearm flap based on an extended dissection of the cephalic vein. The longest venous pedicle? Case report. *Br J Plast Surg* 1986;39:454.
33. Otsuka T, Terauchi M: An anomaly of the radial artery-relevance for the forearm flap. *Br J Plast Surg* 1991;44:390.
34. Reid CD, Moss ALH: One stage repair with vascularized tendon grafts in a dorsal hand injury using the "Chinese" forearm flap. *Br J Plast Surg* 1983;36:473.
35. Sadove R, Luce E, McGrath P: Reconstruction of the lower lip and chin with the composite radial forearm-palmaris longus free flap. *Plast Reconstr Surg* 1991;88:209.
36. Sanger J, Ye Z, Yousif N, Matloub H: The brachioradialis forearm flap: anatomy and clinical application. Presented at the 8th Annual Meeting of the American Society for Reconstructive Microsurgery, Scottsdale, Arizona, November 8, 1992.
37. Small J, Miller R: The radial artery forearm flap: an anomaly of the radial artery. *Br J Plast Surg* 1985;38:501.

38. Song R, Gao Y, Song Y, Yu Y, Song Y: The forearm flap. *Clin Plast Surg* 1982;9:21–26.
39. Soutar D: Radial forearm flaps. In: Baker S, ed. *Microsurgical Reconstruction of the Head and Neck*. New York: Churchill Livingstone; 1989.
40. Soutar DS, McGregor IA: The radial forearm flap in intraoral reconstruction: the experience of 60 consecutive cases. *Plast Reconstr Surg* 1986;78:1.
41. Soutar DS, Scheker LR, Tanner NSB, McGregor IA: The radial forearm flap: a versatile method for intraoral reconstruction. *Br J Plast Surg* 1983;36:1.
42. Soutar DS, Widdowson WP: Immediate reconstruction of the mandible using a vascularized segment of radius. *Head Neck* 1986;8:232.
43. Swanson E, Boyd J, Mulholland R: The radial forearm flap: a biomechanical study of the osteotomized ramus. *Plast Reconstr Surg* 1990;85:267.
44. Tahara S, Susuki T: Eye socket reconstruction with free radial forearm flap. *Ann Plast Surg* 1989;23:112.
45. Takada K, Sugata T, Yoshiga K, Miyamoto Y: Total upper lip reconstruction using a free radial forearm flap incorporating the brachioradialis muscle: report of a case. *J Oral Maxillofac Surg* 1987;45:959.
46. Taylor GI, Ham FJ: The free vascularized nerve graft. A further experimental and clinical application of microvascular techniques. *Plast Reconstr Surg* 1976;57:413.
47. Thoma A, Archibald S, Jackson S, Young J: Surgical patterns of venous drainage of the free forearm flap in head and neck reconstruction. *Plast Reconstr Surg* 1994;93:54.
48. Timmons M: The vascular basis of the radial forearm flap. *Plast Reconstr Surg* 1986;77:80.
49. Urken ML: Composite free flaps in oromandibular reconstruction; review of the literature. *Arch Otolaryngol Head Neck Surg* 1991;117:724.
50. Urken ML, Biller HF: A new bilobed design for the sensate radial forearm flap to preserve tongue mobility following significant glossectomy. *Arch Otolaryngol Head Neck Surg* 1994;120:26–31.
51. Urken ML, Futran N, Moscoso J, Biller HF: A modified design of the buried radial forearm free flap to exteriorize a monitoring segment. *Arch Otolaryngol Head Neck Surg* 1994;[in press].
52. Urken ML, Weinberg H, Vickery C, Biller HF: The neurofasciocutaneous radial forearm flap in head and neck reconstruction: a preliminary report. *Laryngoscope* 1990;100:161.
53. Vaughan ED: The radial forearm free flap in orofacial reconstruction. *J Craniomaxillofac Surg* 1990;18:2.
54. Wakrhouse N, Moss A, Townsend PL: Lower limb salvage using an extended free radial forearm flap. *Br J Plast Surg* 1984;37:394.
55. Yang G, Chen B, Gao Y, et al.: Forearm free skin flap transplantation. *Natl Med J China* 1981;61:139.
56. Yousif NJ, Ye Z: Analysis of cutaneous perfusion: an aid to lower extremity reconstruction. *Clin Plast Surg* 1991;18:559.

FREE FLAPS
Fascial and Fasciocutaneous Flaps

Lateral Arm

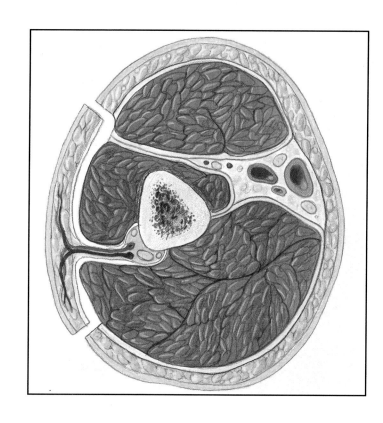

Michael J. Sullivan, M.D., and
Mark L. Urken, M.D.

With the expansion of new donor sites for cutaneous and fasciocutaneous free flaps that has occurred during the past two decades, the upper arm seemed to be a logical choice for expendable quality skin. A variety of different flaps have been described. The medial arm flap, however, was found to have an unreliable vascularity. The variability in the size of the nutrient septocutaneous perforators arising from the superior ulnar collateral artery along the medial intermuscular septum (3) was the principal concern. The deltoid flap was introduced by Franklin (4) and is based on the arteria deltoidea subcutanea, a constant branch of the posterior circumflex humeral artery. However, a deep dissection with limited exposure is necessary to obtain an adequate pedicle length. The vascular pedicle also rests dangerously close to the axillary nerve. In 1982, Song et al. (17) introduced the lateral arm fasciocutaneous flap, which has become a workhorse free flap in head and neck and extremity reconstruction. The lateral arm flap may be transferred with a segment of the humerus, triceps tendon, and two nerves, one of which serves as a sensory supply and the other, as a vascularized nerve graft. It has similarities to the radial forearm flap but offers the distinct advantages that its nutrient artery, the profunda brachii, is not essential to the vascularity of the distal upper extremity, and the donor defect can be closed with a linear scar.

FLAP DESIGN AND UTILIZATION

The territory of the lateral arm flap has been investigated through dye-injection studies. The maximum dimensions of the cutaneous paddle have not been determined; however, flaps as large as 18 × 11 cm have been reported (14). Rivet et al. (14) described a "zone of security" that extended 12 cm proximal to the lateral epicondyle and included one third of the circumference of the arm. They advised that flaps should incorporate this zone to ensure vascularity and a successful reconstruction. Katsaros et al. (7) reported areas of staining that ranged from 8 × 10 cm to 15 × 14 cm. In a review of 150 lateral arm flaps, Katsaros et al. (8) reported the successful transfer of skin flaps that extended both 10 cm proximal to the deltoid insertion and 10 cm distal to the lateral epicondyle. These authors also speculated that the profunda brachii pedicle could support a complete tube of skin from the shoulder to the mid-forearm. In most cases, the width of the harvested skin is limited to 6 to 8 cm, or one third of the arm's circumference, to allow primary closure. However, larger flaps have been harvested, with a skin graft placed over the donor site. The axis on which the flap is usually designed is a line drawn from the insertion of the deltoid to the lateral epicondyle. Alternatively, a line connecting the tip of the acromion and the lateral epicondyle has been advocated (Figure 12-1) (20).

The blood supply to the skin of the lateral arm flap is derived from a series of four to five septocutaneous perforators that arise from the posterior branch of the radial collateral artery in the lateral intermuscular septum. Katsaros et al. (7) described a technique to achieve a wider flap by harvesting a long flap and dividing it transversely, as long as adequate perforators are present to perfuse both the proximal and distal portions. The additional width was achieved by folding the distal segment so that it lay adjacent to the proximal one thereby doubling the width while still achieving primary closure.

Kuek and Chuan (9) investigated the distal limits of the skin paddle through eosin injections and found that the area of staining extended an average of 7.9 cm (4.5 to 10.0 cm) distal to the lateral epicondyle. The additional length of the flap not only

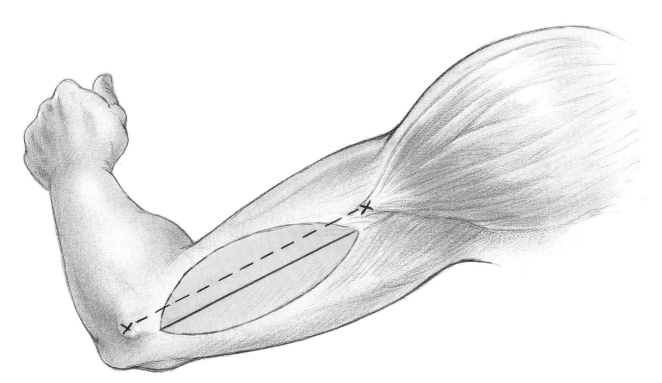

Figure 12-1. The topographical anatomy of the lateral arm flap is illustrated. Although a line drawn between the deltoid insertion and the lateral epicondyle is classically used to make the axis of the flap, the lateral intermuscular septum is actually located 1 to 2 cm posteriorly. The central axis of the flap should be adjusted for this as shown.

allows the flap to be used for wider defects by folding it on itself, but it also permits a distal skin paddle to be harvested that effectively lengthens the vascular pedicle. In addition, the skin of the distal portion of the upper arm tends to be thinner than the skin in the more proximal portion of this region.

The lateral arm flap may be harvested as a fascial flap or as a fasciocutaneous flap. The use of a vascularized fascial flap allows a much larger surface area of tissue to be harvested without having an impact on the primary closure of the donor site. A split-thickness skin graft may be applied to the flap to achieve epithelial coverage. This is also an effective means to harvest thin tissue from this donor site in patients who have a thicker adipose layer in this region. Large segments of well-vascularized fascia measuring 12 × 9 cm have been harvested while still achieving primary donor site closure. Small islands of skin may be included to facilitate postoperative monitoring (21). The fascial subcutaneous free flap has been used to augment contour defects of the maxillofacial region (18). This donor site usually provides a layer of adipose tissue that is intermediate in thickness between that of the radial forearm flap and the scapular flap. Yousif et al. (21) reported detailed descriptions of the fascial envelope that surrounds the triceps, brachialis, and brachioradialis. Portions of this layer fuse to form the intermuscular septum. The superficial layer of this envelope is continuous with the fascial sheath that covers the entire arm. The two layers are separated by adipose tissue. The fascia anterior to the intermuscular septum averages 0.41 mm in thickness compared with the 0.21-mm average thickness of fascia posterior to the septum.

Shenaq (16) reported an alternative solution to the limited dimensions of the lateral free flap by using pretransfer tissue expansion. He was able to harvest an 11 × 18-cm flap from a child's arm and still achieve primary closure. The ability to tailor donor-site properties through staged pretransfer expansion is a technique with significant potential that has not been extensively explored.

An osteocutaneous flap may be harvested by including a segment of humerus measuring 1 × 10 cm. Septal perforators extend to the periosteum in a manner similar to the blood supply to the radius in an osteocutaneous radial forearm flap. A muscular cuff of triceps and brachioradialis is left attached to the lateral intermuscular septum to protect the blood supply (8,10). This segment of bone has been used in mandibular reconstruction, but its limited bone stock imposes restrictions on the capacity to insert endosteal implants for dental rehabilitation. Although limited in dimensions because of concern about pathologic fracture of the residual humerus, this segment of bone may be useful in midface reconstruction.

The posterior cutaneous nerve of the arm (PCNA) and the posterior cutaneous nerve of the forearm (PCNF) provide the potential for reneurotized lateral arm flaps. Sensation can be restored to the transferred skin by anastomosing the PCNA to a suitable recipient nerve in the head and neck (19). Matloub et al. (11) reported on six patients who underwent sensate lateral arm flap restoration of the oral cavity. Two patients who underwent reconstruction of partial glossectomy defects were reportedly able to differentiate light and deep touch and hot and cold stimuli. The PCNF has been described by Rivet et al. (14) as a "nerve in transit". This nerve travels in the intermuscular septum to supply sensation to the skin of the lateral forearm. It receives its blood supply from the branches of the posterior radial collateral artery (PRCA) and, therefore, may be used as a vascularized nerve graft. Katsaros et al. (8) reported using this nerve to bridge facial nerve gaps in four cases.

Katsaros et al. (7) reported harvesting a segment of vascularized triceps tendon for use in extremity reconstruction. The use of this tissue in head and neck reconstruction is limited.

NEUROVASCULAR ANATOMY

The profunda brachii artery is the largest branch of the brachial artery in the arm. It runs a course on the posterior aspect of the arm that parallels the radial nerve as it

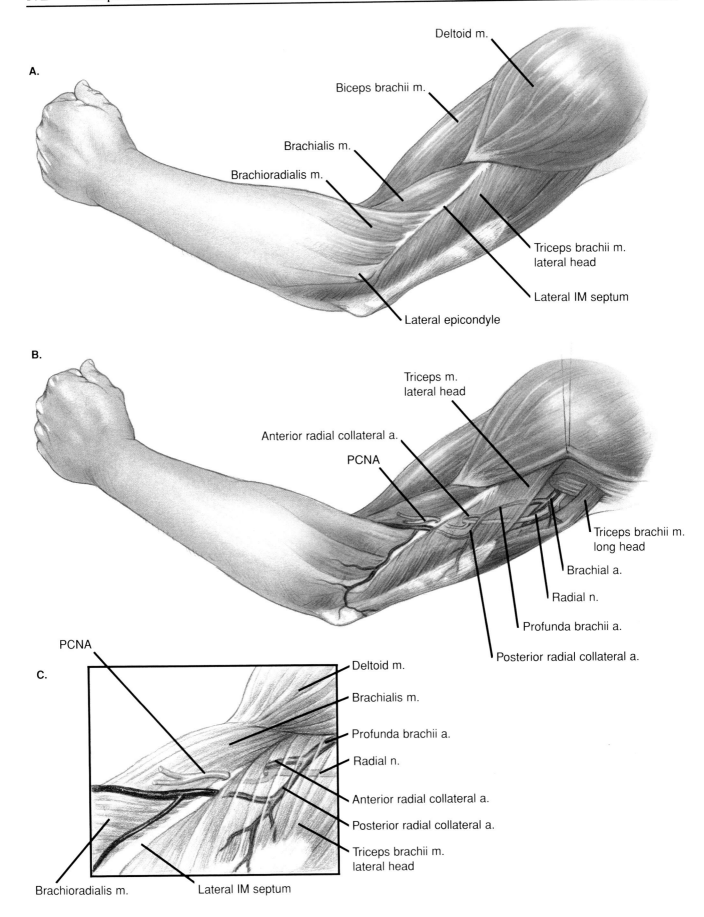

A.

Deltoid m.

Biceps brachii m.

Brachialis m.

Brachioradialis m.

Triceps brachii m.
lateral head

Lateral IM septum

Lateral epicondyle

B.

Triceps m.
lateral head

Anterior radial collateral a.

PCNA

Triceps brachii m.
long head

Brachial a.

Radial n.

Profunda brachii a.

Posterior radial collateral a.

PCNA

C.

Deltoid m.

Brachialis m.

Profunda brachii a.

Radial n.

Anterior radial collateral a.

Posterior radial collateral a.

Triceps brachii m.
lateral head

Brachioradialis m.

Lateral IM septum

spirals around the humerus medially to laterally. The profunda brachii divides into two terminal branches (Figure 12-2). The nomenclature of these branches is somewhat confusing. The PRCA, which is the main nutrient artery of the lateral arm flap, has also been referred to as the middle collateral artery. This vessel passes through the lateral intermuscular septum and anastomoses with the interosseous recurrent artery. This "flow-through" system of the PRCA to interosseous recurrent artery is the physiologic basis for the reverse-flow lateral upper arm flap that has been used for coverage of the elbow region. In this flap, the PRCA is ligated proximally, and flow to the lateral arm flap is achieved through the anastomotic channels of the interosseous recurrent artery (2). The anterior radial collateral artery, which has also been referred to as the radial collateral artery, runs a divergent course along with the radial nerve between the origins of the brachialis and brachioradialis muscles. The anterior radial collateral artery anastomoses with the radial recurrent artery. In the classic description, the profunda brachii also supplies the main nutrient artery of the humerus, the deltoid, and the three heads of the triceps muscles (Figure 12-3).

The average diameter of the profunda brachii was found to be 2.45 mm (range, 1.75 to 2.7 mm) at a distance of 1 cm below its origin from the brachial artery (14). In the region of the deltoid insertion, where it enters the lateral intermuscular septum, the artery has an average diameter of 1.55 mm (range, 1.25 to 1.75 mm) (14). Moffett et al. (12) described a technique to lengthen the vascular pedicle by 6 to 8 cm by extending the dissection proximally between the lateral and long heads of the triceps muscle. In this technique, the standard dissection is performed until the fibers of the lateral head of the triceps limit further dissection along the spiral groove. A tunnel is created underneath the triceps insertion by working both from below and above through the exposure gained by splitting the lateral and long heads of the triceps. The takeoff of the profunda brachii from the brachial artery can usually be exposed by this approach. The authors caution that the muscular branches from the radial nerve to the triceps muscle must be identified and preserved. They tested triceps strength following the extended approach in four patients at 3- and 6-month intervals (12). There was a slight deficit in both extension and flexion relative to the nonoperated arm. This slight discrepancy could be attributed to postoperative disuse of the operated arm and to the fact that the flaps were harvested from the nondominant arm.

The lateral arm flap has both a superficial and deep venous system. The superficial system drains through the cephalic vein; the deep system drains through the paired venae comitantes, which are about 2.5 mm in diameter (8). Inoue and Fujino (6) reportedly transferred a lateral arm flap based on an extended dissection of the cephalic vein, without its interruption, while performing a conventional microarterial anastomosis to a recipient artery in the neck. This flap was used to resurface a defect

Figure 12-2. A: Anatomy of lateral arm musculature. The lateral intermuscular septum is located between the triceps posteriorly and the brachialis and the brachioradialis anteriorly. The actual position of the lateral intermuscular (IM) septum can be seen to lie 1–2 cm behind the deltoid insertion. **B:** The profunda brachii artery arises from the brachial artery and winds its way in the spinal groove along with the radial nerve. Splitting of the long and the lateral heads of the triceps provides extended exposure of the neurovascular pedicle. As the pedicle proceeds in the septum, the profunda brachii divides into the anterior and posterior radial collateral arteries. The anterior radial collateral artery runs an anterior course with the radial nerve between the insertions of the brachioradialis and the brachialis. **C:** A close-up view of the neurovascular anatomy of the lateral intermuscular septum. The radial nerve and the anterior branch of the radial collateral artery are seen diverging anteriorly between the brachialis and brachioradialis. The posterior branch of the radial collateral artery supplies the lateral arm flap; the posterior cutaneous nerve of the arm (PCNA) provides sensation to the flap.

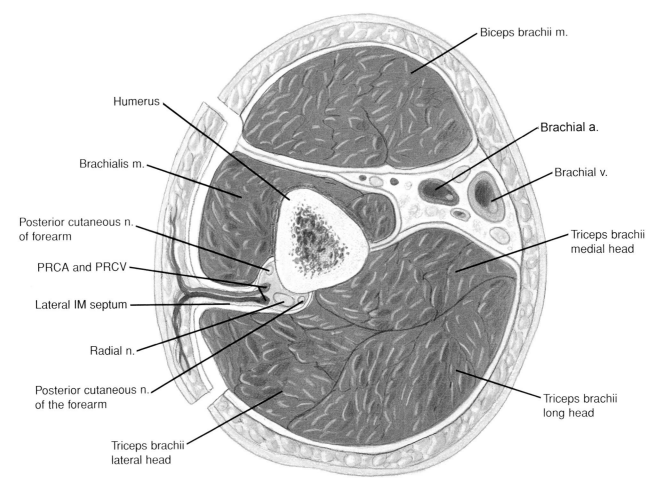

Biceps brachii m.

Humerus

Brachialis m.

Posterior cutaneous n. of forearm

PRCA and PRCV

Lateral IM septum

Radial n.

Posterior cutaneous n. of the forearm

Triceps brachii lateral head

Brachial a.

Brachial v.

Triceps brachii medial head

Triceps brachii long head

Figure 12-3. Cross-sectional anatomy of the upper arm reveals the lateral intermuscular (IM) septum with the neurovascular pedicle running in close proximity to the humerus. PRCA, posterior radial collateral artery; PRCV, posterior radial collateral vein.

in the temporal region. Nakayama et al. (13) described a similar technique for a radial forearm flap in which the cephalic vein was dissected to the level of the clavicle, with a separate arterial anastomosis performed for the radial artery.

There are two sensory nerves that course through the lateral intermuscular septum. The nomenclature of these sensory nerves in the literature is also confusing. The nerve that supplies sensation to the skin of the lateral arm flap is the PCNA, a branch of the radial nerve. The PCNA ramifies into four to five fascicles within the subcutaneous tissue (7). This nerve has also been referred to as the inferior lateral brachial cutaneous nerve, the upper branch of the posterior antebrachial cutaneous nerve (5), or the lower lateral cutaneous nerve of the arm (15). The PCNF, which runs through the septum *en route* to the forearm, does not supply sensation to the lateral arm flap. As noted previously, this nerve can be used as a vascularized nerve graft. It too has been referred to by a variety of names, including the posterior antebrachial cutaneous nerve (5). Reportedly, the PCNF can be preserved to avoid the sensory loss, but it requires meticulous dissection in the septum to do so (Figure 12-4).

Brandt and Khouri (1) described a lateral arm–proximal forearm flap that extended up to 12 cm distal to the lateral condyle. The vascular supply to the forearm component was based on the rich vascular plexus that was located over the posterior

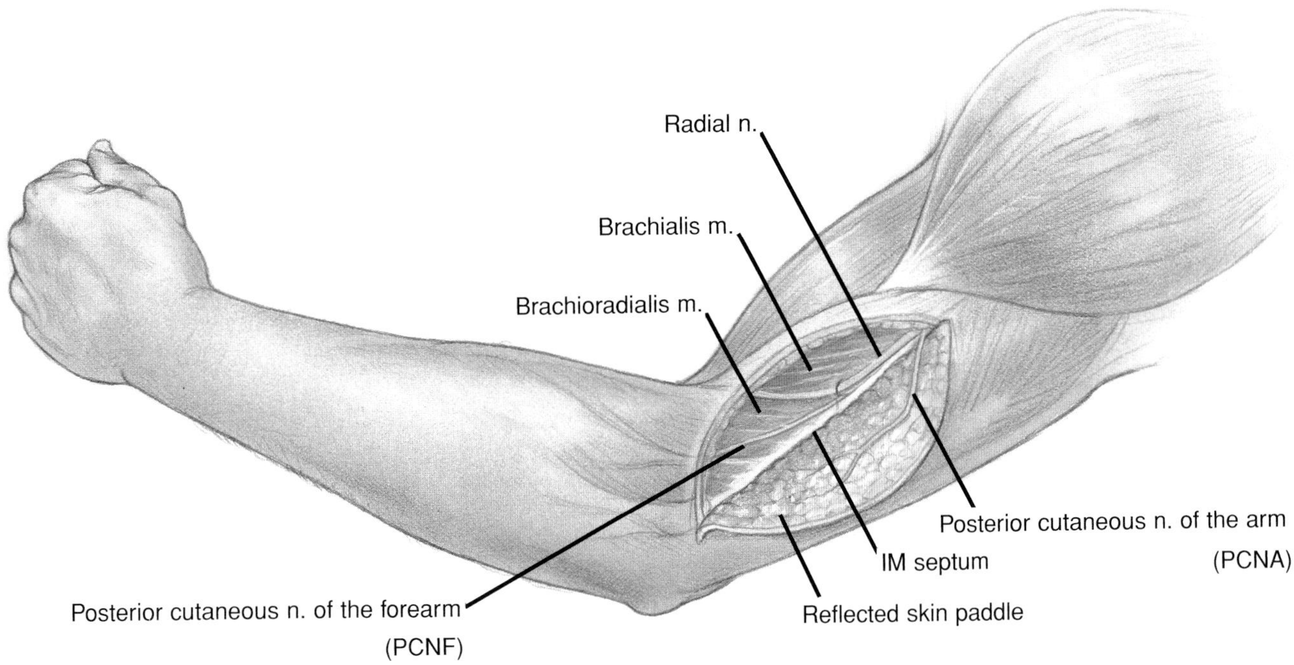

Figure 12-4. The lateral arm flap has been elevated from an anterior approach to show the PCNA ramifying in the subcutaneous tissue of the flap. This nerve can be traced proximally to provide additional length for anastomosis to a suitable recipient nerve in the head and neck. The PCNF, also a branch of the radial nerve, provides no sensation to the lateral arm flap but may be used as a vascularized nerve graft. It is imperative to differentiate these two nerves to reinnervate the lateral arm flap successfully. Interruption of the PCNF leads to an area of anesthesia distal to the lateral epicondyle.

elbow and that was fed by the PRCA. The primary sensory nerve supply in this extended flap was the PCNF.

ANATOMIC VARIATIONS

Unlike the radial forearm flap, there is no concern in harvesting the lateral arm flap for the integrity of the collateral circulation to the distal portion of the limb. The profunda brachii may be interrupted without ischemic sequelae. Most of the anatomic variations that have been reported are related to duplication of the vascular pedicle within the septum. The incidence of double profunda brachii arteries has been reported to be 4% (7), 8% (12), and 12% (14) in different studies. Moffett et al. (12) recommended temporary occlusion of each of the arteries to determine whether one or both should be revascularized. Scheker et al. (15) reported a single case of duplication of the PRCA, which required two arterial anastomoses to achieve total revascularization of the flap.

POTENTIAL PITFALLS

Postoperative radial nerve palsies have been reported and were attributed to compressive dressings or tight wound closure (8). Split-thickness skin grafts can be applied when wound closure is difficult. A light compressive dressing should be applied to avoid iatrogenic injuries.

Flap Harvesting Technique

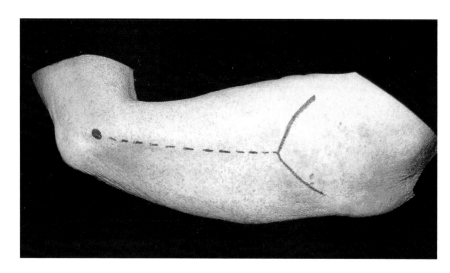

Figure 12-5. The topographical anatomy of the lateral arm flap is outlined. The key landmarks are the V-shaped point of insertion of the deltoid into the humerus and the lateral epicondyle. The *dashed line* represents the intersection of these two points.

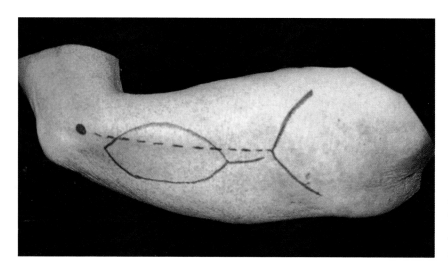

Figure 12-6. The lateral intermuscular septum is located approximately 1 cm posterior to the line drawn from the insertion of the deltoid and the lateral epicondyle. The central axis of the flap design is based on the intermuscular septum. The territory of skin may extend distal to the epicondyle and proximal to the deltoid.

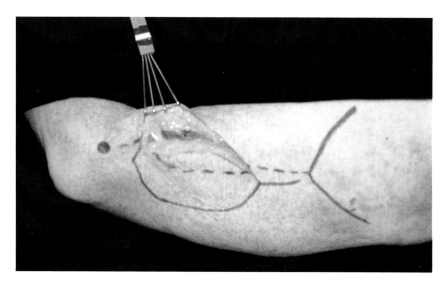

Figure 12-7. Harvest of the lateral arm flap may be performed either with or without tourniquet control. The dissection begins with an anterior incision through the skin and subcutaneous tissue down to the brachioradialis and brachialis.

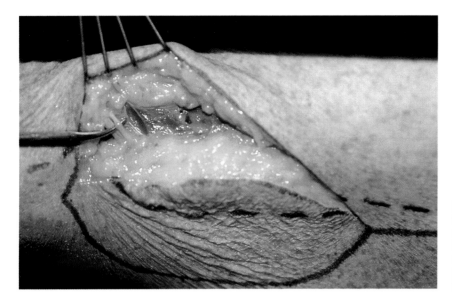

Figure 12-8. The PCNF is identified in the soft tissue of the flap as it courses distally to supply sensation distal to the flap. This nerve may be preserved by meticulous dissection but usually is cut, leaving an area of anesthesia in the forearm.

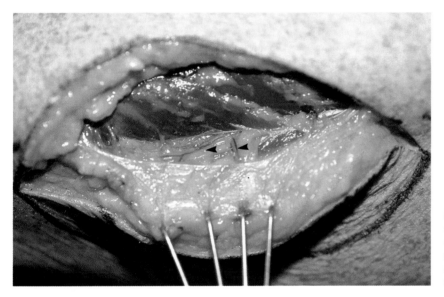

Figure 12-9. Dissection proceeds in a subfascial plane toward the intramuscular septum; at this point, a number of septocutaneous perforators *(arrows)* are identified coursing up into the subcutaneous tissue.

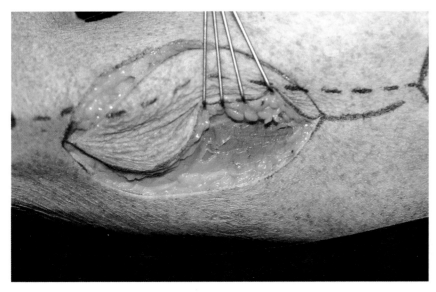

Figure 12-10. Then, attention is turned to the posterior incision, which is carried through the skin and subcutaneous tissue and the deep fascia overlying the triceps muscle.

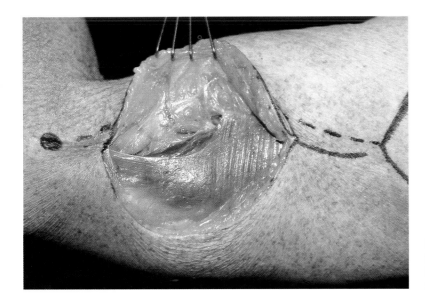

Figure 12-11. The posterior approach to the intermuscular septum is easier because, unlike the brachioradialis, the triceps muscle does not originate from the septum itself.

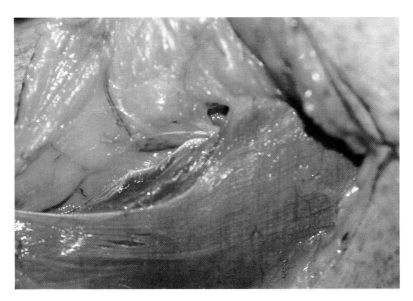

Figure 12-12. As the septum is approached, the septocutaneous perforators are easily identified. These perforators lead to the PRCA.

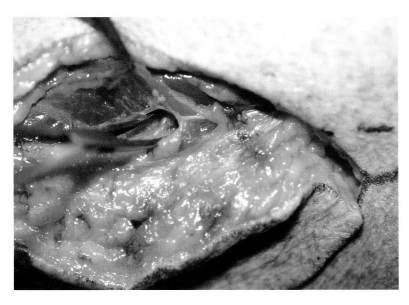

Figure 12-13. Having identified the main vascular pedicle from the posterior approach, attention is then returned to finding the PRCA and posterior radial collateral vein (PRCV) from the anterior approach. This is done by blunt dissection along the fibers of the brachioradialis, which must be separated from the septum.

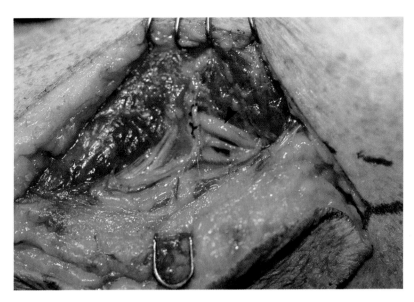

Figure 12-14. Continued dissection along the anterior aspect of the intermuscular septum leads to the radial nerve *(arrow)*, which is easily identified because of its large caliber and its course between the origins of the brachialis and brachioradialis. The anterior branch of the radial collateral artery travels with the radial nerve.

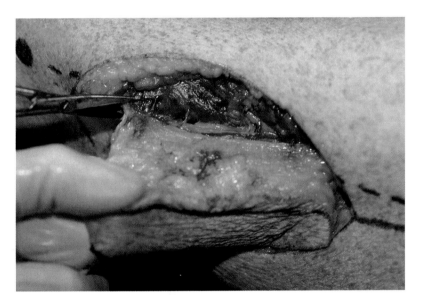

Figure 12-15. Flap elevation proceeds distally to proximally by sharply transsecting the fascial and vascular connections to the humerus.

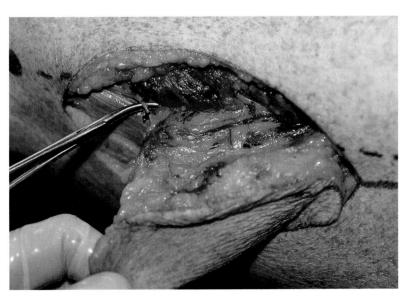

Figure 12-16. The continuation of the PRCA, which anastomoses with the interosseous recurrent artery, must be identified in the soft tissue and ligated.

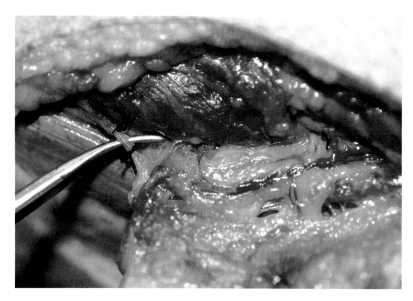

Figure 12-17. After ligation of the distal portion of PRCA, the dissection proceeds along the depth of the intermuscular septum. The PCNA and PCNF are closely associated with the PRC vascular pedicle.

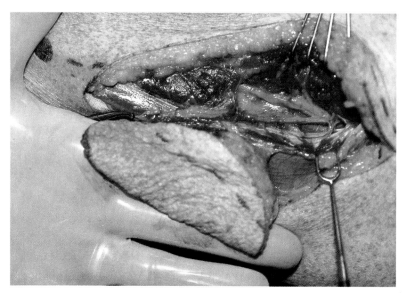

Figure 12-18. The neurovascular pedicle is followed with the radial nerve toward the spinal groove. Extreme care is taken not to injure the radial nerve.

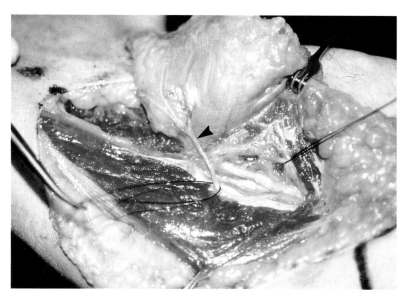

Figure 12-19. Posterior dissection of the flap reveals the PCNA *(arrow)*, which can be seen to ramify in the subcutaneous tissue of the flap.

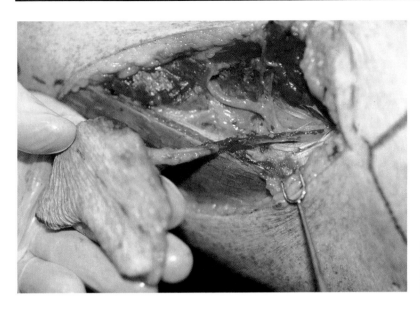

Figure 12-20. The neurovascular pedicle is skeletonized as it passes in the spiral groove. Blunt dissection and retraction may improve visualization of its course.

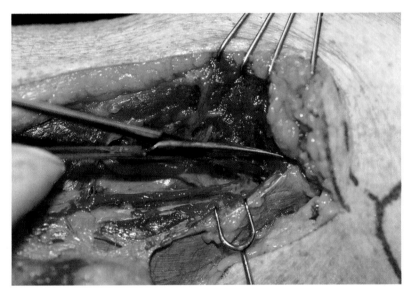

Figure 12-21. A few centimeters of attachment of the deltoid to the humerus may also be divided to improve visualization in the spiral groove. The vascular pedicle is ligated at a comfortable point in the spiral groove. More proximal dissection of the pedicle may be achieved by creating a tunnel deep to the lateral head of the triceps and then separating the long head from the lateral head.

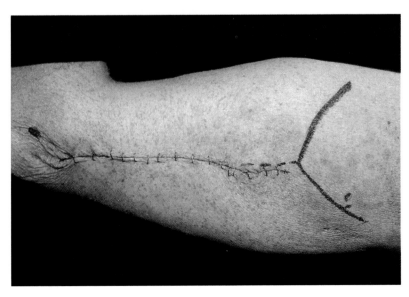

Figure 12-22. Closure is accomplished by suturing the fascia of the brachialis to the triceps. A layered soft tissue closure is accomplished routinely. A light pressure dressing is applied for several days following the procedure.

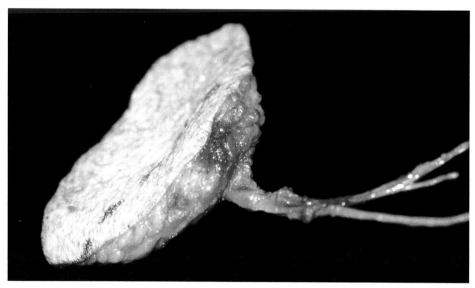

Figure 12-23. The lateral arm flap has been harvested. The neurovascular pedicle can be lengthened by more proximal dissection and by designing the flap more distally in the arm and proximal forearm.

REFERENCES

1. Brandt K, Khouri R: The lateral arm/proximal forearm flap. *Plast Reconstr Surg* 1993;92:1137.
2. Culbertson J, Mutumer K: The reverse lateral upper arm flap for elbow coverage. *Ann Plast Surg* 1987;18:62–68.
3. Daniel R, Terzis J, Schwarz G: Neurovascular free flaps: a preliminary report. *Plast Reconstr Surg* 1975;56:13–20.
4. Franklin J: The deltoid flap: anatomy and clinical applications. In: Buncke HJ, Furnas H, eds. *Symposium on Frontiers in Reconstructive Microsurgery, vol. 24.* St. Louis: Mosby Year Book; 1984.
5. Hollinshead WH: *Anatomy for Surgeons.* 3rd ed. vol. 3. Philadelphia: JB Lippincott; 1982.
6. Inoue T, Fujino T: An upper arm flap, pedicled on the cephalic vein with arterial anastomosis for head and neck reconstruction. *Br J Plast Surg* 1986;39:451–453.
7. Katsaros J, Schusterman M, Beppu M, Banis J, Acland R: The lateral upper arm flap: anatomy and clinical applications. *Ann Plast Surg* 1984;12:489–500.
8. Katsaros J, Tan E, Zoltie N, Barton M, Venugopalsrinivasan, Venkataramakrishnan: Further experience with the lateral arm free flap. *Plast Reconstr Surg* 1991;87:902–910.
9. Kuek L, Chuan T: The extended lateral arm flap: a new modification. *J Reconstr Microsurg* 1991;7:167–173.
10. Martin D, Mondie J, BeBiscop J, Selott H, Peri G: The osteocutaneous outer arm flap: a new concept in microsurgical mandibular reconstructions. *Rev Stomatol Chir Maxillofac* 1988;89:281–287.
11. Matloub H, Larson D, Kuhn J, Yousif J, Sanger J: Lateral arm free flap in oral cavity reconstruction: a functional evaluation. *Head Neck* 1989;11:205–211.
12. Moffett T, Madison S, Derr J, Acland R: An extended approach for the vascular pedicle of the lateral arm free flap. *Plast Reconstr Surg* 1992;89:259–267.
13. Nakayama Y, Soeda S, Iino T: A radial forearm flap based on an extended dissection of the cephalic vein. The longest venous pedicle? *Br J Plast Surg* 1986;39:454–457.
14. Rivet D, Buffet M, Martin D, Waterhouse N, Kleiman L, Delonca D, Baudet J: The lateral arm flap: an anatomic study. *J Reconstr Microsurg* 1987;3:121–132.
15. Scheker L, Kleinert H, Hanel D: Lateral arm composite tissue transfer to ipsilateral hand defects. *J Hand Surg [Am]* 1987;12A:665–672.
16. Shenaq S: Pretransfer expansion of a sensate lateral arm free flap. *Ann Plast Surg* 1987;19:558–562.
17. Song R, Song Y, Yu Y, Song Y: The upper arm free flap. *Clin Plast Surg* 1982;9:27–35.
18. Sullivan M, Carroll W, Kuriloff D: Lateral arm free flap in head and neck reconstruction. *Arch Otolaryngol Head Neck Surg* 1992;118:1095–1101.
19. Urken ML, Vickery C, Weinberg H, Biller HF: The neurofasciocutaneous radial forearm flap in head and neck reconstruction—a preliminary report. *Laryngoscope* 1990;100:161–173.
20. Waterhouse N, Healy C: The versatility of the lateral arm flap. *Br J Plast Surg* 1990;43:398.
21. Yousif NJ, Warren R, Matloub H, Sanger J: The lateral arm fascial free flap: its anatomy and use in reconstruction. *Plast Reconstr Surg* 1990;86:1138–1145.

13
CHAPTER

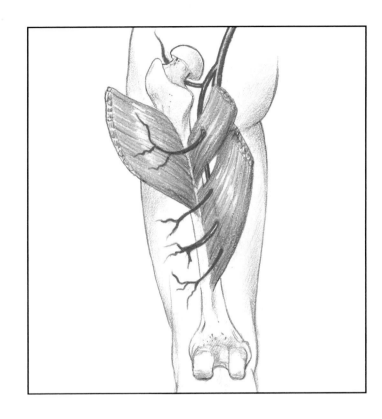

Lateral Thigh

Mark L. Urken, M.D. and
Michael J. Sullivan, M.D.

Surgeons have long recognized the value of the thigh as a reservoir of skin for distant reconstructions. As early as 1976, Harii et al. (4) reported the transfer of the medial thigh skin with a gracilis musculocutaneous flap. In 1978, Hill et al. (6) introduced the tensor fasciae latae musculocutaneous flap as a vehicle for transferring skin from the lateral thigh.

However, the pursuit of thinner cutaneous flaps without the attendant morbidity of removing a functional muscle led Baek (1) to investigate the possibility of basing a thigh flap on a direct cutaneous perforator. In 1983, he introduced two new flaps, the medial and the lateral fasciocutaneous flaps. These were both supplied by septocutaneous vessels, with the former nourished by an "unnamed" artery from the superficial femoral artery and the latter supplied by a perforator of the profunda femoris system. Although Baek reported only two clinical cases using each of these flaps, he pointed out the great potential value of these donor sites. In addition, he noted the capacity for neurosensory restoration using the medial femoral cutaneous and the lateral femoral cutaneous nerves. Although the enthusiasm for these two flaps has been somewhat limited, Hayden (5) popularized the lateral thigh flap and demonstrated its utility in head and neck reconstruction. In selected individuals with a favorable body habitus, this donor site provides a large surface area of expendable tissue with a long vascular pedicle. In addition, the distance from the head and neck allows this flap to be harvested at the same time as the ablative procedure. The loss of skin from this location causes little morbidity.

FLAP DESIGN AND UTILIZATION

The major cutaneous artery of the lateral thigh flap is the third perforator of the profunda femoris artery, which runs in the lateral intermuscular septum between the vastus lateralis and the biceps femoris. As this perforator emerges from the septum, it arborizes over the iliotibial tract to supply large areas of skin over the lateral thigh. Ink-injection studies by Baek (1) revealed that the third perforator supplied an elliptical area of skin with its long axis oriented along the lateral intermuscular septum. This perforator was found to emerge from the septum at about the midpoint of a line drawn from the greater trochanter to the lateral epicondyle of the femur (Figure 13-1). Because anatomic variations in the blood supply to the skin occur along this longitudinal axis, it is advisable to design a longer flap than needed to incorporate these variations should they be encountered after the dissection has begun. Cormack and Lamberty (2) reported that, from their dissections, the septocutaneous perforators arborize in a predominantly anterior direction over the iliotibial tract and, therefore, advised designing a skin paddle with two thirds to three quarters of the surface area anterior to the septum.

Although Hayden (5) reported successful transfer of lateral thigh flaps as large as 25×14 cm, the maximum dimensions of this donor site have not been determined. Primary closure is desirable; however, a split-thickness skin graft may be placed.

The lateral thigh flap is not usually transferred with the tensor fasciae latae. However, Inoue et al. (7) used the lateral thigh flap with a strip of vascularized tensor fasciae latae in the reconstruction of the Achilles tendon. The need for fascia in the head and neck is not common, but it may be useful in static suspension of the lateral commissure following facial paralysis and in support of a paralyzed or reconstructed lower lip.

Preoperative evaluation of the lateral thigh is important to determine the suitability of the skin of this region in each individual patient. The iliotibial tract is the strong lateral layer of the tensor fasciae latae that begins at the greater trochanter and extends across the lateral knee joint. The transition from the firm iliotibial tract to the fleshy biceps femoris (located posteriorly) marks the location of the lateral intermuscular septum. It is common for the subcutaneous tissue of this region to be thicker in the more cephalad aspect of the thigh and to be thicker in female than male patients. It is also important to assess the presence of hair-bearing skin in this region and to determine whether this factor will have an adverse impact on the aesthetic or functional outcome of the reconstruction.

The entry of the vascular pedicle into the midportion of the skin paddle allows this flap to be contoured with considerable freedom. The location of this donor site at a distance from the head and neck is suitable for a two-team approach. The dimensions of the flap should exceed the anticipated size of the defect. As noted, secondary contouring can be performed with great ease following transfer to the head and neck. Its thin pliable nature makes it ideally suited for large reconstructions of the pharynx and pharyngoesophagus. Hayden (5) described the use of this flap for resurfacing the gullet following laryngopharyngectomy. In most cases, this flap is readily tubed to create a circumferential lining. The length of tissue that can be harvested allows reconstruction of the upper digestive tract from the thoracic inlet to the nasopharynx. The major advantage of this donor site for use in pharyngoesophageal defects, compared with the tubed radial forearm flap, as described by Harii et al. (3), is the more aesthetic appearance of the donor site following closure. The transfer of a large surface area of lateral thigh skin usually results in a linear scar compared with the skin-grafted radial forearm.

Baek (1) reported the use of the lateral thigh flap to resurface a cutaneous cheek defect. This flap can certainly be utilized for virtually any external defect of the head and neck and, in particular, large defects of the scalp. The potential for sensory reinnervation of this skin through the lateral femoral cutaneous nerve provides an opportunity for improved functional recovery during reconstruction of the pharynx when the larynx is intact.

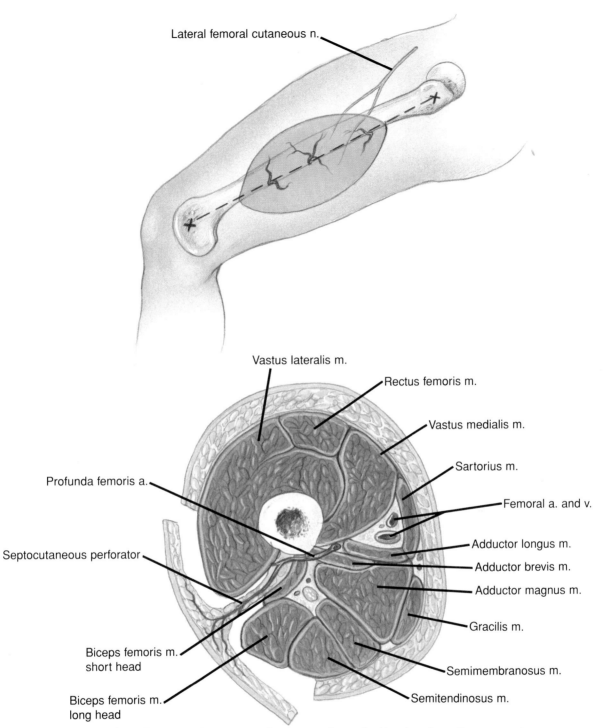

Figure 13-1. The lateral intermuscular septum is marked by drawing a line connecting the greater trochanter to the lateral epicondyle of the femur. This line denotes the posterior aspect of the iliotibial tract and is the central axis for designing the cutaneous paddle of the lateral thigh flap. The lateral femoral cutaneous nerve supplies sensation to the skin of this region. The septocutaneous perforator to this flap, which is usually the third perforator of the profunda femoris artery, pierces the attachment of the adductor magnus to the linea aspera of the femur. It runs between the vastus lateralis anteriorly and the long and short heads of the biceps femoris posteriorly.

NEUROVASCULAR ANATOMY

Through extensive cadaver dissections, Baek (1) identified the third perforator as the dominant blood supply to the lateral thigh. He reported, however, that the second and fourth perforators may be dominant in a minority of individuals. Cormack and Lamberty (2) also identified a large perforator that exited in the more cephalad aspect of the septum within 3 cm of the lower border of the gluteus maximus. This upper vessel is a branch of the first profunda perforator, and in the series of 50 cadaver dissections, Cormack and Lamberty found it to be the dominant septocutaneous perforator in 60% of cases.

The profunda femoris artery, also known as the deep femoral artery, is the largest branch of the femoral artery (Figure 13-2). It arises from the posterolateral aspect of the femoral artery within the femoral triangle, approximately 5 cm below the inguinal ligament. The profunda femoris runs a circuitous course to lie ultimately in a deeper more posterior plane in close proximity to the femur. In its cephalocaudal course, the artery remains superficial to the pectineus, adductor brevis, and adductor magnus muscles, while passing deep to the adductor longus. The pectineus, adductor brevis, and adductor magnus form a broad sheet of muscles that extends from the pelvis to the linea aspera of the femur. The profunda femoris gives off a number of muscular branches to the adductor muscles in the medial compartment.

There are typically four perforating branches of the profunda femoris that pass into the posterolateral compartment through small openings in the attachment of adductor brevis and adductor magnus to the linea aspera. An understanding of these four branches is critical to the safe harvest of the lateral thigh flap. Although the classic description of the profunda femoris system includes four perforators, of which the fourth is the terminal branch, there may be two to six perforators. Each perforator gives off three types of branches: muscular branches to the hamstrings, branches that run in a cephalocaudal direction to anastomose with branches of the other perforators, and fasciocutaneous branches.

The first perforator gives off a large muscular branch, which is the primary blood supply to the adductors. In addition to giving nutrient branches to adductor brevis, longus, and magnus, its terminal branch is the main vascular pedicle of the gracilis muscle. This adductor branch may arise directly from the profunda femoris and often gives off a cutaneous branch to the upper medial thigh. After supplying branches to the gluteus maximus and the greater trochanter, it terminates as a cutaneous artery.

In 50 cadaver dissections, Cormack and Lamberty (2) found a cutaneous branch of the first perforator to be the dominant blood supply to the posterolateral thigh skin in 60% of cases. Maruyama et al. (8) successfully based a fasciocutaneous flap on this first perforator for the repair of ischial and trochanteric pressure sores.

The second perforator gives off major muscular branches to the semimembranosus, the long and short heads of the biceps femoris, and the vastus lateralis. It may give rise to a larger cutaneous branch, but most importantly, it supplies the nutrient artery of the femur.

The third perforator is most frequently the dominant nutrient supply to the lateral thigh flap. It too supplies muscular branches to the biceps femoris and vastus lateralis. The third perforator passes on or through the short head of biceps femoris in its course through the lateral intermuscular septum. It is imperative that the surgeon carefully look for pulsations within the filmy short head of the biceps femoris to detect the primary blood supply to this flap. The short head of the biceps femoris is a flexor of the knee. A small portion of this muscle is often sacrificed in the process of harvesting the lateral thigh flap. The fourth perforator, which is commonly the terminal portion of the profunda femoris, runs a similar course in the lateral intermuscular septum and may occasionally provide the dominant vascular supply to the lateral thigh skin. This branch is readily sacrificed in the process of harvesting a lateral thigh flap based on the third perforator. It is important to recognize that all four perforators anastomose with each other through a cephalocaudal plexus of connecting branches.

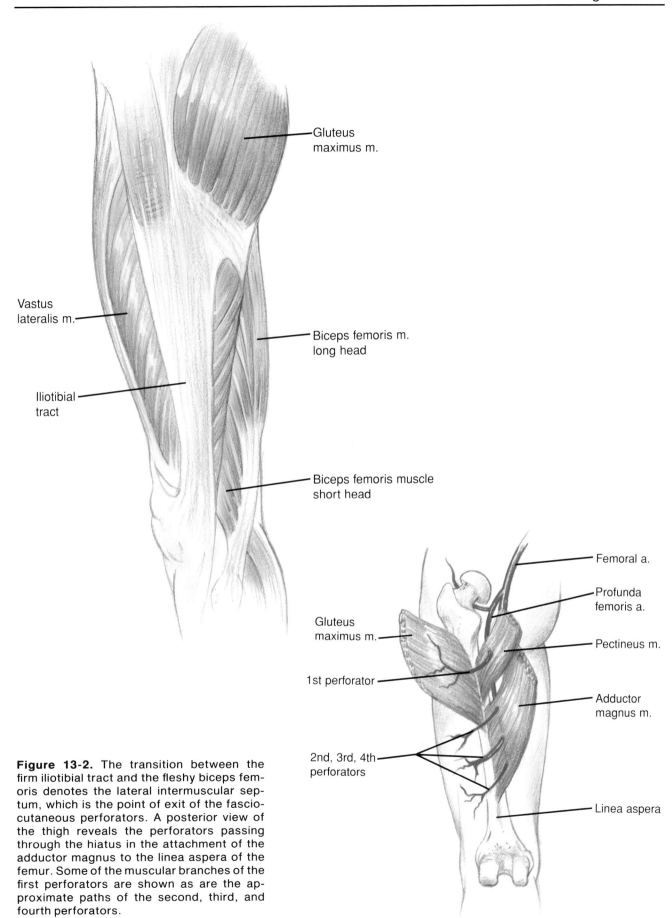

Figure 13-2. The transition between the firm iliotibial tract and the fleshy biceps femoris denotes the lateral intermuscular septum, which is the point of exit of the fasciocutaneous perforators. A posterior view of the thigh reveals the perforators passing through the hiatus in the attachment of the adductor magnus to the linea aspera of the femur. Some of the muscular branches of the first perforators are shown as are the approximate paths of the second, third, and fourth perforators.

The venous drainage of the lateral thigh flap is through paired venae comitantes, which run with the perforating arteries and usually join prior to entering the profunda femoris, or deep femoral vein. The diameter of the parent vein is often in the range of 4 to 5 mm. The profunda femoris usually has a diameter of 3 to 5 mm, but it narrows significantly as it courses toward the lateral aspect of the intermuscular septum where it measures only 1 to 1.5 mm when first identified in the dissection.

The lateral femoral cutaneous nerve is the dominant sensory nerve of the anterior and lateral thigh. This nerve is most commonly a separate branch of the first three lumbar nerves but may arise from the femoral nerve. The lateral femoral cutaneous nerve runs an extraperitoneal course on the surface of the iliacus and the iliopsoas to exit the pelvis below the inguinal ligament just anterior to the anterosuperior iliac spine. It traverses the path of the deep circumflex iliac artery and vein, either superficially or deep to these vessels. The relationship of this nerve to the sartorius is variable, running anteriorly, posteriorly, or through this muscle. In addition, the lateral femoral cutaneous nerve may run through the tensor fasciae latae where it divides and emerges on the anterolateral thigh as multiple small branches. Baek (1) recognized the potential for harvesting a sensate lateral thigh flap. It is often difficult to identify the smaller third- and fourth-generation branches of this nerve in the course of dissecting the anterior aspect of the lateral thigh skin flap. It is far easier to identify the lateral femoral cutaneous nerve more proximally and to harvest a broad cuff of subcutaneous tissues to protect the delicate branches as they course into the anterior border of the flap.

ANATOMIC VARIATIONS

The most important anatomic variations occur along the lateral intermuscular septum and are related to the relative dominance of one of the four perforators of the profunda femoris system. When the fourth perforator is the major source of the blood supply to the skin, the skin paddle is usually centered more distally on the lateral thigh, but the dissection of the pedicle is usually unaffected. The major problem arises when the second perforator is the major arterial supply of the lateral thigh flap. A proximal dissection of the second perforator must stop at the takeoff of the large muscular branches to ensure the vascular supply to the muscles and the femur. Hayden (5) noted a 15% incidence of one of these variations in which the third perforator is not the dominant cutaneous supply to the skin. He also advised inclusion of a large fourth perforator to augment the cutaneous blood supply, even when the third perforator is the dominant vessel.

The constancy of the vascular supply to the lateral thigh skin is reflected by the fact that there has been only one reported dissection with a significant anatomic variation. Baek (1) described one cadaver in which the dominant vascular supply to the lateral thigh skin arose from a branch of the superficial femoral artery. In this cadaver, the profunda femoris was rudimentary and did not give off a third or fourth cutaneous branch.

POTENTIAL PITFALLS

Occasionally, the fourth or second perforator is found to provide a significant vascular contribution to the flap. The flap's design must take these possibilities into consideration. As noted previously, when the second perforator is the dominant artery, the pedicle is dissected proximally only as far as the takeoff of the muscular branch of the second perforator. The major problem we have encountered with this donor site is the prevalence of atherosclerosis in the profunda femoris and its branches. Preoperative angiography is not routinely performed. However, if a patient has a history of lower extremity ischemic symptoms or overt signs of atherosclerotic disease, then an alternative donor site should be selected.

Finally, the surgeon should be aware of the proximity and potential vulnerability of the sciatic nerve after the adductor muscles are detached from the linea aspera to expose the profunda femoris artery and vein. Heavy-handed retraction and electrocautery should be minimized to prevent injury to this vital structure.

POSTOPERATIVE CARE

The donor-site defect is closed by wide undermining. Suction drainage is usually required. Skin grafting of the lateral thigh can be done but should be avoided by carefully limiting the flap's dimensions. Ambulation in the early postoperative period is encouraged.

Flap Harvesting Technique

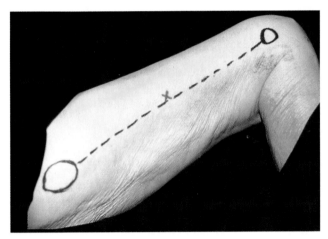

Figure 13-3. The topographical anatomy of the lateral thigh flap is shown with the major landmarks to the intermuscular septum being the greater trochanter superiorly and the lateral epicondyle of the femur inferiorly. The *dashed line* connecting these two points indicates the intermuscular septum. The third perforator of the profunda femoris passes through the intermuscular septum midway between these two bony landmarks.

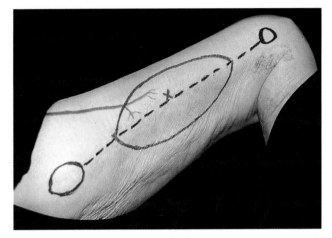

Figure 13-4. A fusiform skin paddle has been outlined. The approximate location of the lateral femoral cutaneous nerve, as it runs over the upper third of the sartorius muscle, is drawn in red. A counterincision near the anterosuperior iliac spine is made to identify the nerve prior to bifurcation. This will be demonstrated in a subsequent dissection.

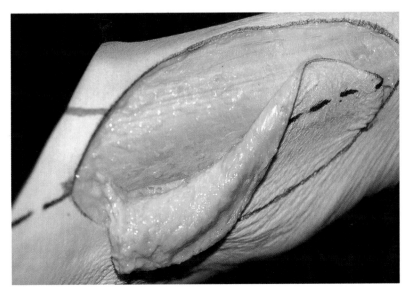

Figure 13-5. After making a circumferential incision around the skin flap, the plane of dissection is between the subcutaneous tissue and the iliotibial tract. The thinness and pliability of this tissue can be seen.

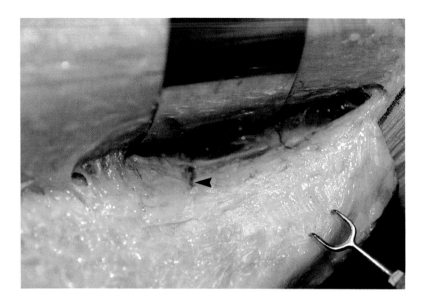

Figure 13-6. As long as the plane of dissection remains superficial to the fascia, the distal branches (*arrow*) of the pedicle can be identified coursing in the subcutaneous tissue.

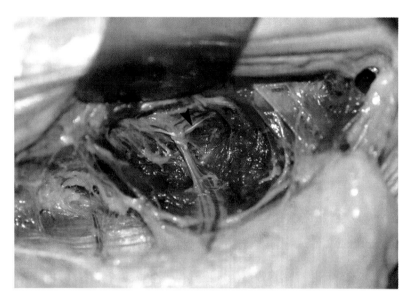

Figure 13-7. The third perforator has been traced through the short head of biceps femoris. The insertion of the adductor magnus to the linea aspera has been detached. In so doing, the profunda femoris artery and vein (*arrow*) are exposed.

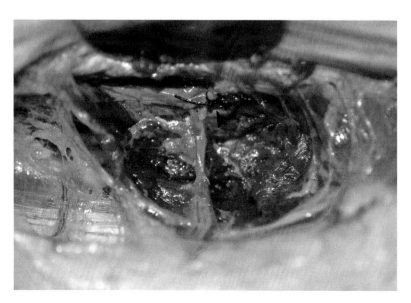

Figure 13-8. The continuation of the profunda femoris pedicle to give off the fourth perforator must be ligated (*arrow*), unless the fourth perforator is identified as a significant contributor to the vascular supply of the flap.

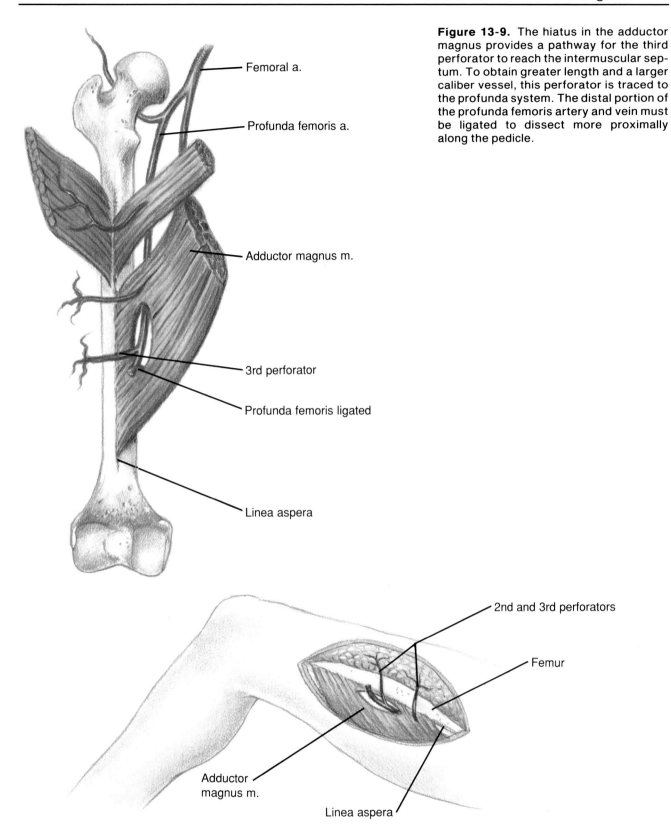

Figure 13-9. The hiatus in the adductor magnus provides a pathway for the third perforator to reach the intermuscular septum. To obtain greater length and a larger caliber vessel, this perforator is traced to the profunda system. The distal portion of the profunda femoris artery and vein must be ligated to dissect more proximally along the pedicle.

Femoral a.

Profunda femoris a.

Adductor magnus m.

3rd perforator

Profunda femoris ligated

Linea aspera

2nd and 3rd perforators

Femur

Adductor magnus m.

Linea aspera

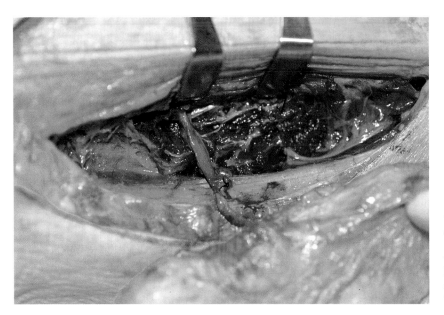

Figure 13-10. The caliber and length of the vascular pedicle can be seen following further mobilization of the profunda femoris system. With the vascular pedicle in full view, the posterior skin incision and dissection can be performed.

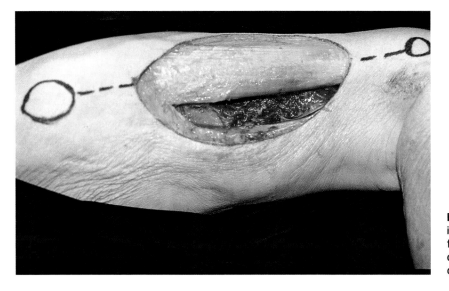

Figure 13-11. The defect in the thigh is closed by approximating the biceps femoris to the iliotibial tract and then closing the skin through wide undermining.

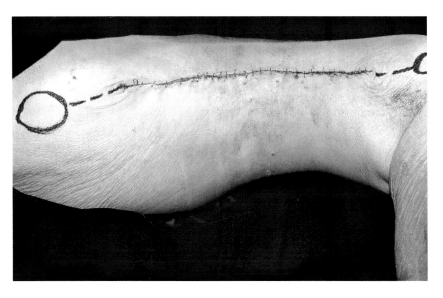

Figure 13-12. A linear closure can usually be achieved. A suction drain should be inserted into the wound. Lateral thigh closure may require a skin graft.

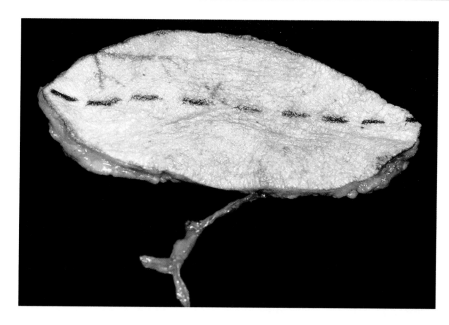

Figure 13-13. The lateral thigh flap is a thin pliable segment of tissue with a long pedicle. Larger flap dimensions may be harvested as needed.

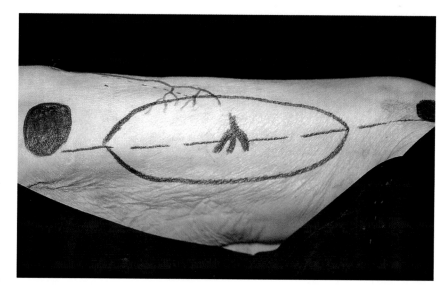

Figure 13-14. When harvesting the lateral femoral cutaneous nerve to supply sensation to this flap, the anterior incision is made only through the dermis.

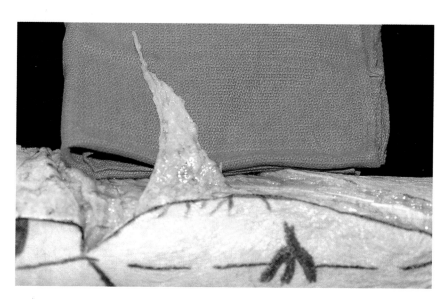

Figure 13-15. The lateral femoral cutaneous nerve is identified in the region of the anterosuperior iliac spine coursing either superficial or deep to the sartorius muscle. A wide cuff of subcutaneous tissue is then harvested between the main trunk of the nerve and the anterior limb of the skin flap. The arborization of the nerve makes this technique more successful than dissecting the distal branches.

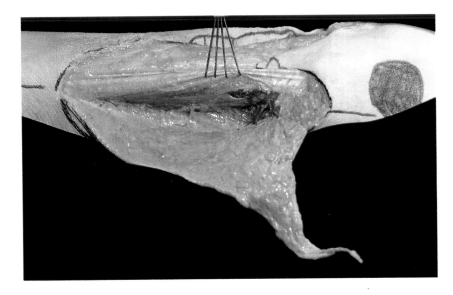

Figure 13-16. The pedicle is approached in a similar fashion by dissecting along the plane of the iliotibial tract.

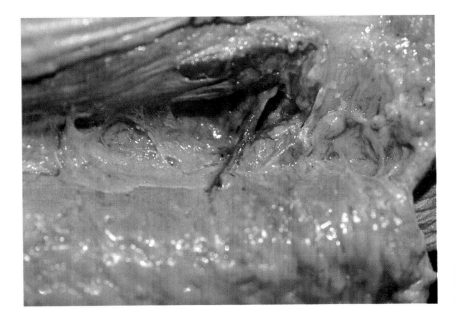

Figure 13-17. A longer vascular pedicle is obtained by dissecting along the profunda femoris system.

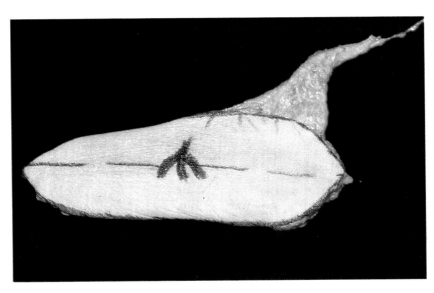

Figure 13-18. The sensate flap has a long nerve pedicle, which can reach virtually any recipient nerve in the head and neck.

REFERENCES

1. Baek SM. Two new cutaneous flaps: the medial and lateral thigh flaps. *Plast Reconstr Surg* 1983;71: 354.
2. Cormack G, Lamberty B. The blood supply of thigh skin. *Plast Reconstr Surg* 1985;75:342.
3. Harii K, Ebihara S, Ono I, Saito H, Terui S. Takato T. Pharyngoesophageal reconstruction using a fabricated forearm free flap. *Plast Reconstr Surg* 1985;75:463–476.
4. Harii K, Ohmori K, Sekiguchi J. The free musculocutaneous flap. *Plast Reconstr Surg* 1976;57:294.
5. Hayden RE. Lateral cutaneous thigh flap. In: Baker S, ed. *Microsurgical Reconstruction of the Head and Neck.* New York: Churchill Livingstone; 1989:211.
6. Hill HL, Nahai F, Vasconey LO. The TFL myocutaneous free flap. *Plast Reconstr Surg* 1978;61:517.
7. Inoue T, Tanaka I, Imai K, Hatoko M. Reconstruction of Achilles tendon using vascularized fascia with free lateral thigh flap. *Br J Plast Surg* 1990;43:728.
8. Maruyama Y, Ohnishi K, Takeuchi S. The lateral thigh fascio-cutaneous flap in the repair of ischial and trochanteric defects. *Br J Plast Surg* 1984;37:103.

14

Temporoparietal Fascia

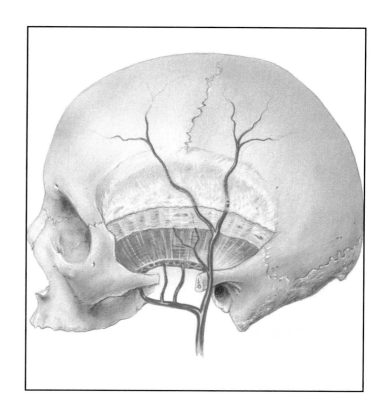

Mack L. Cheney, M.D.

Nearly one century ago, Monks (41) and Brown (11) separately reported cases in which the temporoparietal fascia, based on the superficial temporal vessels, was used for eyelid and auricular reconstruction. More recently, the temporoparietal fascial flap (TPFF) has become popular as a pedicled flap for use in periorbital (25,40) and auricular reconstruction and also as a free flap for the management of a variety of defects (20,28,52,55). During the last two decades, the flap has been reported as a valuable tool in the reconstruction of a variety of extremity defects (30,33,59). As experience with this flap has accumulated, it has become clear that it has several features that make it particularly useful in head and neck reconstruction (18,50). It is ultrathin, highly vascular, and exhibits a significant degree of flexibility, which allows it to drape around grafts and into cavities while, at the same time, maintaining its durability. It is particularly resistant to infection when transferred into infected or irradiated tissue beds. In head and neck reconstruction, the fascia is most commonly transferred as a pedicled flap, but it may also be used as a free flap when the arc of rotation is not adequate. This flap offers the advantage of a well-concealed donor site in the hair-bearing scalp (18,45).

FLAP DESIGN AND UTILIZATION

The TPFF is based on the superficial temporal artery and vein. It may be transferred independently or in combination with skin (9,10,15,18,19,31,45,46,49,51) and calvarial bone (Figure 14-1) (38,39). The key feature of the TPFF is its rich vas-

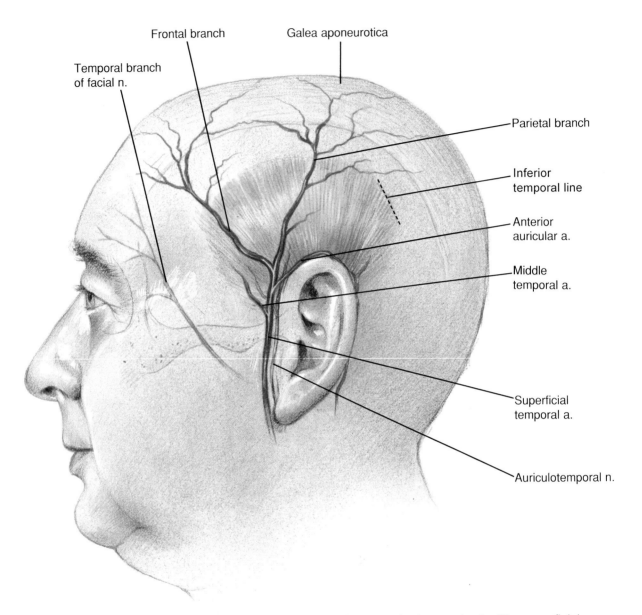

Figure 14-1. The TPFF is supplied by the superficial temporal artery and vein. The superficial temporal vessels divide into the parietal and frontal branches at approximately the superior limit of the helix. Prior to crossing the arch, the superficial temporal vessels usually give rise to the middle temporal artery and vein, which supply the temporalis muscular fascia. In addition, there are cutaneous branches that are given off to the root of the helix that allow transfer of a composite graft from this region. The temporal branch of the facial nerve crosses the zygoma and is at risk to injury during the anterior dissection of the flap.

cularity and pliability, making it an important tool for the rehabilitation of problem cavities (36) and for coverage of cartilage grafts used in head and neck reconstruction (8–10,18,36). A number of authors have commented that this tissue may be used in the face, hand, or lower extremity when a skin graft is preferable to a bulky flap but a suitable recipient bed is lacking (10,18,45,51).

The TPFF may be harvested with dimensions in the range of 17 × 14 cm without extensive scalp undermining. The thickness of the flap ranges from 2 to 4 mm. In most cases, a split-thickness skin graft is applied to the fascia after its transfer. How-

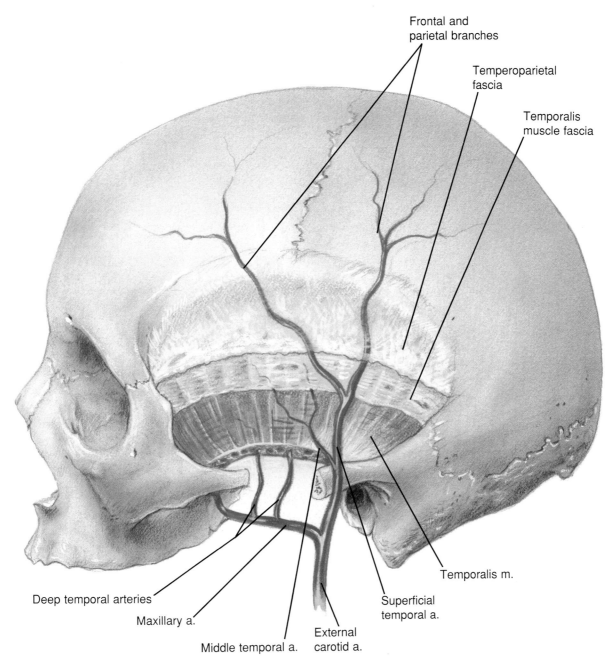

Frontal and
parietal branches

Temperoparietal
fascia

Temporalis
muscle fascia

Temporalis m.

Deep temporal arteries

Maxillary a.

Middle temporal a.

External
carotid a.

Superficial
temporal a.

Figure 14-2. The muscular and fascial layers of the temporal fossa are shown. The deepest plane is the temporalis muscle, which is supplied by the anterior and posterior deep temporal arteries, which arise from the internal maxillary artery. The temporalis muscular fascia is supplied by the middle temporal artery, which arises from the superficial temporal artery below the zygomatic arch. The terminal branches of the superficial temporal artery and vein supply the temporoparietal fascia.

ever, I have used this flap in the oral cavity without a skin graft, and it has provided a watertight seal and a surface for remucosalization.

The temporoparietal fascia may be transferred as a fascial tissue plane for a variety of purposes in head and neck reconstruction (5,12,18,37,45). Brent and others (8–10) carefully outlined the use of this flap for auricular reconstruction in conjunction with autogenous costal cartilage (7) and silastic (44) frameworks. The pliability of this flap makes it ideally suited for dependable coverage of a convoluted auricular framework in which the success of the surgery depends largely on the quality of the soft tissue lining which is critical to allow the detail of the sculpted cartilage to be seen. Others have advocated its use in the acutely traumatized auricle as a method of providing immediate auricular cartilage coverage (21,35,58).

Acland et al. (2) identified the middle temporal artery as the primary vascular supply to the temporalis muscular fascia (Figure 14-2). This vascular pattern provides the opportunity to transfer two separate leaves of vascularized fascia simultaneously. East et al. (25) used this composite flap in a case of post-traumatic tracheomalacia in which a nasal septal cartilage graft was sandwiched between the two leaves of fascia and then inset into the anterior tracheal wall.

The TPFF may also be used in the management of difficult temporal bone and orbital cavities (24,56). Its vascularity and pliability make it a valuable tool to achieve reliable coverage when the bony walls of these cavities have been affected by irradiation. The flap has also been noted to be particularly useful when reconstructing contour defects of the midface and orbital region (39).

In addition to its traditional application as a fascial flap, the tissue may also be used to transfer overlying scalp skin and hair, thereby making it applicable for scalp and lip reconstruction (32,36,42,43). By extending the vascular pedicle with an interposed vein graft, the flap can be mobilized by using a V–Y technique to close full-thickness defects of the scalp (30).

The versatility of this flap is further revealed by a series of reports in which the superficial temporal artery and vein were used to transfer skin and cartilage from the root of the auricular helix. This composite graft may be used to reconstruct sizable defects of the nasal ala (46,47,54). Duplication of the thin natural contour of the nasal ala with its cartilage covered by skin, both on the inside and outside, is one of the most challenging aspects of nasal reconstruction. The root of the helix matches the ala perhaps better than any other tissue in the body and is unique as a donor site for this particular defect.

Calvarial bone may also be harvested in conjunction with this flap. Bone from the outer table of the calvarium may be transferred as a vascularized bone graft from the parietal area above the superior temporal line where the temporoparietal fascia joins the galea. McCarthy and Zido (39) described the elevation of temporoparietal fascia in conjunction with outer calvarial bone and documented the contribution of the superficial temporal artery to the vascularity of this bone (16,23,48). Experimental work by Antonyshyn et al. (3) suggested that the vascularized calvarial bone transfers are superior to standard calvarial bone grafts in terms of early viability and new osteoid formation. The reliability and long-term results of vascularized calvarial bone grafts in craniofacial defects have been demonstrated in large clinical series (6,47). If bone is to be transferred with the flap, a generous cuff of fascia and pericranium must be preserved at the periphery of the graft. The outer table of the skull is harvested as a split cranial graft (17). The temporoparietal fascia is fixed to the bone with a suture to prevent shearing of the delicate vessels that perforate the pericranium (50). By combining the bone graft with the temporoparietal fascia, studies have documented that the surviving osseous mass is increased compared with that of conventional non-vascularized calvarial grafts (13,14,23). An additional benefit of this technique is that it allows the bone graft to be harvested through the same operative field as the soft tissue; therefore, sparing the patient the discomfort of a separate donor site.

The TPFF is dependably vascularized to the midline of the calvarium and may be extended to this point if the flap is to be used for intraoral reconstruction (29). Transfer of the pedicled TPFF, with or without attached calvarial bone, will reach the malar, orbital, and mandibular regions in most patients. It has been my experience that the pedicle's length is often inadequate when transposing the TPFF into the oral cavity. Several options may be considered to improve the arc of rotation, including the temporary removal of the zygomatic arch or the proximal dissection of the pedicle below the tragus. It should be noted that mobilization of the vascular pedicle below the tragus places the facial nerve at risk and requires identification of the main body of the facial nerve in the parotid gland. An incision can be made through the buccal sulcus to allow access for intraoral placement of the flap.

Because of the flap's ease of transfer and thickness, it is often useful in augmenting soft tissue defects of the face. I have used this technique extensively for recontouring defects in the parotid bed and in the midfacial region.

NEUROVASCULAR ANATOMY

A review of the recent medical literature reveals that inconsistent nomenclature is used in the description of the anatomic layers of the temporoparietal region (Figure 14-3) (1,34,57). The temporoparietal scalp consists of five distinct layers. The temporoparietal fascia lies in the central position between two tissue planes in the area below the superior temporal line. It lies deep to the skin and subcutaneous tissue to which it is firmly bound. The temporoparietal fascia should not be confused with the temporalis muscular fascia, which envelops the temporalis muscle. The temporoparietal fascia is a superior extension of the superficial musculoaponeurotic system, both of which attach to the zygomatic arch. The temporalis muscular fascia passes deep to the arch to insert on the coronoid process of the mandible (40). Above the superior temporal line, the temporoparietal fascia becomes the galea aponeurotica. Below the superior temporal line, the tissue planes deep to the temporoparietal fascia consist of loose areolar tissue and temporalis muscular fascia. Loose areolar tissue separates the temporoparietal fascia from the muscular fascia of the temporalis, which gives the scalp its natural mobility. When the scalp is moved, the temporoparietal fascia moves with it, but the muscular fascia and periosteum remain stable. In the area above the temporal line, the temporalis muscular fascia and the periosteum converge and continue cephalad as the pericranium of the superior scalp (Figure 14-3).

The superficial temporal artery and vein are moderate-sized vessels that are best isolated approximately 3 cm superior to the root of the helix where they branch into frontal and parietal divisions (Figure 14-1). These branches anastomose freely with the supraorbital and supratrochlear vessels over the forehead (4). The flap is most commonly based on the parietal branch, with its base centered over the middle third of the superior auricular helix. The frontal branch is routinely ligated approximately 3 to 4 cm distal to its separation from the parietal branch. Dissection beyond this point risks injury to the frontal branch of the facial nerve.

At its origin, the superficial temporal artery has an average diameter of 1.89 mm and lies deep to, or within, the parotid gland (52). In the first part of its course, approximately 15 mm, it ascends behind the ramus of the mandible and then pierces the superficial fascia 4 to 5 mm in front of the tragus (26). In the second, or superficial, part of its course, it crosses the posterior part of the zygomatic process of the temporal bone, lying anterior to the auriculotemporal nerve and the superficial temporal vein where it can be easily palpated. It may lie beneath the anterior auricular muscle and may have a tortuous course, which is significant because, if this is "released," it may increase the length of the pedicle of an island flap by up to 1.5 cm. The middle temporal branch of the artery, which supplies the temporalis muscular fascia, is given off in this region. At a point 2 to 4 cm above the zygomatic arch (range, 0 to 5 cm), the superficial temporal artery divides into two terminal branches: the frontal and the parietal. A delayed division is commonly associated with a well-developed zygomatico-orbital branch from the main stem of the superficial temporal artery and occurs in 80% of cases (48). The frontal branch is generally slightly larger (1.2 mm in diameter) than the parietal branch (1.1 mm in diameter) (20). The frontal branch runs tortuously upward and forward, supplying all layers of the scalp, and anastomoses with the corresponding vessel of the opposite side and also with the ipsilateral supraorbital and supratrochlear arteries.

The parietal branch passes vertically upward toward the vertex. In approximately 7.5% of patients, it may be double, with the two branches roughly parallel to each other. Its course lies within a 2-cm strip centered on the auditory meatus and passing upward to the vertex. Within this band, the artery inclines from the anterior to the

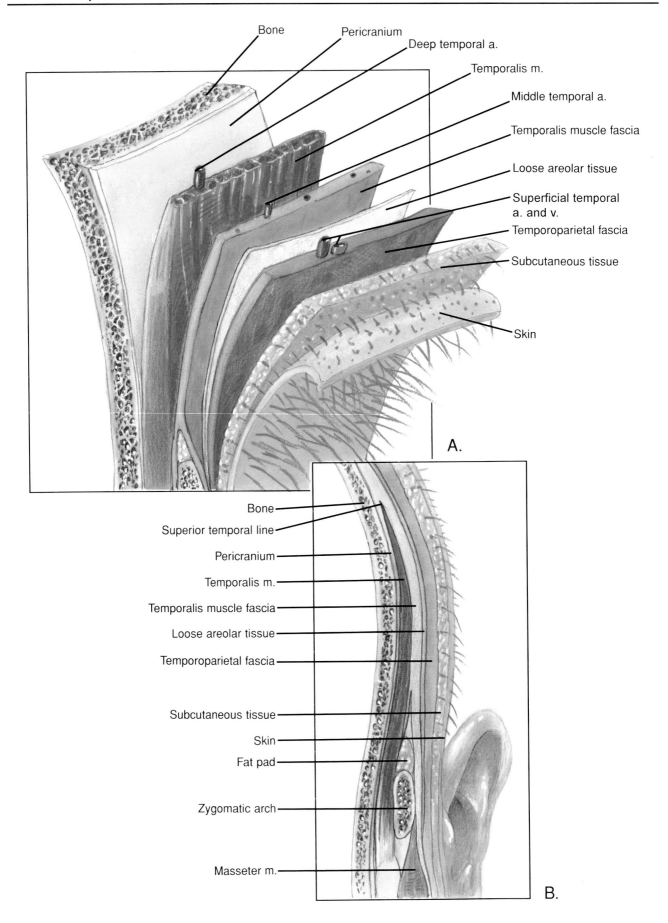

Bone

Pericranium

Deep temporal a.

Temporalis m.

Middle temporal a.

Temporalis muscle fascia

Loose areolar tissue

Superficial temporal a. and v.

Temporoparietal fascia

Subcutaneous tissue

Skin

A.

Bone

Superior temporal line

Pericranium

Temporalis m.

Temporalis muscle fascia

Loose areolar tissue

Temporoparietal fascia

Subcutaneous tissue

Skin

Fat pad

Zygomatic arch

Masseter m.

B.

posterior margins. The superficial temporal vein may be single or duplicate. In most cases, the vein runs with the artery but superficial to it. In 20% to 30% of cases, however, the vein takes a divergent course above the level of the root of the helix and may travel up to 3 cm posterior to the arterial pedicle (50,55). The parietal branch anastomoses with its opposite member, which arises from the contralateral superficial temporal system and with the ipsilateral posterior auricular and occipital arteries (20).

The middle temporal artery arises from the proximal superficial temporal artery at the level of zygomatic arch and supplies the temporalis muscular fascia. Because of this branching vascular pattern, a two-layered fascial flap can be raised on a single vascular pedicle (Figure 14-12) (21).

The superficial temporal system gives off several branches to the skin of the face. The transverse facial artery arises deep to the parotid gland and runs forward over the masseter. In 35% of cases, the transverse facial artery arises from the external carotid artery directly. It runs forward and is accompanied by branches of the facial nerve in the region between the zygomatic arch and the parotid duct, often crossing the duct. It supplies the parotid gland and duct, the masseter muscle, and the skin. A large cutaneous branch is consistently found at the point of intersection of a vertical line drawn 2 cm laterally to the lateral canthus with a horizontal line through the alar base. The transverse facial artery anastomoses superiorly with the lacrimal and infraorbital arteries, anteriorly with the premasseteric and facial arteries, and deeply with the buccal artery. This artery primarily supplies muscle, but it may also make a significant contribution to the blood supply of the skin over the masseter and the parotid and, to a lesser extent, to the skin of the inferior orbital and nasolabial regions (20).

The superficial temporal artery supplies three groups of auricular branches: (a) an inferior group supplies the lobule and tragus; (b) two or three branches in a superior group often form a common trunk and run onto the upper part of the helix, its crura, and triangular fossa (45); and (c) the superficial temporal or its parietal branch gives off a small branch that runs down behind the ear for a short distance, supplies the uppermost part of the cranial surface of the ear, and anastomoses with the posterior auricular artery (20).

The zygomatico-orbital artery may branch from the superficial temporal artery, the middle temporal branch, or the frontal branch. It runs along the upper border of the zygomatic arch between the two layers of the temporalis muscular fascia to the lateral aspect of the orbit. It supplies branches to the orbicularis oculi, anastomoses with the lacrimal and palpebral branches of the ophthalmic artery, and completes the periorbital ring with the infra- and supraorbital vessels (20).

There are various motor and sensory nerves that traverse the temporoparietal donor site. The auriculotemporal nerve, a sensory branch of the trigeminal nerve, lies posterior to the superficial temporal artery, within the temporoparietal fascia, and supplies the regional scalp skin. The frontal branch of the facial nerve courses obliquely across the zygomatic arch and lies approximately 1.5 cm lateral to the orbital rim. This nerve runs within the temporoparietal fascia and represents the anterior limit of flap elevation.

◄ ────────────────────

Figure 14-3. The different layers of the scalp in the temporal fossa are shown extending from the calvarial bone to the skin. The temporalis muscular fascia splits into two layers approximately 2 cm above the zygomatic arch. These two fascial leaves are separated by fat, which provides a natural plane of dissection. The temporalis muscular fascia is continuous with the masseter muscular fascia below the arch; the temporoparietal fascia is continuous with the superficial muscular aponeurotic system below the arch. The temporalis muscular fascia and the TPFF are separated by a loose areolar plane, which also separates the pericranium from the galea in the region cephalad to the superior temporal line.

ANATOMIC VARIATIONS

The superficial temporal artery, the smaller terminal division of the external carotid, consistently branches into two separate vascular systems approximately 3 cm above the root of the helix (30). Five distinct branching patterns have been described (27). However, in all cases, the course of the posterior parietal branch can be traced with Doppler sonography to ensure that the planned territory of the TPFF is well vascularized.

POTENTIAL PITFALLS

Although the TPFF is a highly reliable technique for head and neck reconstruction, there are a number of donor-site problems that should be reviewed (18). The anterior dissection of the flap is limited by the frontal branch of the facial nerve, which also runs in the temporoparietal fascia. Careful identification of this branch during the dissection of the flap will prevent injury to the nerve.

The most common complication after the elevation of this flap is secondary alopecia. This has been noted around the incision site for up to 2 cm. As mentioned previously, prior radiation therapy or surgery in this area predisposes the overlying scalp to ischemic injury after raising the flap. In addition to this, a poor plane of surgical dissection can result in direct injury to the hair follicles and lead to large areas of secondary alopecia. As is true in virtually all flap transfers, it is imperative to include both the nutrient artery and vein. The surgeon must be aware of the potential divergent course of the superficial temporal vein from the artery and be certain to identify both vessels before incising the outlines of the fascial flap.

PREOPERATIVE ASSESSMENT

Many factors can influence the viability of the TPFF and limit its use in the reconstruction of the selected head and neck defect. Preoperative radiation, neck surgery, or external carotid embolization may affect the vascular pedicle and is considered a relative contraindication to the elevation of this tissue. Exposure of the temporoparietal fascia requires that the scalp be elevated in a subfollicular plane, thereby endangering the hair follicles. Therefore, alopecia is a potential risk. This risk is increased if the patient has a history of previous surgery or radiation to the area. The most important preoperative test to determine the reliability of this flap is Doppler ultrasonography, which should be performed in the office before finalizing the surgical plan.

POSTOPERATIVE WOUND CARE

After transfer of the TPFF, careful hemostasis is obtained with bipolar cautery. A special effort is made to avoid thermal injury to the hair follicles. A suction drain is routinely used and should be placed in a superior position to avoid inadvertent contact with the vascular pedicle when a transposition flap has been performed. The wound is closed in layers, and a bulky compressive dressing is applied for 24 hours. The suction drain is kept in place for 24 to 48 hours.

Flap Harvesting Technique

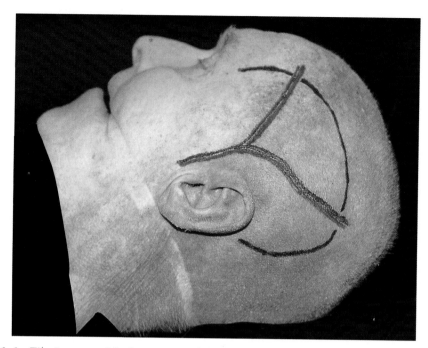

Figure 14-4. The topographical anatomy of the TPFF is outlined on the lateral scalp. The approximate course of the superficial temporal artery and vein has been drawn with the division of the pedicle into anterior and posterior branches at a point approximately 3 cm above the tragus. The venous pedicle may run concurrently with the artery or may separate from the artery and run 2–3 cm posteriorly. The superior temporal line has also been drawn. This bony ridge begins at the zygomatic process of the frontal bone and curves upward and backward across the frontal bone along the lateral margin of the forehead. It passes over the parietal bone and ends by joining the supramastoid crest. The most cephalic origin of the temporalis is at the inferior temporal line. This is an important landmark because it is at this point that the temporoparietal fascia becomes confluent with the galea aponeurotica. The superior temporal line denotes the point where the temporalis muscular fascia joins with the periosteum that covers the calvarium.

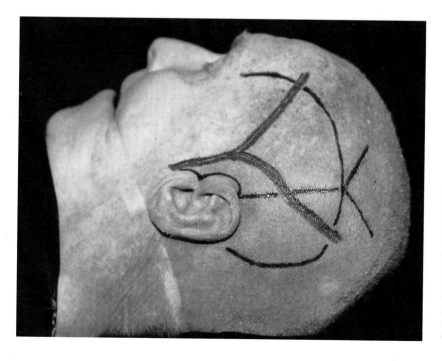

Figure 14-5. A vertical incision extending from the root of the helix to the superior temporal line is used in harvesting the temporoparietal fascia. A V-extension at the superior aspect of the incision is used to gain full access to the fascial layers in this region. Inferiorly, the incision is placed in the preauricular crease adjacent to the root of the helix. In most cases, the vascular pedicle is located anterior to the initial incision; however, the dominant venous system may travel a more posterior course than the artery.

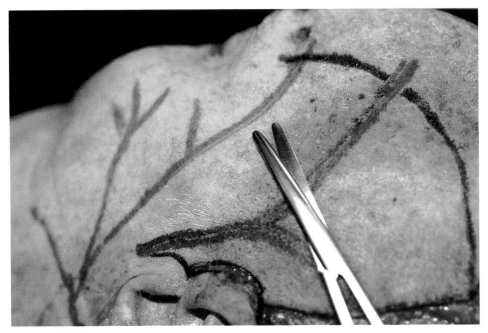

Figure 14-6. The approximate course of the frontal branch of the facial nerve has been drawn as it courses from the main trunk, over the zygoma, and toward the lateral aspect of the forehead. The dissection must remain posterior to this region to avoid injury to this nerve.

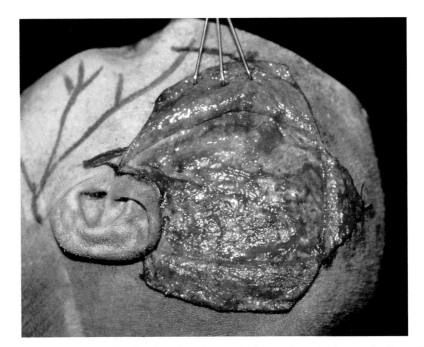

Figure 14-7. The dissection begins by elevating anterior and posterior scalp flaps. Particular attention is given to avoiding injury to the hair follicles as these flaps are elevated. The frontal branch of the superficial temporal artery is ligated at the anterior limits of the flap.

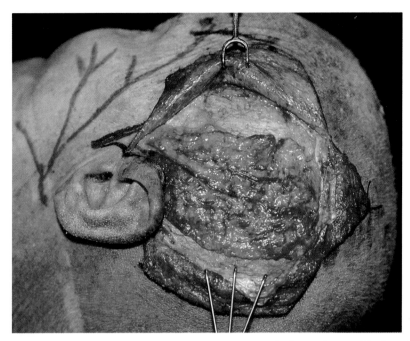

Figure 14-8. With the posterior, superior, and anterior scalp flaps elevated in the plane superficial to the temporoparietal fascia, the deep dissection and elevation of the flap is performed. This elevation is best initiated at the superior temporal line. Identification of the temporalis muscular fascia assures the surgeon of the proper plane for deep elevation of the flap. The layer of loose areolar tissue that separates the temporoparietal fascia from the muscular fascia at this level permits a straightforward nonvascular dissection.

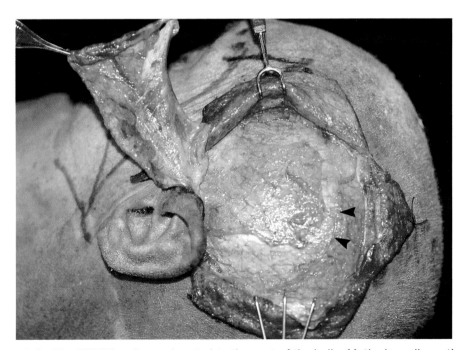

Figure 14-9. The TPFF has been elevated to the root of the helix. Meticulous dissection must be performed in this region to avoid injury to the vascular pedicle. If the temporalis muscular fascia (*arrows*) is to be harvested, the plane of dissection is performed along the surface of the temporalis muscle.

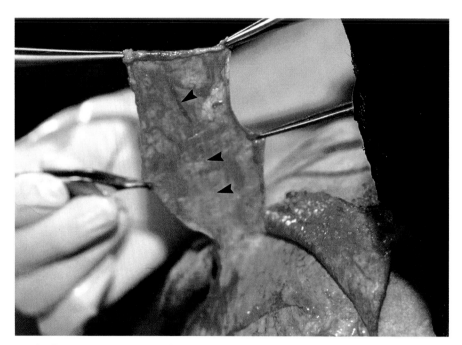

Figure 14-10. The temporoparietal fascia is elevated, and the superficial temporal artery and vein (*arrows*) are isolated. The width of the flap base is normally 2.0–2.5 cm. As demonstrated, the flap is flexible, thin, and highly vascular, and it exhibits exceptional "draping" characteristics.

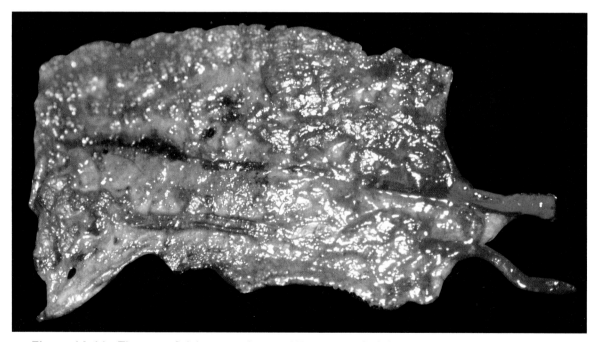

Figure 14-11. The superficial temporal artery (diameter, 1.8–2.2 mm) and vein (diameter, 2.0–3.0 mm) are limited in length by the dangers of extending the caudal dissection in the vicinity of the main trunk of the facial nerve.

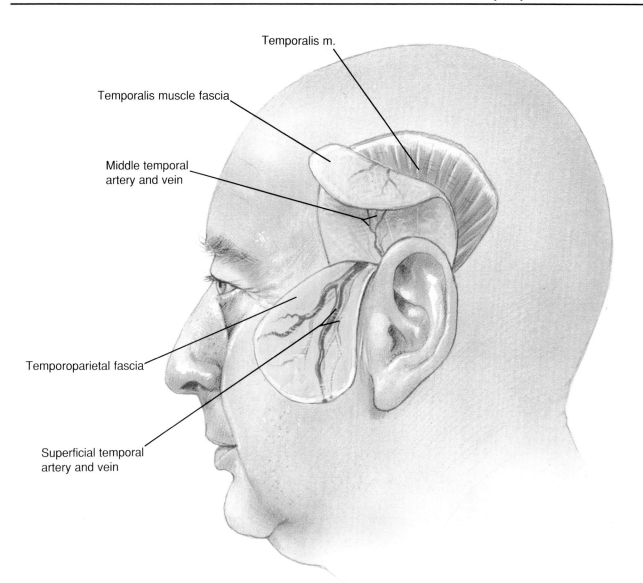

Temporalis m.

Temporalis muscle fascia

Middle temporal artery and vein

Temporoparietal fascia

Superficial temporal artery and vein

Figure 14-12. If two layers of vascularized fascia are required for reconstruction, the TPFF may be harvested along with the temporalis muscular fascia. The two separate nutrient vascular systems allow two independent thin layers of tissue to be harvested, which makes this donor site unique. Careful dissection of the middle temporal artery in the region of the zygomatic arch is required to harvest these two fascial leaves as a microvascular free flap.

REFERENCES

1. Abul-Hassan HS, von Drasek-Ascher G, Acland RD. Surgical anatomy and blood supply of the fascial layers of the temporal region. *Plast Reconstr Surg* 1986;77:17.
2. Acland RD, Abul-Hassan H, Ulfe E. Superficial and deep temporal fascia flap: an anatomic approach. Videotape presentation at the Annual Meeting of the American Society of Plastic and Reconstructive Surgeons. Las Vegas, Nevada, October 12, 1983.
3. Antonyshyn O, Colcleugh RG, Hurst LN, Anderson C. The temporalis myo-osseous flap: an experimental study. *Plast Reconstr Surg* 1986;77:406.
4. Antonyshyn O, Gruss JS, Birt BD. Versatility of temporal muscle and fascial flaps. *Br J Plast Surg* 1988;41:118.
5. Avelar JM, Psillakis JM. The use of galea flaps in craniofacial deformities. *Ann Plast Surg* 1981;6:464.
6. Bite U, Jackson IT, Wahner HW, Marsh RW. Vascularized skull bone grafts in craniofacial surgery. *Ann Plast Surg* 1987;19:3.
7. Boudard PH, Benassayag CL, Alvarez FL, Portmann O, Bebear JP, Portmann M. Temporoparietal fascial flap in difficult total ear reconstruction. *Rev Laryngol* 1989;110:219.
8. Brent B. Auricular repair with autogenous rib cartilage grafts: two decades of experience with 600 cases. *Plast Reconstr Surg* 1992;9:355.
9. Brent B, Byrd HS. Secondary ear reconstruction with cartilage grafts covered by axial, random, and free flaps of temporoparietal fascia. *Plast Reconstr Surg* 1983;72:141.
10. Brent B, Upton J, Acland RD, Shaw WW, Finseth FJ, Rogers C, Pearl RM, Hentz VR. Experience with the temporoparietal fascial free flap. *Plast Reconstr Surg* 1985;76:177–188.
11. Brown WJ. Extraordinary case of horse bite: the external ear completely bitten off and successfully replaced. *Lancet* 1898;1:1533.
12. Byrd HS. The use of subcutaneous axial fascial flaps in reconstruction of the head. *Ann Plast Surg* 1980;4:191:
13. Canalis RF. Further observation of the fate of pedicle osseocutaneous grafts. *Otolaryngol Head Neck Surg* 1979;87:763.
14. Canalis RF, Saffouri M, Mirra J, Ward PH. The fate of pedicle osseocutaneous grafts. *Laryngoscope* 1977;87:895.
15. Carstens MH, Greco RJ, Hurwitz DJ, Tolhurst DE. Clinical applications of the subgaleal fascia. *Plast Reconstr Surg* 1991;87:615.
16. Casanova R, Cavalcante D, Grotting JC, Vasconez LO, Psillakis JM. Anatomic basis for vascularized outer-table calvarial bone flaps. *Plast Reconstr Surg* 1986;78:300.
17. Cheney ML, Gliklich RE. The use of calvarial bone in nasal reconstruction. *Arch Otolaryngol Head Neck Surg* 1994;[*in press*].
18. Cheney ML, Varvares MA, Nadol JB Jr. The temporoparietal fascial flap in head and neck reconstruction. *Arch Otolaryngol Head Neck Surg* 1993;119:618.
19. Chiarelli A, Baldelli A, Vincenzo AD, Martini G. Utilization of the superficial temporoparietal fascia in reconstructive plastic surgery. *Ophthal Plast Reconstr Surg* 1989;5:274.
20. Cormac GC, Lamberty BGH. *The Arterial Anatomy of Skin Flaps.* New York: Churchill Livingstone; 1986.
21. Cotlar SW. Reconstruction of the burned ear using a temporalis fascial flap. *Plast Reconstr Surg* 1983;71:45.
22. Cutting CB, McCarthy JG. Comparison of residual osseous mass between vascularized and nonvascularized onlay bone transfers. *Plast Reconstr Surg* 1983;72:672.
23. Cutting CB, McCarthy JG, Berenstein A. Blood supply of the upper craniofacial skeleton: the search for composite calvarial bone flaps. *Plast Reconstr Surg* 1984;74:603.
24. East CA, Brongh MD, Grant HR. Mastoid obliteration with the temporoparietal fascial flap. *J Laryngol Otol* 1991;105:417.
25. East C, Grant H, Jones B. Tracheal reconstruction using a composite microvascular temporoparietal fascia flap and nasal septal graft. *J Laryngol Otol* 1992;106:741.
26. Esser JFS. Uber eine gestielte Ueberpflanzung eine senrecht angelegten Kells aus dem oberen Augenlid in das gleichseitige Unterlid oder umgekehrt. *Klin Monatsbl Augenheilkd* 1919;63:379.
27. Busthianos NA. Étude anatomique sur les artères temporales superficielles. *Ann Anat Pathol (Paris)* 1932;9:678.
28. Fox JW, Edgerton MT. The fan flap: an adjunct to ear reconstruction. *Plast Reconstr Surg* 1976;58:663.
29. Godfrey PM. Sinus obliteration for chronic oro-antral fistula: a case report. *Br J Plast Surg* 1993;46:341.
30. Hallock GG. The extended temporoparietal fascia "non free" flap. *Ann Plast Surg* 1988;21:65.
31. Hallock GG. Scalp fascia for the extremities. *Contemp Orthop* 1990;21:542.
32. Harii K, Ohmori K, Ohmori S. Hair transplantation with free scalp flaps. *Plast Reconstr Surg* 1974;53:410.
33. Hing DN, Buncke HJ, Alpert BS. Use of temporoparietal free fascial flap in the upper extremity. *Plast Reconstr Surg* 1988;81:534.
34. Horowitz JH, Persing JA, Nichter IS, Morgan RF, Edgerton MT. Galeal-pericranial flaps in head and neck reconstruction: anatomy and application. *Am J Surg* 1984;148:489.
35. Jenkins AM, Finucan T. Primary nonmicrosurgical reconstruction following ear avulsion using the temporoparietal fascial island. *Plast Reconstr Surg* 1989;83:148.
36. Lyons GB, Milroy BC, Lendvay PG, Teston LM. Upper lip reconstruction: use of the free superficial temporal artery hair-bearing flap. *Br J Plast Surg* 1989;42:333.
37. Maillard FG, Gumener R, Montandon D. Correction of depressed supratarsal sulcus by an arterial subcutaneous composite flap. *Plast Reconstr Surg* 1984;74:362.

38. McCarthy JG, Cutting CB, Shaw WW. Vascularized calvarial flap. *Clin Plast Surg* 1987;14:37.

39. McCarthy JG, Zido BM. The spectrum of calvarial bone grafting: introduction of the vascularized calvarial bone graft. *Plast Reconstr Surg* 1984;74:10.

40. Mitz V, Peyronie M. The superficial musculoaponeurotic system (SMAS) in the parotid and cheek area. *Plast Reconstr Surg* 1976;58:80.

41. Monks GH. The restoration of a lower lid by a new method. *N Engl J Med* 1898;139:385.

42. Ohmori K. Free scalp flap. *Plast Reconstr Surg* 1980;65:42.

43. Ohmori K. Free scalp flap surgery. *Ann Plast Surg* 1980;5:17.

44. Ohmori S. Reconstruction of microtia using the Silastic frame. *Clin Plast Surg* 1978;5:379.

45. Panje R, Morris MR. The temporoparietal fascial flap in head and neck reconstruction. *Ear Nose Throat J* 1991;70:311.

46. Parkhouse N, Evans D. Reconstruction of the ala of the nose using a composite free flap from the pinna. *Br J Plast Surg* 1985;38:306.

47. Pribaz JJ, Falco N. Nasal reconstruction with auricular microvascular transplant. *Ann Plast Surg* 1993;31:289.

48. Psillakis JM, Grotting JC, Casanova R, Cavalcante D, Vasconez LO. Vascularized outer-table calvarial bone flaps. *Plast Reconstr Surg* 1986;78:309.

49. Rieboung B. Mitz, Lassau JP. Artère temporale superficielle. *Ann Chir Plast Esthet* 1975;20:197.

50. Rose EH, Norris MS. The versatile temporoparietal fascial flap: adaptability to a variety of composite defects. *Plast Reconstr Surg* 1990;85:224.

51. Smet HT. Fascial flaps. In: *Tissue Transfers in Reconstructive Surgery*. Part 2. New York: Raven Press; 1989:51.

52. Smith RA. The free fascial scalp flap. *Plast Reconstr Surg* 1980;66:204.

53. Stock AL, Collins HP, Davidson TM. Anatomy of the superficial temporal artery. *Head Neck* 1980;2:466.

54. Tanaka Y, Tojima S, Tsuijiguchi K, Fukea E, Ohmiya Y. Microvascular reconstruction of the nose and ear defects using composite auricular free flaps. *Ann Plast Surg* 1993;31:298.

55. Tegtmeier RE, Gooding RA. The use of a fascial flap in ear reconstruction. *Plast Reconstr Surg* 1977;60:406.

56. Teichgraeber JF. Temporoparietal fascial flap in orbital reconstruction. *Laryngoscope* 1993;103:931.

57. Tolhurst DE, Carstins MH, Graco RJ, Hurwitz DJ. The surgical anatomy of the scalp. *Plast Reconstr Surg* 1991;87:603.

58. Turpin JM, Altman OI, Cruz G, Acjaver BM. Salvage of the severely injured ear. *Ann Plast Surg* 1988;21:170.

59. Upton J, Rogers C, Durham-Smith G, Swartz W. Clinical applications of free temporoparietal fascial flaps in hand reconstruction. *J Hand Surg [Am]* 1986;11a:475.

15
CHAPTER

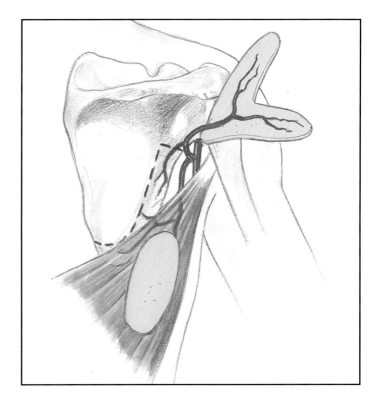

Subscapular System

Michael J. Sullivan, M.D.

The subscapular system of flaps is unique among all available donor sites for free tissue transfer because of the diversity of tissue type, the potential surface area of tissue that can be transferred, and the mobility of the various flaps relative to each other. One of the earliest free flaps that was harvested from the axillary region was the lateral thoracic flap, which is based on the lateral thoracic artery or the accessory lateral thoracic artery (2,4,7). The variability in the vascular anatomy to this flap, in addition to the emergence of the subscapular system of flaps, soon relegated the lateral thoracic flap to one of historical interest only.

The branching pattern of the subscapular artery and vein permits the transfer of the following flaps on a single pedicle (Figure 15-1):

1. Scapular fasciocutaneous flap.
2. Parascapular fasciocutaneous flap.
3. Scapular–parascapular osteofasciocutaneous flap (*e.g.*, angular branch osteocutaneous flap with two pedicles).
4. Latissimus dorsi flap.
5. Latissimus dorsi musculocutaneous flap.
6. Latissimus dorsi rib osteomusculocutaneous flap.
7. Serratus anterior flap.
8. Serratus anterior musculocutaneous flap.
9. Serratus anterior rib flap.

Although the necessity to transfer more than one flap to the head and neck is rare, there are occasions on which this is necessary. Harii et al. (6,8) reported the combi-

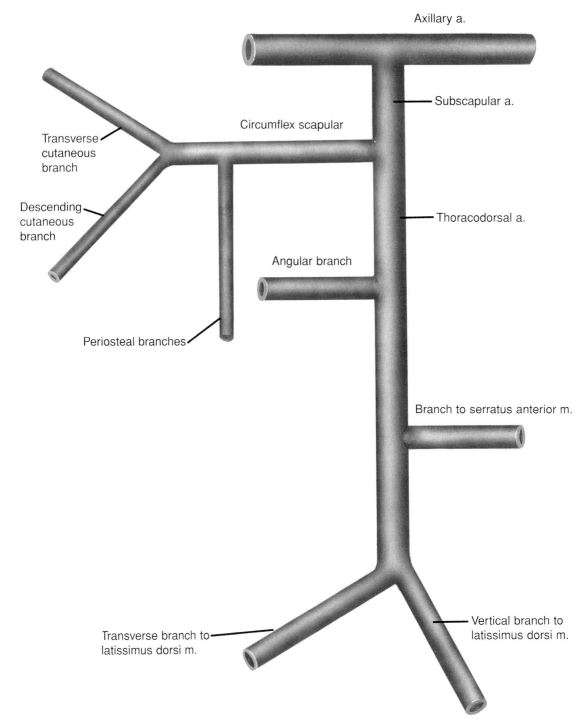

Figure 15-1. The multiple branches of the subscapular artery are the key to understanding the range of flaps with independent pedicles that can be harvested with this system. The subscapular artery divides into the circumflex scapular and the thoracodorsal arteries. The former supplies the periosteum of the lateral scapular border and the scapular and parascapular fasciocutaneous flaps. The thoracodorsal artery gives off the angular branch to the tip of the scapular bone and the muscular branch to the serratus anterior. It terminates in the transverse and vertical branches which supply the latissimus dorsi muscle.

nation of a latissimus dorsi musculocutaneous flap with a serratus anterior musculocutaneous flap to provide inner and outer linings for through-and-through defects of the cheek. In 1984, Batchelor and Tully (3) reported on the resurfacing of a total scalp defect with a single cutaneous flap that included the territories of the scapular, parascapular, latissimus dorsi, and lateral thoracic flaps. In their patient, the thoracodorsal and subscapular arteries had a separate origin and required two arterial anastomoses. Richards (10) used the combination of the latissimus dorsi and the serratus anterior muscles to resurface a scalp and calvarial defect. A vascularized segment of the sixth rib was included with the serratus muscle to reconstruct the superior and lateral orbital rims.

In a large series using the scapular osteocutaneous flap for head and neck reconstruction, Swartz et al. (11) included the latissimus dorsi musculocutaneous flap for reconstruction of a composite defect of the oral cavity. The symphysis was restored with the lateral scapular border, and the floor of mouth was closed with the scapular skin paddle. The latissimus dorsi flap provided coverage of the external cutaneous defect. Similarly, Granick et al. (5) transferred the latissimus dorsi scapular osteocutaneous flap to close a composite defect but skin grafted the latissimus dorsi because of the the bulk of its cutaneous island. These authors also reported that the use of this composite flap with an innervated latissimus dorsi muscle improves lower lip competence. The muscle was suspended from the orbicularis oris on both sides, and the thoracodorsal nerve was anastomosed to the lower division of the facial nerve. The overlying skin of the latissimus dorsi was used to reconstruct the cutaneous defect of the mentum. The restoration of dynamic activity and the degree of oral competence could not be assessed because the patient had an anoxic cerebral injury following surgery.

However, the concept of using the dynamic potential of the latissimus dorsi muscle remains an intriguing one. This is particularly true when reconstructing composite defects of the cheek in which the mimetic muscles are removed but the proximal portion of the facial nerve remains intact. In this situation, a portion of the latissimus dorsi muscle can be inset to restore upward and lateral movement to the corner of the mouth by anastomosing the thoracodorsal nerve to the facial nerve. Complex reconstructions that include the mandible, inner and outer linings, and facial reanimation can be achieved by the transfer of a variety of flaps based on the subscapular pedicle (1).

Composite defects of the midface often provide very complex problems because of the three-dimensional nature of the reconstruction. Replacement of the palate with vascularized bone must often be accompanied by restoring oral lining, nasal lining, and cutaneous defects of the cheek. The freedom to move the multiple soft tissue flaps of the subscapular system relative to the bone has been extremely beneficial (1,9).

The latissimus dorsi and its musculocutaneous flap and the scapular–parascapular fasciocutaneous and osteofasciocutaneous flaps are the most commonly used components of the subscapular system of flaps. In Chapters 16 and 17, these flaps are discussed in detail.

REFERENCES

1. Aviv JE, Urken ML, Vickery C, Weinberg H, Buchbinder D, Biller HF. The combined latissimus dorsi-scapular free flap in head and neck reconstruction. *Arch Otolaryngol Head Neck Surg* 1991;117:1242.
2. Baker S. Free lateral thoracic flap in head and neck reconstruction. *Arch Otolaryngol Head Neck Surg* 1981;107:409.
3. Batchelor A, Tully L. A multiple territory free tissue transfer for reconstruction of a large scalp defect. *Br J Plast Surg* 1984;37:76.
4. Baudet J, Guimberteau JC, Nascimento E. Successful clinical transfer of two free thoracodorsal axillary flaps. *Plast Reconstr Surg* 1976;58:680.
5. Granick MS, Newton ED, Hanna DC. Scapular free flap for repair of massive lower facial composite defects. *Head Neck Surg* 1986;8:436–441.

6. Harii K, Ono I, Ebihara S. Closure of total cheek defects with two combined myocutaneous free flaps. *Arch Otolaryngol Head Neck Surg* 1982;108:303.

7. Harii K, Torii S, Sekiguchi J. The free lateral thoracic flap. *Plast Reconstr Surg* 1978;62:212.

8. Harii K, Yamada A, Ishihara K, Miki Y, Itoh M. A free transfer of both latissimus dorsi and serratus anterior flaps with thoracodorsal vessel anastomosis. *Plast Reconstr Surg* 1982;70:720.

9. Jones N, Hardesty R, Swartz W, Ramasastry S, Heckler F, Newton E. Extensive and complex defects of the scalp, middle third of the face, and palate: the role of microsurgical reconstruction. *Plast Reconstr Surg* 1988;82:937.

10. Richards M. Free composite reconstruction of a complex craniofacial defect. *Aust N Z J Surg* 1987;57:129.

11. Swartz W, Banis J, Newton D, Ramasastry S, Jones N, Acland R. The osteocutaneous scapular flap for mandibular and maxillary reconstruction. *Plast Reconstr Surg* 1986;77:530.

16
CHAPTER

Scapular and Parascapular Fasciocutaneous and Osteofasciocutaneous

Mark L. Urken, M.D. and
Michael J. Sullivan, M.D.

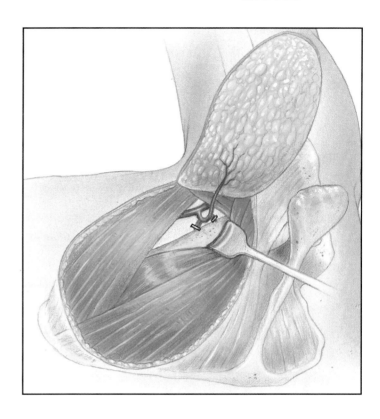

Saijo (20) should be credited with being the first to recognize the potential for transfer of a vascularized cutaneous free flap based on the circumflex scapular artery (CSA) and vein (CSV). Dye-injection studies of the CSA caused staining of the skin overlying the scapula. Saijo hypothesized that separate axial pattern flaps based on the CSA and the thoracodorsal artery and vein could be successfully harvested as free flaps. Lucinda dos Santos (10,11) made significant contributions to our understanding of this donor site through a large series of cadaver dissections and performed the first clinical transfer of a free scapular flap along with Gilbert and Teot (13). The next major milestone in the evolution of this donor site was reported by Teot et al. (25) in 1981 when a series of cadaver dissections demonstrated the area of vascularized bone that could be harvested from the lateral scapular border based on the circumflex scapular pedicle. In addition, they described the various cross-sectional shapes and dimensions of bone that were present at different points along the lateral border from the glenohumeral joint to the tip. The technical aspects of harvesting a composite flap from this region were described along with three successful clinical cases of free scapular osteocutaneous flap transfers that included one case of orbital floor and one case of mandibular reconstruction. The use of this composite flap for head and neck reconstruction was popularized by the work of Swartz et al. (23) in the latter part of the 1980s.

In 1982, Nassif et al. (18) reported a longitudinally oriented skin paddle referred to as the parascapular flap. This fasciocutaneous flap was based on the descending branches of the CSA and CSV. An additional major contribution to the clinical usefulness of this donor site was made by Coleman and Sultan (6) in 1991 who described an alternative vascular supply to the tip of the lateral scapular border through the angular branch of the thoracodorsal artery and vein.

FLAP DESIGN AND UTILIZATION

The unique features that make the scapular system of flaps so useful for head and neck reconstruction are as follows:

1. The long length and large caliber of the vascular pedicle.
2. The abundant surface area of relatively thin skin that can be transferred.
3. The separation of the soft tissue and bone flaps, which provides the most freedom for three-dimensional insetting of any composite free flap.
4. The ability to combine the latissimus dorsi and the serratus anterior muscles, along with overlying skin, and adjacent segments of rib.

The dimensions of the territory supplied by the circumflex scapular pedicle have grown since the earliest description. Based on the results of her dye injection studies, dos Santos (10,11) placed the following limitations on the skin flap supplied by the CSA: 10 cm in the vertical dimension, 13 cm in the horizontal dimension, no further cephalad than the scapular spine, no further caudal than 3 cm above the inferior scapular spine, no further medial than 2 cm from the vertebral column, and no further lateral than the posterior axillary line. Other authors placed similar or even more stringent restrictions (2,14,29). Urbaniak et al. (29) proposed the "rule of twos" to define the skin territory. They advised that the upper limit should be 2 cm inferior to the scapular spine, and the inferior limit should be 2 cm superior to the tip of the scapula. They also limited the medial intent to a point 2 cm lateral to the vertebral processes.

In 1982, Nassif et al. (18) introduced the parascapular flap, which is based on the descending branch of the CSA. This vertical skin paddle, oriented over the lateral scapular border, markedly expanded the dimensions of the cutaneous territory of the CSA (4). Successful parascapular flaps have been reported with lengths up to 25 cm (5). An anatomic study of the dorsal thoracic fascia by Kim et al. (16) provided justification for referring to the scapular and parascapular flaps as fasciocutaneous flaps. Their study also demonstrated rich vascular communications between branches of the CSA and the musculocutaneous perforators of the trapezius and latissimus dorsi, suggesting that much of the skin overlying the latissimus dorsi muscle could be transferred based on the CSA by including the dorsal thoracic fascia. Kim et al. also showed that the CSA runs within the layers of the posterior thoracic fascia, which could therefore be transferred by itself as a thin vascularized tissue layer. De-epithelialized scapular and parascapular flaps have been used extensively for soft tissue augmentation to restore the facial contour in a wide range of disorders, including hemifacial microsomia; atrophy; and deformities caused by radiation, trauma, and ablative cancer surgery (28). The anatomic features of the dorsal thoracic fascia and the transverse and descending branches of the CSA provide the basis for designing multiple skin paddles when needed. Scapular and parascapular skin flaps may be simultaneously transferred based on a single CSA. Alternatively, the dorsal thoracic fascia allows the transfer of multiple skin paddles that are separated by a considerable distance and connected only by this fascial layer (26).

The medial extent of the scapular skin flap has been traditionally limited by the midline of the back. This concept was challenged by Thoma and Hiddle (27) who reported their experience in five patients who required "extended free scapular flaps," which crossed the midline and measured up to 39 cm in length. The basis for their work was a report by Batchelor and Bardsley (3) of a scapula flap with two pedicles that spanned the entire width of the back and was based on the anastomosis of both CSAs. However, after the release of the clamps on the anastomosis of the first CSA and CSV and prior to performing the second set of anastomoses, the entire skin paddle was noted to be well vascularized. The reliability of the extended scapular flap can be examined by invoking the angiosome concept of Taylor and Palmer (24). The vascular anatomy of the back can be separated into longitudinally divided zones based on different source arteries. The regions over each scapula represent the primary angiosomes of the CSA. On either side of the midline, there are two trapezius angiosomes, each supplied by the transverse cervical artery and vein. Hence, as the transverse dimensions of a scapular flap are extended, it is necessary to cross three successive angiosomes (Figure 16-1). Taylor and Palmer suggested that the source artery of a single angiosome can reliably capture the territory of an adjacent angiosome, but that the angiosome once removed (i.e., zone III) is less predictable. The dynamics of the flow across angiosomes through the connecting choke vessels can be altered by prior ligation of the source artery that supplies the adjacent territory. This maneuver essentially produces a delay phenomenon by opening up the choke vessels and achieving a more favorable hemodynamic situation by which to capture more distant angiosomes. It is tempting to speculate that such a delay phenomenon may be achieved when harvesting an extended scapular flap on the side of the back on which a radical neck dissection was previously performed. Prior interruption of the transverse cervical vessels should allow the scapular flap to be more reliably extended across the midline.

Regardless of the design or dimensions of the distal portions of the scapular–parascapular flaps, it is critical that the base of the flap is centered over the infraspinatus fossa, which is the dorsal extent of the triangular space. That space may be found by palpation of the muscular hiatus along the lateral scapular border or by Doppler sonographic localization of the CSA as it emerges from its origin in the axilla. The infraspinatus fossa has been roughly localized to a point either halfway (14) or two fifths of the way (18) along the lateral scapular border when measuring from the spine to the tip (Figure 16-2).

The successful transfer of vascularized bone from the lateral scapular border dramatically expanded the versatility of the subscapular donor site and the range of applications to the head and neck. The length of bone that can be harvested ranges from 10 to 14 cm, depending on the sex and size of the patient (Figures 16-3 and 16-4). It is limited in its cephalad extent by the glenohumeral joint, which must be protected. The variations in thickness of the bone allow it to be used for different purposes in the head and neck. The thin blade of the midportion of the scapula is useful for reconstructing the orbital floor and the palate. The greatest application of this composite flap is in restoring the bone and soft tissue components of oromandibular defects. The periosteal blood supply derived from the CSA permits osteotomies to be made to contour the bone to the shape of the mandible. The vascularity to distal segments is maintained as long as the periosteum and a cuff of muscle are preserved when providing exposure to perform the osteotomy (23). The separation of the scapular and parascapular skin flaps from the bone provides a unique capacity to restore the complex three-dimensional defects of the head and neck. Extensive experience with the composite scapular flap has demonstrated its utility in reconstructing the oral cavity following trauma and ablative surgery (21,22).

Swartz et al. (23) described an extension of the bone harvest along the medial aspect of the scapular tip to provide an additional 3 to 4 cm of bone. However, the blood supply to distal portions of the scapular bone was somewhat suspect, especially after the creation of an osteotomy. This was evident by the findings on postoperative bone scans, the occurrence of nonunions, and the necessity to perform sequestrectomies. In 1991, Coleman and Sultan (6) reported their experimental and clinical findings using a separate vascular supply to the caudal portion of the lateral scapular border based on the angular branch of the thoracodorsal artery and vein (Figure 16-5). They credited Deraemaecher et al. (9) for the initial discovery and report of this branch in

Text continues on page 225.

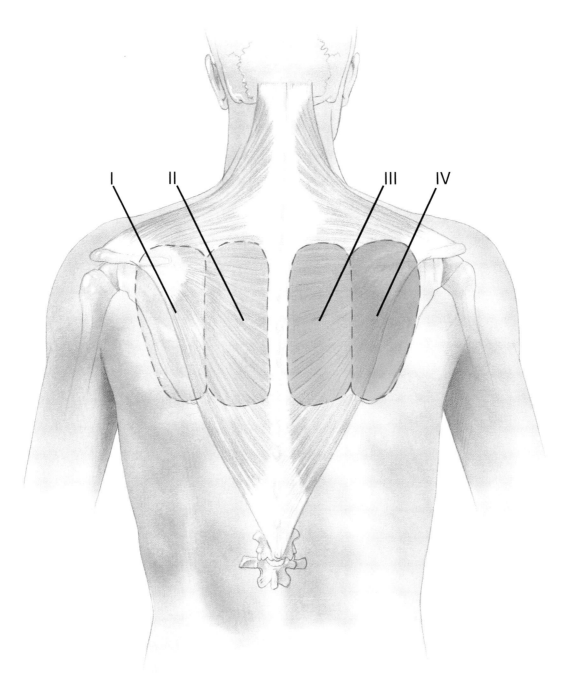

Figure 16-1. The vascular zones of the scapular system have been labeled I through IV. When harvesting a transverse scapular flap based on the left CSA, the skin paddle extends from the primary angiosome (I) into the angiosome of the transverse cervical artery and vein (II). As this transverse flap crosses the midline, the third angiosome in the series, that of the contralateral trapezius flap, is entered (III). Finally, the fourth angiosome in the series is the one primarily supplied by the contralateral CSA (IV). By performing a radical neck dissection on the left side and interrupting the transverse cervical artery, the skin overlying zone II may be partially or totally delayed so as to make it, and the skin of zone III, more reliably captured in the transfer of the left scapular flap.

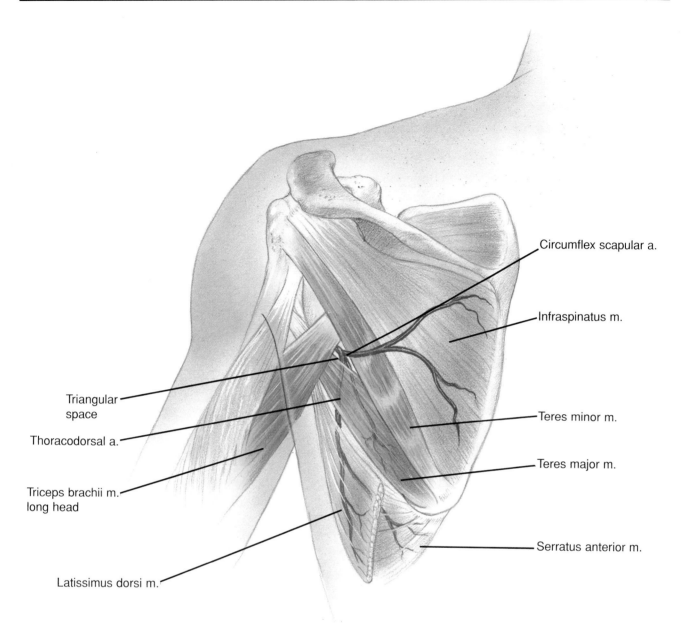

Circumflex scapular a.

Infraspinatus m.

Triangular space

Thoracodorsal a.

Teres minor m.

Teres major m.

Triceps brachii m. long head

Serratus anterior m.

Latissimus dorsi m.

Figure 16-2. The muscles that make up the posterior axillary and scapular region are critical to the understanding of the subscapular system of flaps. The circumflex scapular artery and vein traverse the triangular space before reaching the infraspinatus fossa. The triangular space is bounded by the teres major, teres minor, and the long head of the triceps muscles. The teres minor originates from the upper two thirds of the lateral scapular border and inserts into the greater tuberosity of the humerus. Its action is opposite to that of the teres major, which arises from the inferior aspect of the lateral scapular border and inserts into the bicipital groove of the humerus. The terminal branches of the CSA anastomose with the suprascapular and transverse cervical vessels.

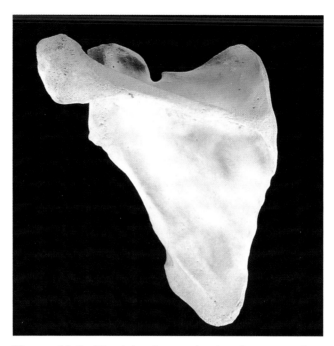

Figure 16-3. The lateral scapular border, extending from the glenohumeral joint to the scapular tip, may be transferred as a vascularized bone flap based on the CSA and CSV. The thick bicortical bone of the lateral border becomes markedly thinner in the midsection of the blade of the scapula. Approximately 10 to 14 cm in length can be harvested from the lateral border. The bone cuts may be extended to include the inferomedial border.

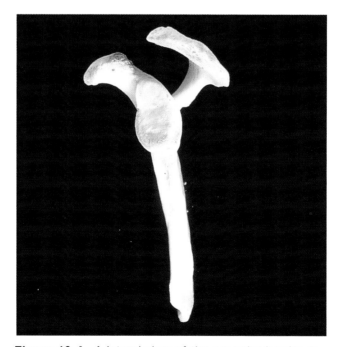

Figure 16-4. A lateral view of the scapular border reveals that the bone is fairly straight. Contouring of this bone to fit the shape of bone defects in the maxillomandibular skeleton requires ostectomies to be performed, while preserving the nutrient periosteal layer.

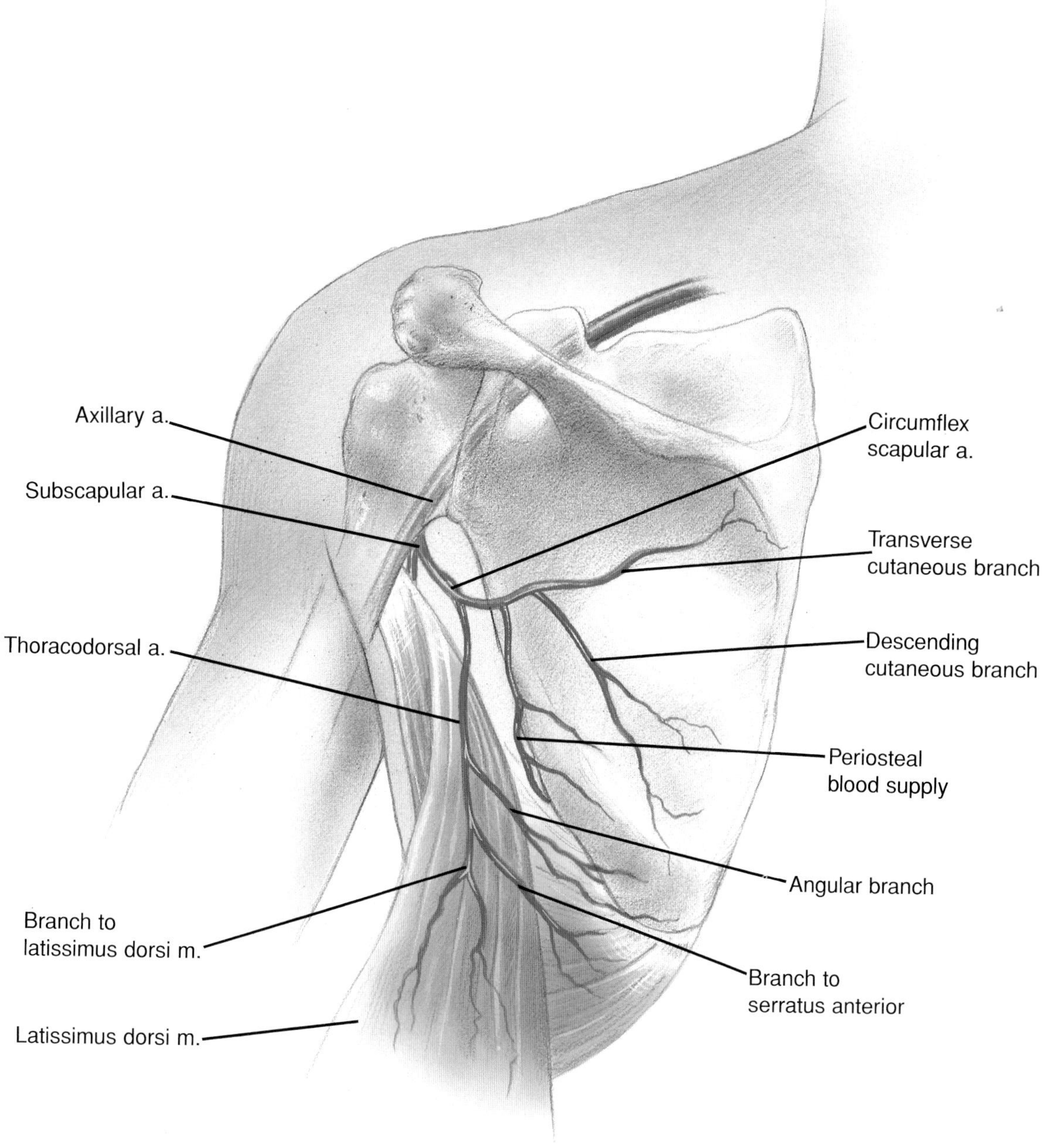

Figure 16-5. With the overlying muscles removed, the blood supply to the scapular bone is shown arising from periosteal feeders of the CSA that supply the upper portions of the lateral scapula and the angular branch that supplies the periosteum of the caudal scapular border.

A.

B.

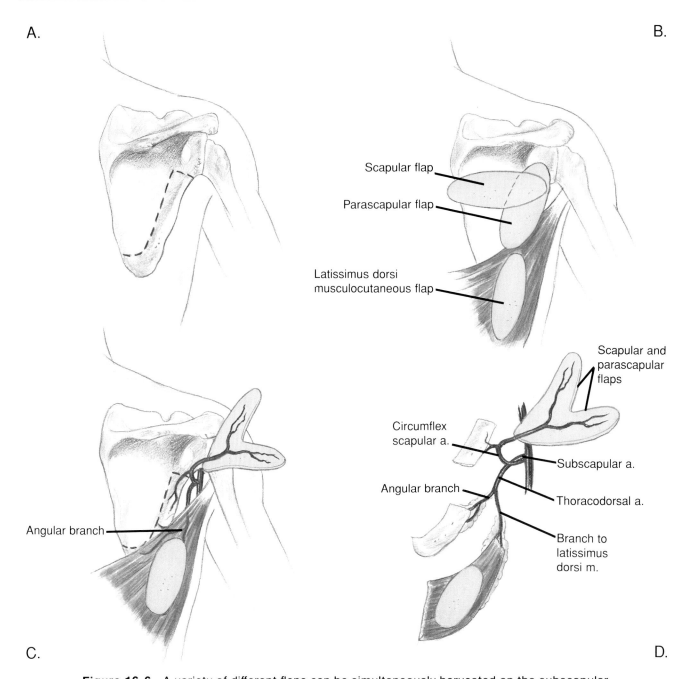

Scapular flap

Parascapular flap

Latissimus dorsi
musculocutaneous flap

Scapular and
parascapular
flaps

Circumflex
scapular a.

Subscapular a.

Angular branch

Thoracodorsal a.

Angular branch

Branch to
latissimus
dorsi m.

C.

D.

Figure 16-6. A variety of different flaps can be simultaneously harvested on the subscapular artery and vein. **A:** The bone of the lateral scapular border can be transferred with a small cuff of muscle for pure bony reconstructions. The caudal tip can be used to reconstruct the angle of the mandible. Alternatively, the thin central portion of the bone can be used as a shelf to replace the hard palate. **B:** The most common varieties of subscapular soft tissue flaps are shown. These flaps can be harvested separately or in concert. In addition, the serratus anterior muscle and musculocutaneous flaps can be included with this vascular axis. **C:** The bone of the lateral scapular border can be divided on two separate vascular pedicles: the circumflex scapular and the angular. A scapular–parascapular cutaneous flap has been reflected to show the periosteal vascular supply. **D:** The multiple different soft tissue and osseous components that can be harvested on the subscapular system are shown. Intramuscular bifurcation of the thoracodorsal artery allows splitting of the latissimus dorsi muscle. Both the latissimus dorsi and the serratus anterior muscles can be transferred with their nerve supply for restoration of dynamic motor activity.

1988. The identification of a separate blood supply to the tip of the scapula is important for a number of reasons.

1. Osteotomies can be made in the lateral scapula without concern about devascularization of the distal bone because of the preservation of the angular branch.
2. Two separate segments of bone with their own vascular supply can be used to reconstruct bone defects that are separated in space.
3. The tip of the scapula can be transferred alone without requiring the intervening bone of the lateral scapula. The tip provides an excellent shape to reconstruct the hard palate.
4. Maximum separation between the soft and hard tissues can be achieved by transferring a scapular or parascapular flap based on the CSA and a segment of bone supplied by the angular branch. These two components may be separated by as much as 15 cm. This contrasts with the 2.5 cm that separates the skin and bone segments when transferring both on the CSA (Figure 16-6).

Coleman and Sultan (6) reported the successful transfer of segments of the scapula measuring up to 8 cm in length. They used the osteocutaneous flap with two pedicles to advance the symphysis in a patient with a hypoplastic mandible by performing bilateral mandibular osteotomies and inserting two vascularized bone segments to maintain the advanced symphysis. They also reported using the scapular tip to reconstruct the orbital floor. We have had experience in using the scapular tip supplied by the angular branch to reconstruct partial and total hard palate defects.

Thoma et al. (26) transferred the medial scapular border, based on the CSA's supply of the dorsal thoracic fascia. The vascularity of this segment of bone is entirely dependent on preserving the fascial attachments to it. The rationale for designing this composite flap is that it lengthens the vascular pedicle to the bone and avoids disruption of the muscular attachments to the lateral scapula. The disadvantages of this flap are that the bone of the medial scapular border is thinner than that of the lateral border, the relationship of the bone to the undersurface of the skin must be maintained to preserve the fascial blood supply, and the tolerance of this bone to contouring through osteotomies is uncertain.

NEUROVASCULAR ANATOMY

The parent vessels of the scapular flap are the subscapular artery and vein, which arise from the third part of the axillary artery and vein (Figure 16-6). However, depending on the length of the vascular leash that is required, the CSA and CSV may also be used, thereby, preserving the vascular supply to the latissimus dorsi through the thoracodorsal vessels. The CSA runs through the triangular space where it supplies muscular branches to the teres major and minor and the periosteal branches to the lateral border of the scapula. The CSA terminates in the transverse and descending cutaneous branches that supply the scapular and parascapular fasciocutaneous flaps. In its course, the CSA is accompanied by paired venae comitantes. These two veins are usually different sizes, with the larger having a diameter in the range of 2.5 to 4.0 mm. In the majority of cases, the two venae comitantes join with the thoracodorsal vein. In approximately 10% of cases, the CSV enters the axillary vein separate from the thoracodorsal vein. The average diameter of the CSA at its origin from the subscapular artery is 4 mm (range, 2 to 6 mm). At its origin from the axillary artery, the subscapular artery has an average diameter of 6 mm (range, 4 to 8 mm) (19). Dos Santos (11) reported the diameter of the CSA to be slightly smaller (average, 2.8 mm).

As noted previously, the vascular pedicle length varies depending on the extent of proximal dissection. If only the cutaneous branch of the CSA is used, then a pedicle length of 4 to 6 cm is obtained. When the CSA is harvested at its takeoff from the subscapular vessels, then the fasciocutaneous flaps have a pedicle length of 7 to 10 cm. A maximum pedicle length in the range of 11 to 14 cm is obtained by transsecting the subscapular vessels at their junction with the axillary artery and vein (18).

The CSA and CSV run in the fascial septum between the teres major and minor, and then they divide into the transverse and descending branches, which run in the fascial layers and send perforators to the overlying skin and subcutaneous tissue (7). As noted previously, this fascial plexus spreads out over the adjoining muscles and communicates with the musculocutaneous perforators of the latissimus dorsi and trapezius muscles (16).

Coleman and Sultan (6) reported that the angular branch to the tip of the scapula was present in 100% of the cadaver dissections and clinical cases. The angular branch arose from the thoracodorsal artery just proximal to the serratus anterior branch in 58% of cases. In the remaining 42%, it arose from the crossing branch of the thoracodorsal artery to the serratus anterior. In its course toward the scapular tip, the angular branch supplies small feeders to the subscapularis and the serratus anterior muscles prior to its terminal arborization, which supplies the periosteum at a point about 3 cm cephalad to the inferior scapular border. Differentiation of the two patterns of origin of the angular branch is not critical in the flap harvest. Following identification of the CSA, the angular branch is easily isolated by opening the plane between the teres major and the latissimus dorsi. The teres major is then transsected, leaving a small cuff attached to the scapula. The course of the angular branch can then be readily traced (22).

The standard posterior approach to the subscapular pedicle involves working through the triangular space or with the added exposure afforded by transsecting the teres major. An alternative route to the proximal portion of the pedicle involves a counter incision in the axilla that permits a direct visualization of the thoracodorsal, angular, and subscapular vessels. In addition, this maneuver allows the flap to be delivered into the axilla without interrupting the vascular supply during closure of the donor site (12).

The cutaneous nerve supply to the scapular region is derived from the dorsal rami of the spinal nerves. Following an extensive review of the literature, there were no reported cases of a successful sensate scapula or parascapular flap, although Upton et al. (28) noted two unsuccessful cases following the anastomosis of the dorsal rami.

ANATOMIC VARIATIONS

There has been no reports in which the CSA has not been identified in the triangular space. There was some variability in the course of the descending branch of the CSA that supplies the parascapular flap. In 7 of 30 dissections, the descending branch assumed a course that was deep to the teres major and ascended to the fascial layer to supply the skin by running in the plane between the teres major and latissimus dorsi muscle. Upton et al. (28) reported on two clinical cases involving this variant and detached the teres major to maintain continuity of the vascular supply to the parascapular skin. Because of the rich vascularity to the dorsal thoracic fascia, it is unclear that such a maneuver and the integrity of the descending branch are critical to successful parascapular flap transfer.

In a series of 100 cadaver dissections, Rowsell et al. (19) reported that the subscapular artery arose from the axillary artery in 97% of cases. In 81%, it arose from the third part, and in 13%, it was a branch of the second part. In 3%, the subscapular artery arose from the first part, and in 3%, it was absent. In the latter group, the CSA was a direct branch of the axillary artery. Hitzrot (15) divided the branching pattern of the axillary artery into seven different types based on 47 cadaver dissections. He did not report any cases in which the thoracodorsal artery and CSA had a separate origin from the axillary artery. However, in two cases, a large subscapular artery provided the origin for the acromiothoracic trunk, in addition to the usual branches. DeGaris and Swartley (8) performed a much more extensive study of 512 axillary artery dissections and divided the branching patterns into 23 different groups. They noted a common trunk of the subscapular and thoracoacromial arteries in 4.5% of the dissections. A separate origin for the thoracodorsal artery and CSA was rare, noted in 0.8% of cases. In a third anatomic series of 50 dissections, Bartlett et al. (1) reported this variant as occurring with an incidence of 4%. The presence of double CSAs was noted in 8% of cases.

Variations in the venous anatomy are much more common. Separate origins for the CSA and the thoracodorsal vein from the axillary vein were reported to occur in 12% of dissections (1).

POTENTIAL PITFALLS

There are a variety of complications that have been reported in harvesting flaps based on the subscapular vascular system. The potential morbidity to the brachial plexus as a result of arm position during flap harvest is discussed in detail in Chapter 17. Similarly, uncertainty regarding the integrity of the vascular supply in a patient who had undergone prior axillary node dissection would contraindicate against the use of this donor site.

The bone stock of the lateral scapular border is fairly limited when considering placement of endosteal implants for dental rehabilitation. The most favorable quantity of bone is obtained from the caudal aspect of the lateral scapula, and thus, this must be incorporated into the strategy of graft orientation in mandibular reconstruction (17). Particular caution is advised when making the cephalad bone cuts along the lateral scapular border to be certain to stay 1 cm below the glenoid fossa to avoid injury to the joint space.

A variety of muscles in the axilla may be disrupted in the process of harvesting an osteocutaneous scapular flap. Perhaps the most significant of these is the teres major, which is usually detached in whole or in part from its origin to the scapula. In addition, the technique of flap harvest may lead to denervation and devascularization of this muscle. The teres major is an internal rotator, extensor, and adductor of the arm. There is some uncertainty as to whether shoulder function is affected by reattaching the teres major by placing drill holes through the remaining scapular bone. Although reattachment would help to anchor the scapula and prevent winging, a scarred, denervated, fibrotic muscle may actually limit the range of motion of the arm. If there is concern for the vascularity of the teres major at the end of the procedure, it should be excised rather than risk a wound infection as a result of muscle necrosis (6).

The aesthetic appearance of the donor site is usually related to the amount of skin that is removed. Widened scars are not uncommon when large cutaneous flaps are required. A skin graft placed on the back to close this donor site is less favorable and should be avoided by judicious planning. Pretransfer expansion of the scapular region was reported for unusual circumstances (28).

POSTOPERATIVE CARE

The shoulder disability following the harvest of flaps from the scapular region is related to the nature of the tissue that is removed. The use of the scapular and parascapular flaps alone is unlikely to produce significant morbidity. Postoperative rehabilitation is indicated in patients who undergo osteocutaneous flap harvest. Following 3 to 4 days of immobilizing the arm against the trunk, active and passive range-of-motion exercises are begun. A program for strengthening the muscles of the shoulder girdle should be instituted within 2 to 3 weeks after surgery and monitored by a physical therapist on an outpatient basis.

Flap Harvesting Technique follows on page 228.

Flap Harvesting Technique

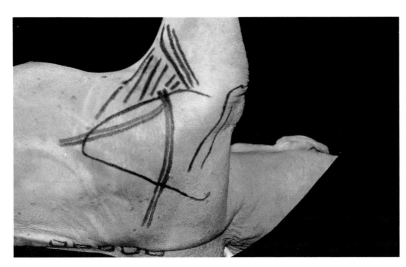

Figure 16-7. The topographic anatomy is outlined on the upper lateral back. The medial and lateral border of the scapula are outlined in black. The muscular triangle anterior to the lateral border of the scapula is composed of the teres major, teres minor, and the long head of the triceps. This triangle can be identified by palpation or Doppler ultrasonography of the CSA. The approximate course of the transverse and descending branches of the CSA is drawn.

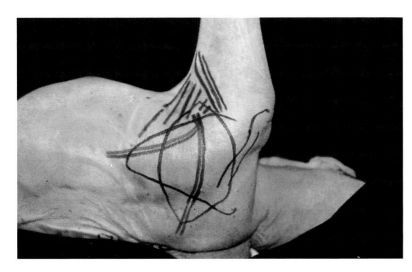

Figure 16-8. The entire arm and shoulder are prepared into the operative field to allow for shoulder mobility during the dissection to improve visualization of the vessels in the axilla. Patients are positioned on their sides with an angulation of approximately 45 degrees. In most cases, this position accommodates both the ablative and reconstructive team. An axillary roll must be placed under the contralateral axilla. A transverse scapular flap has been drawn.

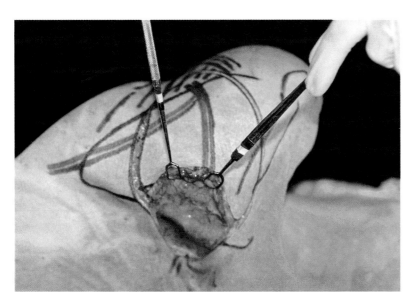

Figure 16-9. The dissection proceeds in a medial to lateral direction. The initial incisions are made through the skin and subcutaneous tissue to the deep fascia overlying the rhomboid and infraspinatus musculature.

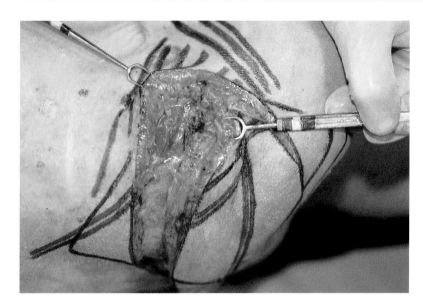

Figure 16-10. The teres major is an important landmark. Careful sharp and blunt dissection along the upper border of this muscle advances the dissection into the muscular triangle.

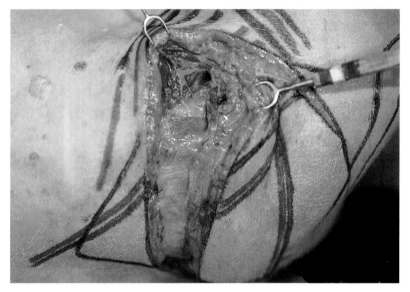

Figure 16-11. The circumflex scapular vessels are easily palpated as they course onto the undersurface of the flap. Branches from the pedicle to the teres major must be ligated.

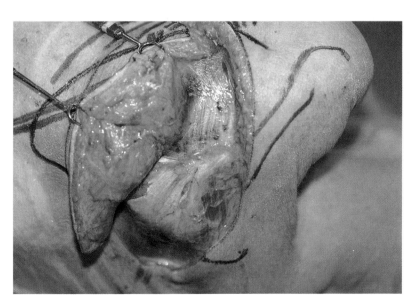

Figure 16-12. The superior incision has been made. The flap is elevated off the deltoid and the teres minor. As the dissection proceeds along the inferior border of the teres minor the CSA and CSV are again visualized.

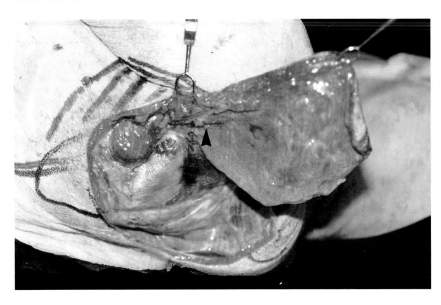

Figure 16-13. As the scapular flap is elevated on its pedicle, care is taken to preserve a cuff of soft tissue attachment of the cutaneous paddle to the fascia of the infraspinatus along the lateral scapular border. The CSA and CSV (*arrow*) are easily visualized on the undersurface of the scapular flap.

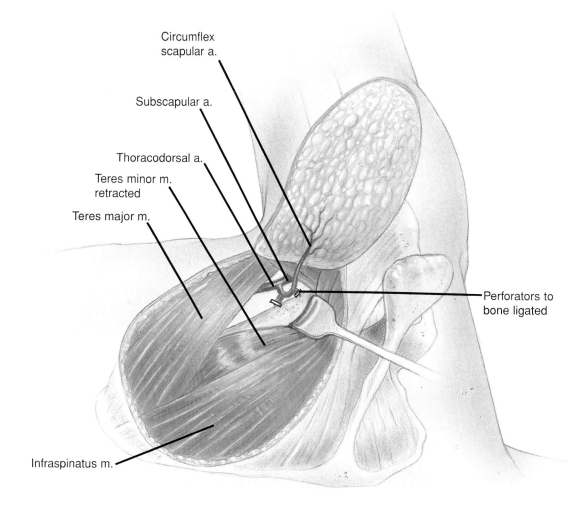

Figure 16-14. The anatomy of the muscular triangle reveals the thoracodorsal artery continuing in its caudal course and the CSA supplying the scapular skin paddle. This illustration shows the periosteal perforators transsected, which must be done if a fasciocutaneous flap without bone is harvested.

Thoracodorsal a.

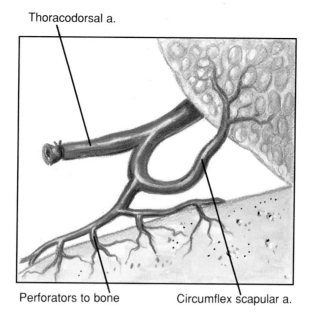

Perforators to bone   Circumflex scapular a.

Figure 16-15. When the bone of the lateral scapula is to be harvested, the periosteal feeders must be preserved. This blood supply to the bone is never skeletonized to the extent shown in this illustration.

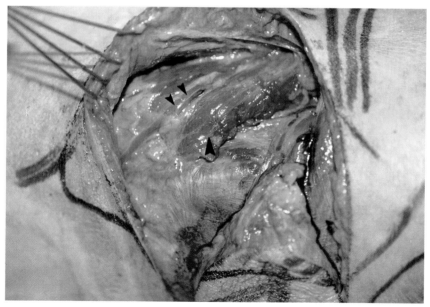

Figure 16-16. The harvest of a composite osteocutaneous flap requires transsection of the teres major (*large arrow*) from the lateral scapular border. A cuff of this muscle is left attached to the bone to protect the periosteal blood supply. The inferior border of the teres major must be separated from the latissimus dorsi (*small arrows*).

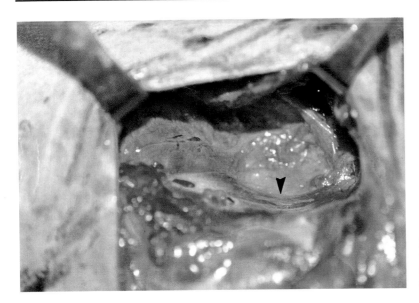

Figure 16-17. Following transsection of the teres major, the thoracodorsal (*arrow*), angular, and proximal circumflex scapular vessels can be visualized.

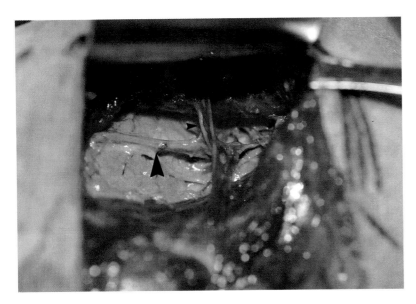

Figure 16-18. With the cut edge of the teres major and the long head of the triceps retracted, the vascular anatomy of the axilla is well visualized. The descending course of the thoracodorsal system is easily seen (*large arrow*). The primary neurovascular pedicle to the teres major (*small arrow*) must usually be transsected to allow further dissection in the axilla.

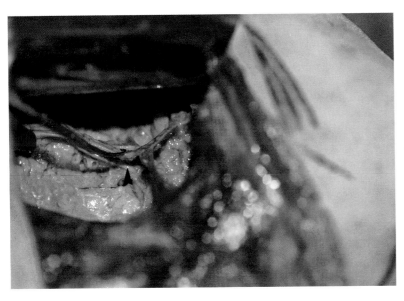

Figure 16-19. The thoracodorsal pedicle must be ligated (*arrow*) and transsected to extend the dissection proximally to the subscapular vessels. The surgeon would not take this step in the dissection if (a) the latissimus dorsi or the angular branch supply to the scapula were to be included in the dissection or (b) the CSA and CSV were of sufficient caliber and length for anastomosis to the recipient vessels. Following division of the thoracodorsal pedicle, the dissection can proceed to the subscapular artery and vein.

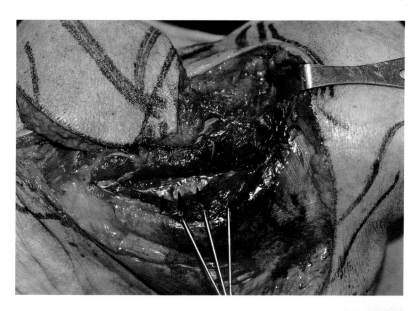

Figure 16-20. Access to the bone to make the osteotomies is achieved by dividing the infraspinatus muscle in a longitudinal direction (*arrows*), leaving a 2- to 3-cm cuff attached to the lateral border. Several muscular branches to this muscle are encountered, which must be ligated and divided.

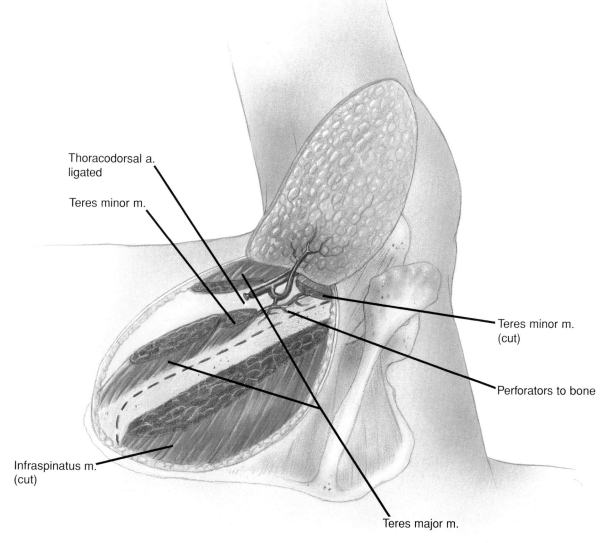

Thoracodorsal a. ligated

Teres minor m.

Teres minor m. (cut)

Perforators to bone

Infraspinatus m. (cut)

Teres major m.

Figure 16-21. The *dotted line* shows the osteotomy that is made to harvest bone from the lateral scapular border. Care must be taken when making the superior transverse cut so that the glenohumeral joint is not violated.

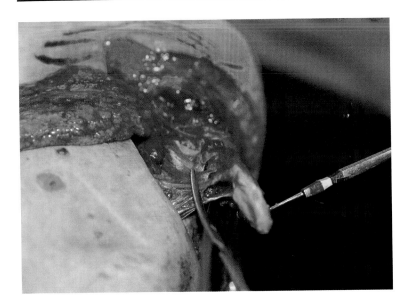

Figure 16-22. This view is taken from the vantage point of the iliac crest looking cephalad toward the scapula following the osteotomy. The subscapularis must be divided, leaving a small cuff of muscle attached to the bone.

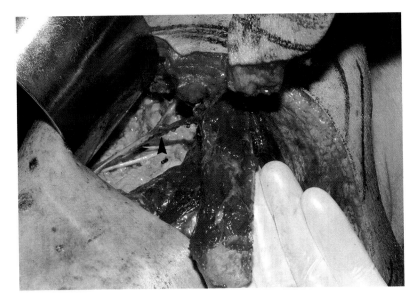

Figure 16-23. In the cephalad portion of the lateral scapular dissection, the CSA and CSV (*arrow*) must be directly visualized while making the final releasing cuts of the subscapularis.

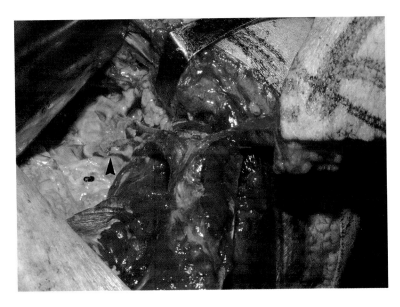

Figure 16-24. With the osteocutaneous flap completely isolated, except for its nutrient supply, the remainder of the dissection along the subscapular vessels can be performed. After this is completed, the vascular pedicle (*arrow*) is transsected. Care is taken during the course of this dissection to avoid injury to the thoracodorsal nerve.

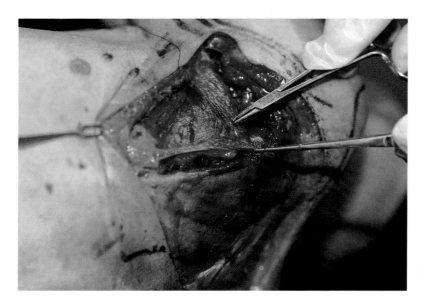

Figure 16-25. Closure of the donor site is accomplished by drilling holes in the lateral scapular border and then reattaching the cut end of the teres major.

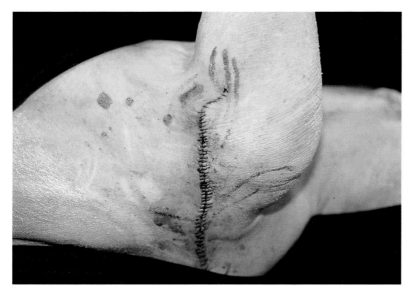

Figure 16-26. Wide undermining of the skin is required to bring the skin edges together for a tension-free closure. Both deep and superficial suction drains are usually placed.

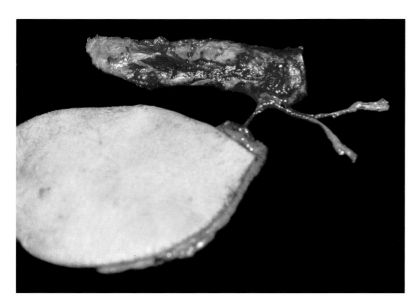

Figure 16-27. The osteocutaneous scapular flap has been harvested. The length of the circumflex scapular and subscapular pedicle is noted as is the freedom of movement of the skin relative to the bone.

REFERENCES

1. Bartlett SP, May JW, Yaremchuk MJ. The latissimus dorsi muscle. A fresh cadaver study of the primary neurovascular pedicle. *Plast Reconstr Surg* 1981;67:631.
2. Barwick W, Goodkind D, Serafin D. The free scapular flap. *Plast Reconstr Surg* 1982;69:779.
3. Batchelor A, Bardsley A. The bi-scapular flap. *Br J Plast Surg* 1987;40:510.
4. Chandrasekhar B, Lorant J, Terz J. Parascapular free flaps for head and neck reconstruction. *Am J Surg* 1990;160:450.
5. Chiu D, Sherman J, Edgerton B. Coverage of the calvarium with a free parascapular flap. *Ann Plast Surg* 1984;12:60.
6. Coleman J, Sultan M. The bipedicled osteocutaneous scapula flap: a new subscapular system free flap. *Plast Reconstr Surg* 1991;87:682.
7. Cormack G, Lamberty B. The anatomical vascular basis of the axillary fasciocutaneous pedicled flap. *Br J Plast Surg* 1983;36:425.
8. DeGaris C, Swartley W. The axillary artery in white and Negro stocks. *Am J Anat* 1928;41:353.
9. Deraemaecher R, Thienen CV, Lejour M, Dor P. The serratus anterior-scapular free flaps: a new osteomuscular unit for reconstruction after radical head and neck surgery (abstract). In: *Proceedings of the Second International Conference on Head and Neck Cancer.* 1988.
10. dos Santos LF. Retalho escapular: um novo retalho livre microcirurgico. *Bras Cir* 1980;70:133.
11. dos Santos LF. The vascular anatomy and dissection of the free scapular flap. *Plast Reconstr Surg* 1984;73:599.
12. Gabhos F, Tross R, Salomon J. Scapular free flap dissection made easier. *Plast Reconstr Surg* 1985;75:115.
13. Gilbert A, Teot L. The free scapular flap. *Plast Reconstr Surg* 1982;69:601.
14. Hamiton S, Morrison W. The scapular free flap. *Br J Plast Surg* 1982;35:2.
15. Hitzrot J. A composite study of axillary artery in man. *Johns Hopkins Bull* 1901;12:136.
16. Kim P, Gottlieb J, Harris G, Nagle D, Lewis V. The dorsal thoracic fascia: anatomic significance with clinical applications in reconstructive microsurgery. *Plast Reconstr Surg* 1987;79:72.
17. Moscoso J, Keller J, Genden E, Weinberg H, Biller HF, Buchbinder D, Urken ML. Vascularized bone flaps in oromandibular reconstruction: a comparative anatomic study of bone stock from various donor sites to assess suitability for enosseous dental implants. *Arch Otolaryngol Head Neck Surg* 1994;120:36.
18. Nassif TM, Vidal L, Bovet JL, Baudet J. The parascapular flap: a new cutaneous microsurgical free flap. *Plast Reconstr Surg* 1982;69:591.
19. Rowsell A, Davies M, Eisenberg N, Taylor GI. The anatomy of the subscapular thoracodorsal arterial system: study of 100 cadaver dissections. *Br J Plast Surg* 1984;37:374.
20. Saijo M. The vascular territories of the dorsal trunk: a reappraisal for potential flap donor sites. *Br J Plast Surg* 1978;31:200.
21. Sullivan M, Baker S, Crompton R, Smith-Wheelock M. Free scapular osteocutaneous flap for mandibular reconstruction. *Arch Otolaryngol Head Neck Surg* 1989;115:1334.
22. Sullivan MJ, Carroll WR, Baker SR. The cutaneous scapular free flap in head and neck reconstruction. *Arch Otolaryngol Head Neck Surg* 1990;116:600.
23. Swartz W, Banis J, Newton D, Ramasastry S, Jones N, Acland R. The osteocutaneous scapular flap for mandibular and maxillary reconstruction. *Plast Reconstr Surg* 1986;77:530.
24. Taylor GI, Palmer J. The vascular territories (angiosomes) of the body: experimental study and clinical applications. *Br J Plast Surg* 1987;40:113.
25. Teot L, Bosse JP, Moufarrege R, Papillon J, Beuregard G. The scapular crest pedicled bone graft. *Int J Microsurg* 1981;3:257.
26. Thoma A, Archibald I, Payk I, Young J. The free medial scapular osteofasciocutaneous flap for head and neck reconstruction. *Br J Plast Surg* 1991;44:477.
27. Thoma A, Hiddle S. The extended free scapular flap. *Br J Plast Surg* 1990;43:712.
28. Upton J, Albin R, Mulliken J, Murray J. The use of scapular and parascapular flaps for cheek reconstruction. *Plast Reconstr Surg* 1992;90:959.
29. Urbaniak J, Komar A, Goldman R, Armstrong N, Nunley J. The vascularized cutaneous scapular flap. *Plast Reconstr Surg* 1982;69:772.

17

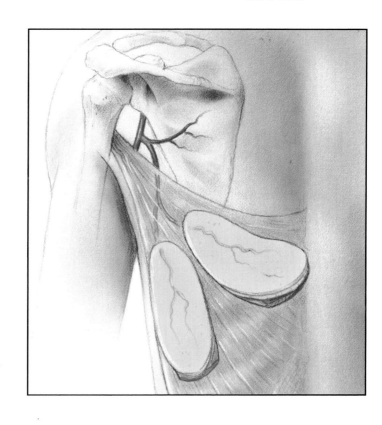

Latissimus Dorsi

Mark L. Urken, M.D. and
Michael J. Sullivan, M.D.

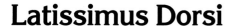

The latissimus dorsi flap was the first musculocutaneous flap described in the medical literature. Tansini (50) reported this technique for chest wall reconstruction following radical mastectomy in 1896. There followed a number of other publications that reported using the latissimus dorsi musculocutaneous flap for primary reconstruction of the postmastectomy defect and the prevention of lymphedema in the ipsilateral arm (9,20). This technique remained buried in the medical literature until the 1970s when it was resurrected by Olivari (34,35) for chest wall reconstruction. More extensive series by Bostwick et al. (5) and Maxwell et al. (31) demonstrated the safety and the reliability of this reconstructive technique.

Quillen et al. (38) are credited with being the first to use the pedicled latissimus dorsi musculocutaneous flap for head and neck reconstruction in 1978. Subsequent reports by Quillen (37) and Barton et al. (4) established the latissimus dorsi musculocutaneous flap as a front-line reconstructive technique for head and neck defects. In 1979, Watson et al. (56) reported the first successful microvascular transfer of a free latissimus flap. The length and caliber of the neurovascular pedicle, the ease of dissection, the large surface area, and the minimal donor site morbidity are the major factors that explain the popularity of this donor site for the transfer of tissue as a pedicled or free flap to the head and neck region.

The latissimus dorsi is a broad flat muscle that covers a large portion of the lower back. It arises from the spinous processes of the lower six thoracic vertebrae and from the thoracolumbar fascia, which attaches to the lumbar and sacral vertebrae (Figure 17-1). Laterally, it arises from the fascia that is attached to the iliac crest. The latissimus also arises from the lower four ribs, where its fibers coalesce with those of the

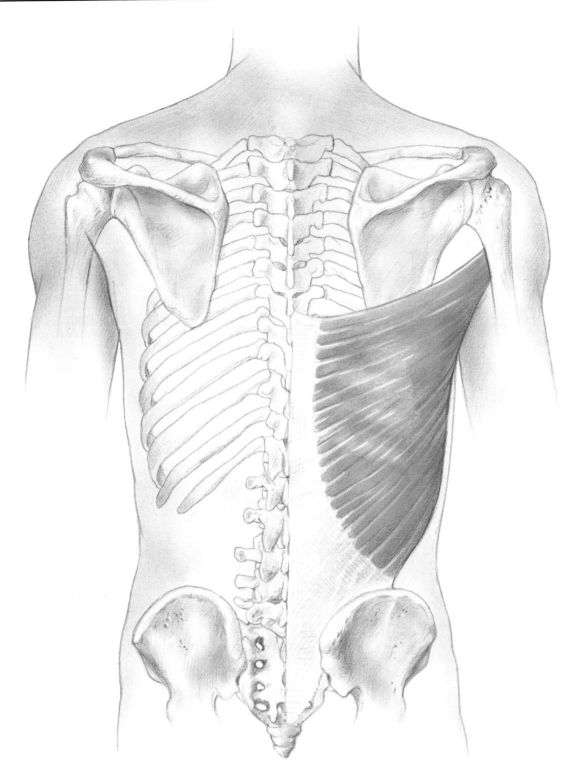

Figure 17-1. The latissimus dorsi muscle covers the entire lower back from the iliac crest to the lower border of the scapula. It arises from the lower six thoracic vertebrae, the thoracolumbar fascia, and the iliac crest. Its free upper border overlaps the inferior angle of the scapula. It forms the posterior axillary fold and then inserts on the medial surface of the humerus.

external oblique muscle. In its upper medial portion, the latissimus is overlapped by the caudal fibers of the trapezius muscle. As it passes laterally and cephalad, the free edge of the latissimus overlies the tip of the scapula, from which it may also take a minor origin. The converging fibers of the latissimus dorsi spiral around the caudal border of the teres major to insert on the medial surface of the humerus. Along with the teres major, the tendon of the latissimus dorsi forms the posterior axillary fold and they insert in close proximity along the intertubercular groove of the humerus.

The major actions of the latissimus dorsi are to adduct, inwardly rotate, and extend the arm. These actions are most easily visualized in the completion of the arm motion performed in the free-style swimming stroke. Through its attachments to the caudal tip of the scapula, the latissimus also stabilizes the scapula and prevents its superior and lateral displacement. This action is most easily visualized in the climbing motion when the arms are raised above the head and the trunk is pulled upward and forward. Following transfer of a latissimus dorsi flap, its major muscular actions are said to be well compensated by the other muscles that act across the glenohumeral joint. However, progressive morbidity to the shoulder occurs when sacrifice of the latissimus dorsi is combined with loss of either the trapezius muscle, following radical neck dissection, or the pectoralis major. This issue is discussed in detail later in this chapter.

FLAP DESIGN AND UTILIZATION

The latissimus dorsi may be used as either a free or pedicled flap. As a pedicled flap, one can reach virtually any site on the head and neck by passing the flap through the axilla between the pectoralis minor and major. The arc of rotation may be improved by exteriorizing the pedicle, which allows the flap to reach most areas of the scalp (29). Excision of the intervening muscle is performed following a delay of several weeks. The arc of rotation of the pedicled latissimus dorsi flap is also enhanced by several maneuvers. Transsection of the branches to the serratus anterior prevents tethering of the thoracodorsal pedicle. Friedrich et al. (12) advised that additional length could also be achieved through division of the circumflex scapular branch. However, others caution that preservation of this branch helps to prevent kinking of the pedicle as it traverses the axilla from posteriorly to anteriorly (4,29). Barton et al. (4) also speculated that the intact circumflex scapular vessels provided collateral flow to the latissimus dorsi. Transsection of the tendon of the latissimus dorsi provides a considerable amount of additional freedom and markedly improves the arc of rotation. Designing the skin paddle over the caudal portion of the muscle also helps to improve the flap's reach. However, the density of the perforators in this region is diminished, and therefore, the blood supply to the skin is more tenuous. Quillen (37) reported a delay procedure to enhance the reliability of the distal muscle and skin, that involved a staged division of the intercostal perforators that run from the chest wall to the deep surface of the muscle approximately 1 week prior to flap transfer.

The dimensions of the total area covered by the latissimus dorsi is in the range of 25 to 40 cm. The maximum size of the skin paddle that can be transferred is limited by the patient's body habitus and the surgeon's ability to achieve primary closure. Although less satisfactory, donor-site closure with a skin graft has been successfully accomplished (35). The reliability of skin paddles designed over different regions of the territory of the latissimus dorsi varies and is discussed later in this chapter. Transfer of the latissimus dorsi muscle with a skin graft provides an alternative solution to the problem of covering massive defects of the head and neck while still achieving primary closure. This technique has been used extensively in reconstruction of the scalp (13).

The latissimus dorsi is one of the thinnest muscles in the body. Denervation atrophy produces an even thinner flap. Primary "thinning" of this muscle has been reported in the reconstruction of the forehead. The location of the vascular pedicle on the deep surface of the muscle permits the superficial muscle layers to be removed prior to coverage with a skin graft (40). Hayashi and Maruyama (19) described the "reduced" latissimus dorsi musculocutaneous flap in which a proximal skin paddle overlying the muscle is transferred with a "reduced" distal fasciocutaneous unit. The blood supply to the fasciocutaneous segments, which measured up to 12 cm in length, was derived from the fascial, subcutaneous, and subdermal vascular plexuses. The authors also transferred cutaneous extension flaps from the region anterior to the border of the muscle. The concept of a reduced flap is an outgrowth of the observation reported by Barton et al. (4) that, although skin islands overlying the distal muscle were unreliable, this territory could be successfully transferred when designed as an extension of a superior skin island. This phenomenon is presumably the result of the capture of the more plentiful musculocutaneous perforators in that location.

The skin overlying the thoracolumbar aponeurosis is notoriously unreliable. However, this fascial sheath may be used in head and neck reconstruction for any number of purposes. Smith et al. (48) described resurfacing a composite defect of the scalp and skull in which the thoracolumbar fascia was used to patch a dural defect and the musculocutaneous unit was used to replace the scalp.

Harii et al. (15) introduced a further modification of this donor site in an effort to increase the surface area and the reach of the transferred skin territory. They described a combined pedicled musculocutaneous and microvascular free flap in which the latissimus dorsi flap was combined with a conventional groin flap. The blood supply to the upper portion of this skin was derived from the thoracodorsal vessels; the groin skin was perfused by either the superficial inferior epigastric vessels or the superficial circumflex iliac vessels. When rotated as a superiorly based flap, the thoracodorsal vessels were left attached, and the blood supply to the groin flap component was anastomosed to recipient vessels in the head and neck. Alternatively, the inferiorly based compound flap could be left attached to the vessels supplying the groin flap and the thoracodorsal pedicle, anastomosed to recipient vessels in the lower extremity (Figure 17-2).

Complex defects of the head and neck region often require two epithelial surfaces to repair the inner mucosal lining and the overlying skin. This can be achieved by folding the latissimus dorsi skin paddle and de-epithelializing the intervening bridge of skin or dividing the subcutaneous tissue to the muscle layer (29). This, however, may compromise the vascularity to the tip of the flap. An alternative solution to this problem was described by Tobin et al. (53,54) who designed two separate musculocutaneous units based on the transverse and the longitudinal intramuscular branches of the thoracodorsal vascular system. The feasibility of splitting the latissimus dorsi was investigated in dogs and then subsequently applied to humans (Figure 17-3).

Another desirable feature of a donor site for head and neck reconstruction is the ability to incorporate vascularized bone and, therefore, design a composite flap that would permit restoration of the calvarium or the maxillomandibular skeleton. Investigative studies performed by Schlenker et al. (43) in dogs suggested that a posterior segment of the rib could be vascularized through the latissimus dorsi. The anatomic basis for this composite flap is the perforating branches of the posterior intercostal artery, which traverse the fifth through the tenth intercostal spaces along the posterior axillary line. Micro-opaque injections of the subscapular vessels revealed retrograde filling of the posterior intercostal perforators. The blood supply to the bone was then hypothesized to occur through the nutrient medullary branch of the posterior intercostal artery. Tetracycline-labeling studies were performed in the dog model and confirmed the bone's vascularity. However, injection studies in fresh human cadavers performed by Friedrich et al. (12) led to the conclusion that the thoracodorsal system did not provide a blood supply to the rib. It is unclear from the latter report whether the authors investigated the possibility of capturing the intercostal vascular system through perforating branches, as described by Schlenker et al. (43). Despite these conflicting views, there are two reports in the literature of successful transfer of the latissimus dorsi–rib composite flap for oromandibular reconstruction. Schmidt and Robson (44) reported three successful cases and described the transfer of either the seventh, eighth, or ninth rib, depending on which intercostal space had the dominant perforator. They transferred this composite flap as a microvascular procedure, in contrast to the report of Maruyama et al. (27) who performed a transfer of a pedicled composite flap. Primary wound healing, radiographic evidence of bone union, and

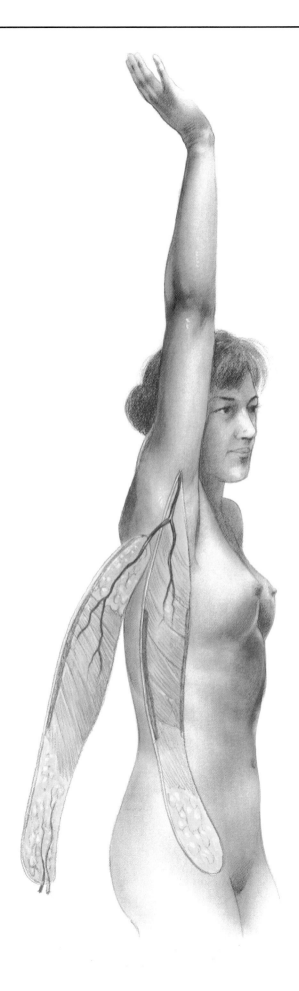

Figure 17-2. Harii et al. (15) described the combined latissimus dorsi and groin flaps transferred in series with one vascularized as a free flap and the other as a pedicled flap. For use in the head and neck, the thoracodorsal vessels remained intact; the vessels supplying the groin flap were interrupted and anastomosed to recipient vessels in the neck.

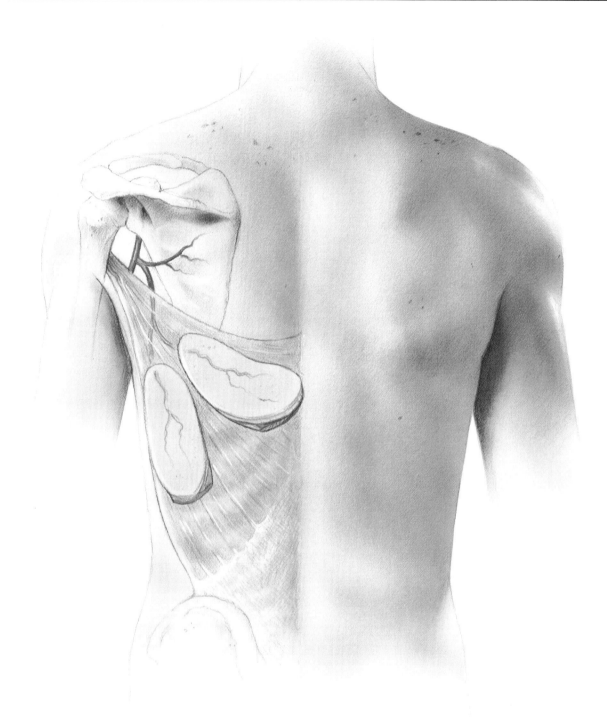

Figure 17-3. Two skin paddles may be harvested overlying the latissimus dorsi based on the transverse and the vertical branches of the thoracodorsal artery. By dissecting on the undersurface of the latissimus dorsi, the surgeon can identify the division of the thoracodorsal vessels and, therefore, totally separate these two musculocutaneous paddles.

early postoperative bone scans were used as evidence of the viability of the osseous component.

Increased concern for maximizing the functional recovery in head and neck reconstruction has heightened the desirability of restoring sensation to the oral cavity and pharynx through the use of sensate free flaps. There are two reports of restoring sensation to the latissimus dorsi musculocutaneous flap. Dabb and Conklin (7) described the sensory supply to the skin of the lower back as arising from two sources: the cutaneous branches of the dorsal rami and the posterior branches of the lateral cutaneous branch of the intercostal nerve. They reported the successful restoration of sensation following reconstruction of the foot. The posterior branches of the lateral cutaneous nerves were anastomosed to the medial plantar branch of the posterior tibial nerve. In addition, the dorsal rami were anastomosed to the anterior tibial nerve. The detection of pressure and pain were reported at 6 months. Gordon et al. (13) described an alternative route to provide sensory nerve ingrowth into the latissimus dorsi flap. They anastomosed the thoracodorsal nerve to a recipient sensory nerve and noted that five of seven patients were able to distinguish sharp from dull stimuli. The mechanism for the recovery of sensation in these patients was uncertain, not only in light of using a motor nerve, but also because the latissimus dorsi muscle flaps were covered with skin grafts.

The latissimus dorsi has been used to restore dynamic activity by either preserving the integrity of the thoracodorsal nerve or anastomosing it to an appropriate recipient motor nerve. Zancolli and Mitre (60) reported the restoration of elbow flexion in patients with poliomyelitis or traumatic loss of such function by transferring the latissimus dorsi so that it crossed the elbow joint.

Dynamic facial reanimation was achieved by the transfer of the latissimus dorsi to the paralyzed face in a two-stage procedure (25). The first stage involves placement of a cross facial nerve graft that is anastomosed to buccal branches on the noninvolved side. By eliciting the Tinel sign, the advancing nerve fibers can be followed and then a free muscle flap transferred and both revascularized and reneurotized. Various different muscles have been used for this purpose, including the gracilis (16), the extensor digitorum brevis (33), the pectoralis minor (52), and the serratus anterior (58,59). The advantages of the latissimus dorsi for this procedure are the length and caliber of the neurovascular pedicle and its division into two segments, which allows the transfer of two separate muscle units. One segment has been used for reanimation of the mouth and the other, for the lower eyelid. Mackinnon and Dellon (25) outlined a number of subtle changes in this procedure that include marking of the resting muscle length at the donor site and then precisely reestablishing that resting tension during insetting of the flap into the face. In addition, they also described a distal dissection of the thoracodorsal nerve so that nerve fibers that extend beyond the muscle segment can be reinserted into the muscle to help increase the dynamic activity.

The latissimus dorsi musculocutaneous flap has also been used for dynamic reconstruction of composite cheek defects that include the loss of the mimetic muscles of the midface. In this situation, a one-stage procedure can be performed whereby the musculocutaneous unit is transferred and revascularized and the thoracodorsal nerve is sutured to the ipsilateral facial nerve. Dynamic activity and electromyographic recordings confirmed the muscle's contraction (26).

The other area in which a dynamic reconstruction is desirable is in restoring function to the mouth following significant or total glossectomy. The complexity of the tongue's musculature, which is composed of both extrinsic and intrinsic muscle, has daunted surgeons for decades. Although it is tempting to try to duplicate the success of free muscle grafting in facial paralysis, the motions of the tongue are far more complex. In considering this problem, it is difficult to decide which of the almost limitless changes in position and shape of the native tongue to try to restore with a free muscle flap composed of unidirectional fibers. Haughey (17) and Haughey and Frederickson (18) described the use of the reinnervated latissimus dorsi musculocutaneous flap for total tongue reconstruction. The muscle fibers were oriented transversely to the long axis of the mouth and sutured to the pterygoid, constrictor, and masseter, depending on which were available. The thoracodorsal nerves were anastomosed to the stumps of the hypoglossal nerve. In this reconstruction, the upward movement of the flap that was observed by the authors was caused by either the contraction of the latissimus dorsi or the muscles to which the flap was sutured.

The pedicled latissimus dorsi musculocutaneous flap has been utilized for a number of reconstructive problems, including mucosal defects of the pharynx and oral cavity and cutaneous defects of the neck and face (4,29,37). Watson and Lendrum (57) reported a one-stage tubed latissimus dorsi flap for circumferential pharyngoesophageal reconstruction. Watson et al. (58) described several technical considerations in using the latissimus dorsi flap for pharyngeal defects. The authors advised transferring a large segment of muscle around the circumference of the skin paddle that is to be tubed. The muscle was sutured to the surrounding tissues to provide a second-layer seal. The large surface area of this donor site has made it particularly suitable for resurfacing very large defects of the face and neck (22,45). Composite defects involving both mucosa and skin can be readily restored by the methods described previously. However, a word of caution is needed regarding the weight of this flap, especially when it is folded on itself for coverage of through-and-through defects. Secondary debulking procedures are often needed (55). The latissimus dorsi flap easily reaches the midline of the lower neck and, therefore, is an excellent alternative donor site to the pectoralis major for defects resulting from resections for stomal recurrent cancer (11).

The free latissimus dorsi musculocutaneous flap has been used for a variety of midface defects that require bulk and freedom to place epithelial surfaces in a number of different three-dimensional planes. Baker (1) reported the suitability of this flap for extensive orbitomaxillary defects. This flap has also been used for closure of palatal and midfacial cutaneous defects. Shestak et al. (47) described using two skin paddles that were obtained by de-epithelializing an intervening strip of skin that permitted their placement in two different planes oriented at 90 degrees to each other. Several reports in the literature demonstrate the efficacy of the latissimus dorsi flap for highly complex and extensive defects of the midface and skull base (14,21).

Scalp defects located in the temporal or occipital regions are readily accessible by a pedicled latissimus dorsi flap. However, when the area to be resurfaced enlarges and/or extends to the vertex, then a free flap is often required. The latissimus dorsi is an excellent choice for this problem because of the surface area of either skin or muscle that is available, the length of the nutrient pedicle (which easily extends to recipient vessels in the neck), and the thinness of the tissue (which matches that of the remaining scalp). The number of reports using this flap for this purpose is testimony to these distinguishing characteristics (2,10,36,39,48,49). Pennington et al. (36) noted their preference for resurfacing the convex contour of the skull with vascularized muscle and a skin graft because of the intrinsic ability of the muscle to stretch and therefore to avoid dog ears, which often occur with skin flaps. In addition, vascularized muscle flaps eliminate the concern for primary donor site closure when large skin paddles are harvested. As noted previously, the thoracolumbar fascia has been used to repair dural defects (48). The efficacy of using the latissimus dorsi flap to achieve a stable wound following débridement of scalp and calvarium for osteoradionecrosis has been reported by Robson et al. (39) in a series of six cases. In one patient, these authors reported the transfer of a latissimus dorsi osteomusculocutaneous flap containing a vascularized segment of the fourth rib to replace a portion of the calvarial defect. The merits of restoring structural support along with soft tissue coverage varies with the size and location of the skull defect. Although protection of the brain and improved cosmesis are the most frequent indications for cranioplasty, some authors espouse the merits of restoring the calvarium to prevent or correct a variety of symptoms, including pain, headache, dizziness, and post-traumatic seizures (49). In addition to vascularized bone, this problem has been solved by using split rib grafts, synthetic cranioplasty, and titanium plates (36,48,49).

NEUROVASCULAR ANATOMY

I noted that some important arterial branches stem from a prominent branch of the subscapular artery and extend to the pedicle of my flap. It is this branch that is called the scapular circumflex, and of this branch, the lower one is the most involved in the feeding of the flap. The arterial branch makes a path toward the surface between the teres major and teres minor and the branch reaches in part to the latissimus dorsi muscle and to the skin. It is also important to note that the latissimus dorsi muscle receives branches straight from the subscapular artery. From this observation, it is understood that in order to ensure the vitality of the flap, it is necessary to include at least the latissimus dorsi muscle: by this method, we not only preserve the flow of blood to the skin that stems from the scapular circumflex, but also that which arrives there by way of the latissimus dorsi muscle.

Tansini, 1906

The degree of Tansini's understanding of the blood supply to the skin of this musculocutaneous flap is truly astounding and boggles the minds of students of medical history who ponder the tremendous time delay between Tansini's discovery and the widespread enthusiasm with which this donor site is presently embraced (30). Although Tansini's description wrongly placed too great an emphasis on the role of the circumflex scapular artery, it is evident that he understood the axial pattern blood supply to the latissimus dorsi and the necessity to include that blood supply to ensure the viability of the skin.

According to the classification system of Mathes and Nahai (28), the latissimus dorsi is a type 5 muscle with one dominant vascular pedicle and a series of smaller segmental pedicles. The dominant pedicle is composed of the thoracodorsal artery and vein, which are the terminal branches of the subscapular artery and vein. There are numerous musculocutaneous perforators over the entire latissimus dorsi, with a particular preponderance located along the anterior border. In addition, there are segmental paraspinal perforators in the medial portion of the muscle (Figure 17-4).

Taylor and Palmer (51) described a system of angiosomes to help explain the vascular basis for reconstructive flaps. They divided the body into three-dimensional territories that are each supplied by a named source artery and vein and connected to each other by a system of choke vessels. The latissimus dorsi is divided into three angiosomes: the proximal portion of the muscle, which is supplied by the thoracodorsal pedicle; the mid and medial portion, which is supplied by the posterior intercostals; and the most caudal portion, which is nourished by the lumbar arteries (Figure 17-5). The intercostal system of perforators are sizable vessels that range from 1 to 1.5 mm in diameter and have been used to support posteromedially based, or "reversed," muscle and musculocutaneous flaps (6). However, the thoracodorsal pedicle is the dominant supply for pedicled or free flap transfers to the head and neck.

The angiosome concept allows us to predict the reliability of muscle and skin transferred from different regions of the latissimus dorsi. Taylor and Palmer (51) hypothesized that muscle and skin can be reliably harvested from an adjacent angiosome by crossing one system of choke vessels. However, the vascularity diminishes when the "tertiary" territory is harvested by crossing the second set of connecting vessels. This has been the experience encountered with the latissimus dorsi flap, which is unreliable in its caudal and medial segments.

The thoracodorsal artery and vein arise from the subscapular vessels, which are branches of the third portion of the axillary artery and vein. The thoracodorsal vessels run in a cephalocaudal direction through the fatty tissue of the axilla prior to entering the hilum of the muscle. In their course, they give off branches to a variety of muscles, including the subscapularis, teres major, and serratus anterior. In addition, they supply a consistent angular branch to the tip of the scapula. The vascular anatomy of the thoracodorsal vessels has been extensively studied. The average diameter of the artery at its origin was 2.7 mm (range, 1.5 to 4.0 mm); the diameter of the vein was 3.4 mm (range, 1.5 to 4.5 mm); the average length of the thoracodorsal pedicle was 9.3 cm (range, 6.0 to 16.5 cm). In the majority of cadaver dissections (92%), the subscapular artery and vein arose in close proximity from the axillary vessels, and the thoracodorsal vessels traversed the axilla together. In the remaining cases, the artery and vein arose at a distance from each other and ran separate courses until joining as far caudal as the takeoff of the branches to the serratus anterior. In the majority of cases, there is a single branch to the serratus anterior (54%), with double (44%) and triple branches (2%) encountered less frequently (3).

At the neurovascular hilum, the vein is situated lateral to the artery, and the nerve runs in between. In 99% of cases, there was a single neurovascular hilum; in the remaining 1%, there were two distinct hila identified (54). In 86% of cases, the thoracodorsal vessels were found to bifurcate into transverse and longitudinal branches. The transverse branch usually paralleled the free upper border, separated from the edge by an average of 3.5 cm. The longitudinal branch was usually slightly smaller

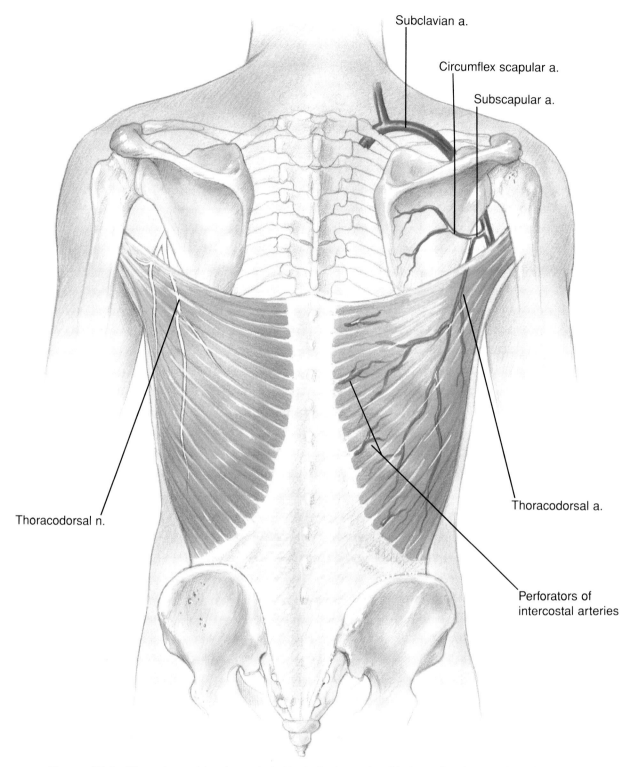

Figure 17-4. The primary blood supply to the latissimus dorsi is from the thoracodorsal artery and vein that arise from the subscapular axis. The thoracodorsal pedicle was consistently divided into transverse and longitudinal branches. The thoracodorsal pedicle can usually be mobilized to achieve a length of 10 to 12 cm. The thoracodorsal artery has a diameter of 1.5 to 4.0 mm prior to branching. The thoracodorsal nerve supplies motor innervation to the muscle and also divides into transverse and longitudinal branches.

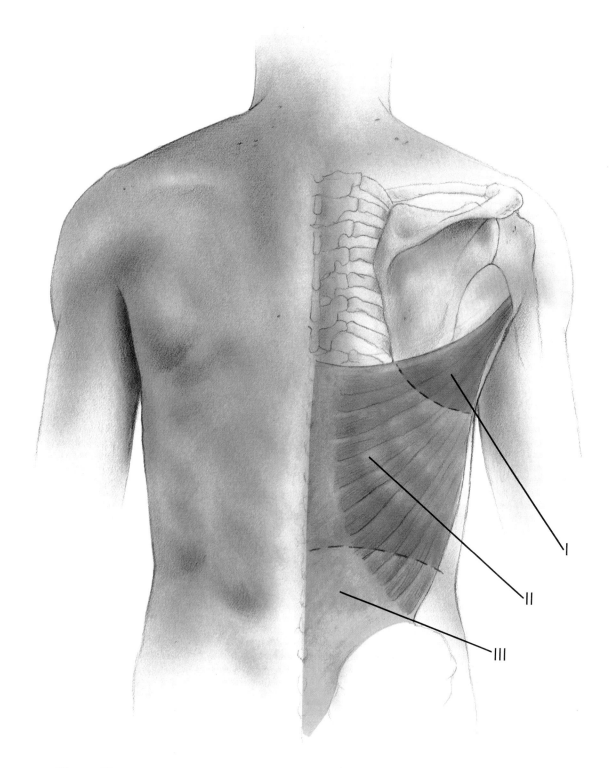

Figure 17-5. The latissimus dorsi may be divided into three primary angiosomes. By doing so, we can better understand the reliability of the different skin paddles overlying this muscle. The upper territory is primarily supplied by the source artery, the thoracodorsal artery (I). The second vascular territory (II) of the latissimus dorsi is supplied by the intercostal perforators that enter both medially in the paraspinal region, as well as laterally. The lower portion of the muscle is supplied by lumbar vessels (III). The skin paddles overlying the third angiosome are less reliable when based entirely on the thoracodorsal system. It is important to realize this factor when using the latissimus dorsi musculocutaneous flap as a pedicled flap. Improving the arc of rotation is often done by placing the skin paddle over the more caudal extent of the muscle but, therefore, incurring a greater risk of skin ischemia.

and ran a course toward the iliac crest at a distance of 2.1 cm from the lateral edge. Dye-injection studies of each of these branches produced staining of the overlying skin and the entire muscle, which reflected the rich anastomoses between the two major branches. The intramuscular branching pattern of the thoracodorsal nerve paralleled the vessels and, therefore, provides the anatomic basis for harvesting two separate vascularized neuromuscular units. It also provides the opportunity to preserve a functional muscle and, therefore, to reduce donor-site morbidity (54).

One of the most appealing characteristics of the latissimus dorsi donor site is the length of the vascular pedicle. There is considerable variation in the combined length of the thoracodorsal and subscapular vessels, which ranged from 7.6 to 14.4 cm (average, 9.7 cm). Differences in length appeared to be more related to the size of the patient rather than to a variation in the point of entry into the muscle (12). In two separate cadaver dissection series, there was little atherosclerosis noted (3,12).

The thoracodorsal nerve supplies the motor innervation to the latissimus dorsi. It arises from the posterior cord of the brachial plexus. It enters the axilla from behind the axillary vessels and then descends with the thoracodorsal artery and vein to the neurovascular hilum. The thoracodorsal nerve usually crosses the axillary vessels approximately 3 cm proximal to the subscapular artery and vein. The length of nerve that can be harvested ranges from 8.5 to 19.0 cm (average, 12.3 cm). Bifurcation of the thoracodorsal nerve was noted in 85% of dissections (3). Earlier in this chapter, the sensory supply to the skin of the back and trunk was discussed. The long thoracic nerve runs on the superficial aspect of the serratus anterior, which it innervates.

ANATOMIC VARIATIONS

There are few significant anatomic variations of the latissimus dorsi itself. As noted previously, the subscapular artery and vein arise in close proximity to each other in the majority of dissections. In those cases in which their origins are separated, the subscapular artery arises proximally in the axilla, by an average of 4.2 cm. The surgeon should be aware of this anatomic variant to avoid confusion when harvesting this flap (3). The thoracodorsal artery, on occasion, may arise as a separate branch from the axillary artery. In a series of 512 cadaver dissections, DeGaris and Swartley (8) reported that this anomaly occurs with an incidence of 0.8%.

POTENTIAL PITFALLS

The latissimus dorsi flap is a safe and reliable reconstructive option, as evidenced by the abundance of reports in the literature. However, marginal flap necrosis is not uncommon and most likely results from improper design over the more distal aspects of the muscle (10). This is usually caused by pushing the limits of the maximum size of this flap or the placement of the skin paddle close to the iliac crest to enhance the arc of rotation. This problem can be avoided by transferring the latissimus dorsi as a free flap.

Passage of the latissimus dorsi as a pedicled flap between the pectoralis major and minor must be done with great caution. The tremendously long course that the vessels traverse place them at risk of occlusion with changes in arm position. Immobilization of the arm in a flexed position across the chest has been advocated (29). If the pectoralis major has not previously been used as a reconstructive flap it is imperative to avoid injury to the thoracoacromial vessels when creating the tunnel. In addition to being cautious about injury to the long thoracic nerve and paralysis of the serratus anterior with winging of the scapula, Baker (1) warned against injury to the medial brachial cutaneous nerve that supplies sensation to the medial aspect of the upper arm. Failure to create an adequate tunnel may lead to compression of the vascular pedicle between the pectoralis major and the clavicle. Watson et al. (58) reported one case of total flap necrosis caused by this problem.

An even greater concern is the reported injuries to the brachial plexus that have occurred as a result of positioning the arm during flap harvest. Quillen (37) noted a single case of temporary radial nerve weakness, and Barton et al. (4) reported four cases of temporary weakness and sensory changes in the upper extremity. The mechanism of injury to the brachial plexus was studied by Logan and Black (24) who described an additional case of brachial plexus injury with a permanent deficit noted at 7 months after latissimus dorsi flap harvest. These authors described impingement of the brachial plexus by the clavicle on extreme elevation of the arm. They advised placing a pad between the shoulder and neck to help prevent the occurrence of this injury.

Sacrifice of the nerve supply of a muscle carries an intrinsic morbidity caused by the loss of its functional activity. Although the deficits resulting from the loss of the latissimus dorsi have been examined, the combined loss of several muscles that act across the glenohumeral joint has not. It is fairly common for patients with head and neck cancer to lose the action of the trapezius following radical neck dissection and the pectoralis major for reconstructive purposes. Harvest of a scapular composite flap may additionally lead to disruption or denervation of the teres major, subscapularis, and infraspinatus. The detrimental effects of radiation therapy on the brachial plexus may add to shoulder and upper extremity morbidity. Laitung and Peck (23) compared shoulder function in a group of 19 male patients who underwent latissimus dorsi transfer with that in a group of matched controls. The range of shoulder motion was normal in 13 of 19 patients who underwent the flap procedure. The disability score diminished with greater time from surgery. Scar contracture had a detrimental effect on the disability score and the range of motion. These authors found that latissimus dorsi sacrifice caused few occupational problems and did not interfere with normal sporting activities. These findings differ from those reported by Russell et al. (42) who noted a change in occupation, household activities, and sporting activities attributable to the loss of the latissimus dorsi muscle in a group of 23 patients. They found a global weakness of virtually all the muscles tested surrounding the operated shoulder. In a small group of patients with an ipsilateral loss of pectoralis major function as a result of either Poland's syndrome or mastectomy, the authors noted an even greater degree of shoulder weakness following latissimus dorsi transfer.

Loss of the latissimus dorsi has been associated with additional donor-site problems in children, which were related to the development of scoliosis and underdevelopment of the paravertebral muscles. Serra et al. (46) described a technique of reneurotizing the residual muscle to preserve latissimus dorsi function. In this procedure, the thoracodorsal nerve is transsected at the point where it enters the muscle. Following transfer of a portion of the muscle, the cut ends of the nerve are reintroduced into the remaining muscle. Follow-up electromyographic studies revealed reinnervation of the muscle. There was no mention, however, of whether the development of the feared sequelae was avoided.

The potential morbidity of transferring the latissimus dorsi in pediatric patients may differ from that in adults. However, with the majority of free flaps transferred to the head and neck occurring in an older population of patients with cancer, the functional shoulder deficits must be studied in a systematic fashion to account for the variables noted.

PREOPERATIVE ASSESSMENT

The anterior border of the latissimus dorsi can be readily palpated by instructing patients to press their hands against their hips while seated. Preoperative localization of the thoracodorsal vessels is rarely necessary because of the consistency of anatomy. In patients who have had a prior axillary lymph node dissection, the situation is more complex because of the likelihood that the thoracodorsal vessels have been ligated. Collateral flow to the muscle is derived through the rich anastomotic network around the scapula, with retrograde flow in the circumflex scapular artery and the branches to serratus anterior (32). Although coverage of the chest wall may be feasible under these circumstances, it is unlikely that the flap could be safely harvested for use in the head and neck unless it is transferred as a free flap. Preoperative angiography has been advocated in this setting (41).

Flap Harvesting Technique

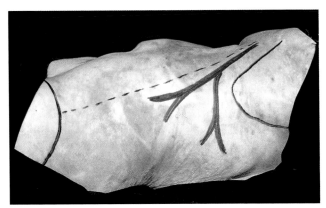

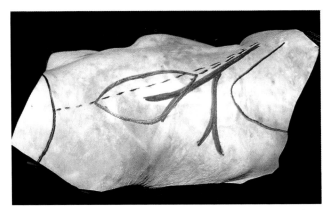

Figure 17-6. The topographical anatomy of the latissimus dorsi flap has been outlined on the lateral back. The important landmarks include the midpoint of the axilla, the iliac crest, and the scapula tip. A *dashed line* is drawn between the midpoint of the axilla and a point midway between the anterior superior iliac spine and the posterior superior iliac spine on the iliac crest. This line represents the anterior border of the latissimus dorsi. Eight to 10 cm below the midpoint of the axilla, along this line, the thoracodorsal artery and vein enter the undersurface of the latissimus dorsi, and the vessels divide into a horizontal branch, which runs a few centimeters below the scapula tip, and a more vertically directed branch, which runs 3–4 cm posterior to the anterior edge of the muscle.

Figure 17-7. The outline for a cutaneous paddle has been drawn based on the vertically oriented branch. The cutaneous paddle is usually drawn as a fusiform shape to assist in closure. The cutaneous paddle has been designed with a few centimeters of random skin anterior to the leading edge of the latissimus dorsi.

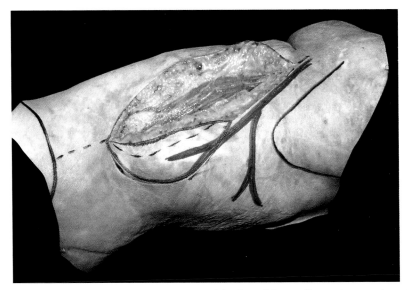

Figure 17-8. The initial incision is made at the midpoint of the axilla and runs along the *dashed line* superiorly and the anterior edge of the cutaneous paddle inferiorly. Through this incision, the anterior leading edge of the latissimus muscle is easily identified.

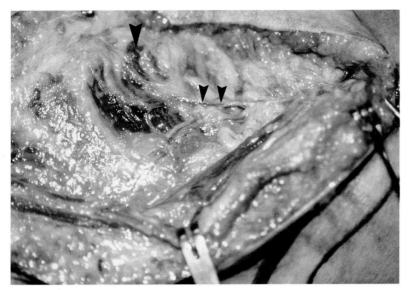

Figure 17-9. The thoracodorsal pedicle runs through the adipose tissue of the axilla, providing branches to the regional muscles and the angular branch to the scapula before entering the hilum of the latissimus dorsi. The branches to the serratus anterior (*double arrows*) are often the first vascular structures to be encountered. These branches lie on the superficial surface of the serratus anterior (*large arrow*) and can be used to find the thoracodorsal vessels from which they arise.

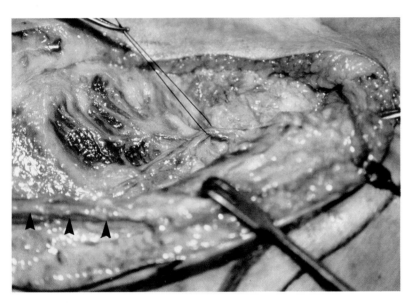

Figure 17-10. With the anterior edge (*arrows*) of the latissimus dorsi retracted posteriorly, a suture has been placed around the branches to the serratus anterior.

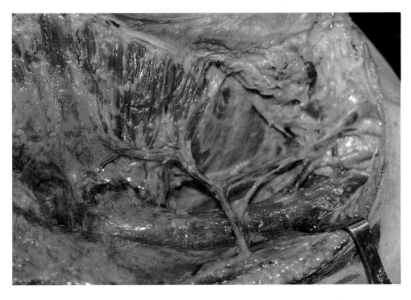

Figure 17-11. In a dissection in which much of the adipose tissue has been removed, the anatomy of the thoracodorsal system consisting of artery, vein, and nerve, can be more clearly visualized.

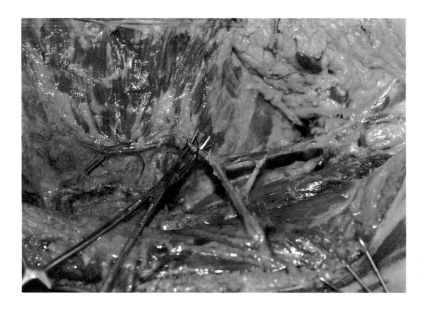

Figure 17-12. Division of the serratus anterior branch allows near-complete mobilization of the thoracodorsal pedicle.

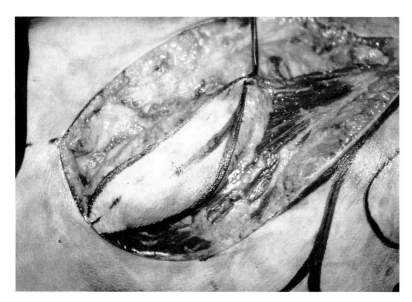

Figure 17-13. An incision is then made circumferentially around the posteromedial portion of the skin paddle. This incision is made to the level of the fascia overlying the muscle. At this juncture, the dissection may proceed by harvesting only a limited portion of the latissimus dorsi underlying the skin paddle or the entire muscle.

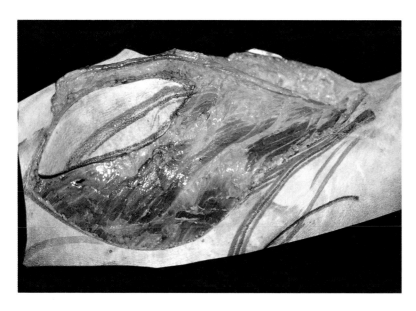

Figure 17-14. Elevation of the back skin off the muscle provides exposure of the latissimus dorsi to the posterior midline.

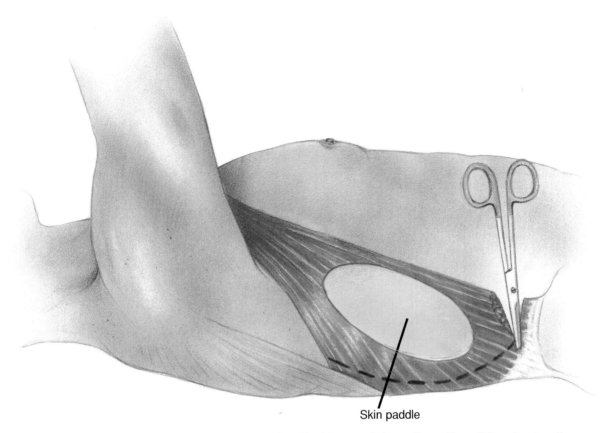

Skin paddle

Figure 17-15. The latissimus dorsi is mobilized by blunt and sharp dissection off the chest wall and the external oblique and serratus anterior muscles. The muscle and aponeurotic attachments to the iliac crest, the vertebrae, and the ribs are sharply transsected. Feeders entering the deep surface of the muscle during the inferior and medial dissection must be ligated and divided.

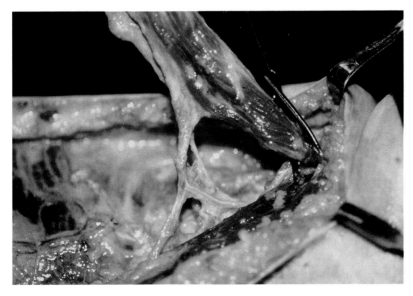

Figure 17-16. As the dissection proceeds distally to proximally, the vascular hilum is identified. Careful dissection along the thoracodorsal neurovascular pedicle toward the axilla requires division of muscular branches and the angular branch.

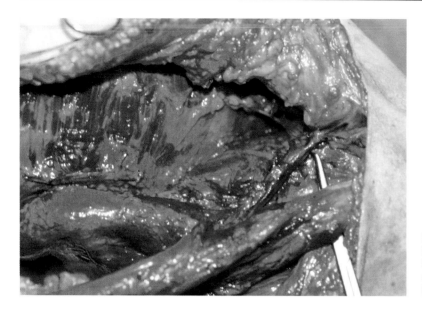

Figure 17-17. Complete mobilization of the latissimus dorsi requires transsection of the tendinous insertion to the humerus. This maneuver is performed carefully while protecting the vascular pedicle.

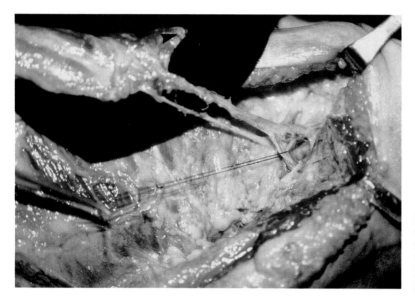

Figure 17-18. The tendon (*arrow*) has been cut, leaving the muscle attached by the neurovascular pedicle. A suture is placed around the circumflex scapular vessels which can be ligated to further mobilize the thoracodorsal pedicle.

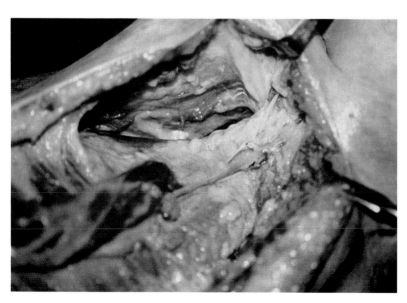

Figure 17-19. Passage of the pedicled flap requires preparation of a tunnel between the pectoralis major and minor. The lateral edge of these muscles is identified in the anterior axilla.

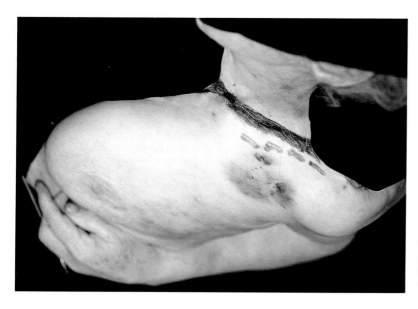

Figure 17-20. An incision parallel and inferior to the clavicle is required to complete the tunnel. The pectoralis major attachments to the clavicle are incised.

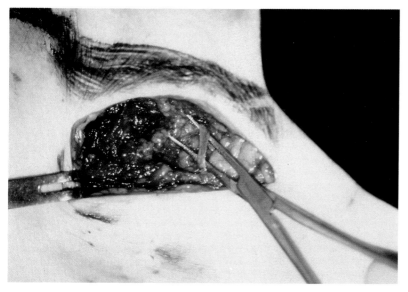

Figure 17-21. The thoracoacromial pedicle is identified and preserved.

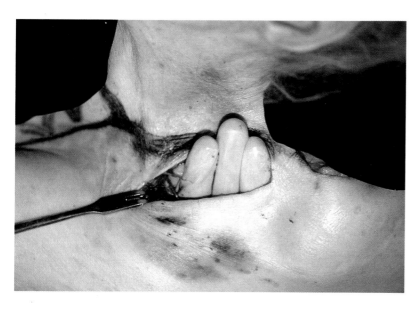

Figure 17-22. A generous tunnel must be created to allow passage of the latissimus dorsi flap. A good guide to an adequate passage is one that accommodates three or four of the surgeon's fingers.

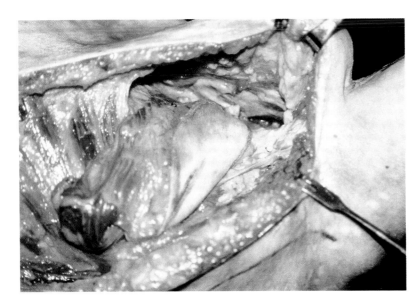

Figure 17-23. Under direct vision, the latissimus dorsi flap is passed through the tunnel while being certain not to twist the pedicle or cause shearing forces between the skin and the muscle.

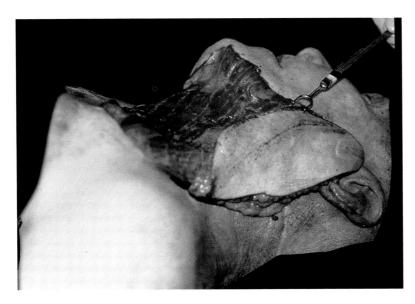

Figure 17-24. The latissimus dorsi flap has been transferred to the temporal region without tension on the vascular leash.

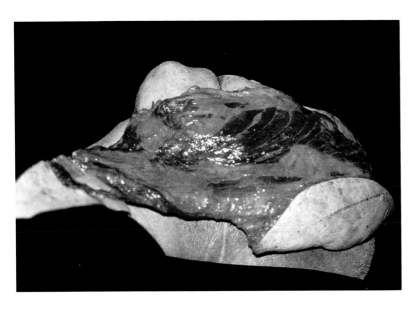

Figure 17-25. The importance of transsecting the tendon of the latissimus muscle to maximize the arc of rotation is illustrated by the position of the flap shown here compared with the previous figure in which the tendon had not yet been cut.

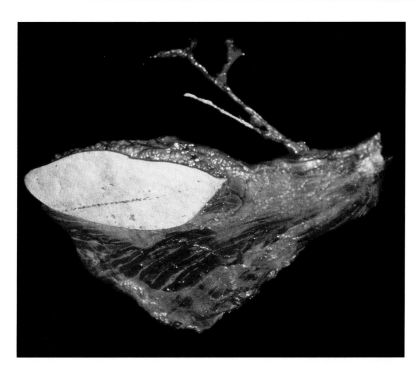

Figure 17-26. Harvest of the free latissimus dorsi musculocutaneous flap reveals the long neurovascular pedicle and the tremendous surface area that can be covered.

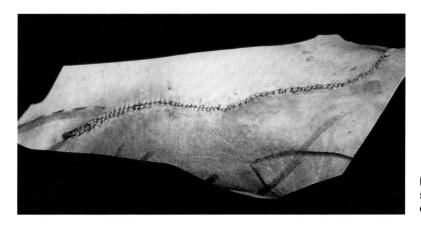

Figure 17-27. Primary closure of the donor site can usually be accomplished by wide undermining to produce a linear scar.

REFERENCES

1. Baker S. Closure of large orbital maxillary defects with free latissimus dorsi myocutaneous flaps. *Head Neck* 1984;6:828.
2. Barrow D, Nahai F, Fleischer A. Use of free latissimus dorsi musculocutaneous flaps in various neurosurgical disorders. *J Neurosurg* 1983;58:252.
3. Bartlett SP, May JW, Yaremchuk MJ. The latissimus dorsi muscle. A fresh cadaver study of the primary neurovascular pedicle. *Plast Reconstr Surg* 1981;67:631.
4. Barton F, Spicer T, Byrd H. Head and neck reconstruction with the latissimus dorsi myocutaneous flap: anatomic observations and report of 60 cases. *Plast Reconstr Surg* 1983;71:199.
5. Bostwick J, Nahai F, Wallace J, Vasconez L. Sixty latissimus dorsi flaps. *Plast Reconstr Surg* 1979;83: 31.
6. Bostwick J, Schiflan M, Nahai F, Jurkiewicz M. The "reverse" latissimus dorsi muscle and musculocutaneous flap: anatomical and clinical considerations. *Plast Reconstr Surg* 1980;65:395.
7. Dabb R, Conklin W. A sensory innervated latissimus dorsi musculocutaneous free flap: case report. *J Microsurg* 1981;2:289–293.
8. DeGaris C, Swartley W. The axillary artery in white and Negro stocks. *Am J Anat* 1928;4:353.
9. D'este S. La technique de l'amputation de la mamelle pour carcinome mammaire. *Rev Chir* 1912;45: 164.
10. Earley MJ, Green M, Milling M. A critical appraisal of the use of free flaps in primary reconstruction of combined scalp and calvarial cancer defects. *Br J Plast Surg* 1990;43:283–289.

11. Fredrickson JM, Jahn AF, Bryce DP. Leiomyosarcoma of the cervical trachea. Report of a case with reconstruction using a latissimus dorsi island flap. *Ann Otol Rhinol Laryngol* 1979;88:463–466.
12. Friedrich W, Berbenhold C, Lierse W. Vascularization of the myocutaneous latissimus dorsi flap. *Acta Anat (Basel)* 1988;131:97.
13. Gordon L, Bunche H, Alpert B. Free latissimus dorsi muscle flap with split-thickness skin graft cover: a report of 16 cases. *Plast Reconstr Surg* 1982;70:173.
14. Hardesty R, Jones N, Swartz N, Ramasastry S, Heckler F, Newton D, Schramm V. Microsurgery for macrodefects: microvascular free-tissue transfer for massive defects of the head and neck. *Am J Surg* 1987;154:399.
15. Harii K, Iwaya T, Kawaguchi N. Combination myocutaneous flap and microvascular free flap. *Plast Reconstr Surg* 1981;68:700. ·
16. Harii K, Ohmori K, Toru S. Free gracilis muscle transplantation with microneurovascular anastomoses for treatment of facial paralysis. *Plast Reconstr Surg* 1976;57:133.
17. Haughey B. Tongue reconstruction: concepts and practice. *Laryngoscope* 1993;103:1132.
18. Haughey B, Fredrickson J. The latissimus dorsi donor site. Current use in head and neck reconstruction. *Arch Otolaryngol Head Neck Surg* 1991;117:1129.
19. Hayashi A, Maruyama Y. The "reduced" latissimus dorsi musculocutaneous flap. *Plast Reconstr Surg* 1989;84:290.
20. Hutchins E. A method for the prevention of elephantiasis. *Surg Gynecol Obstet* 1939;69:795.
21. Jones N, Hardesty R, Swarty W, Ramasastry S, Heckler F, Nauton E. Extensive and complex defects of the scalp, middle third of the face, and palate: the role of microsurgical reconstruction. *Plast Reconstr Surg* 1988;82:937.
22. Krishna B, Green M. Extended role of latissimus dorsi myocutaneous flap in reconstruction of the neck. *Br J Plast Surg* 1980;33:233.
23. Laitung J, Peck F. Shoulder function following loss of the latissimus dorsi muscle. *Br J Plast Surg* 1985;38:375.
24. Logan A, Black M. Injury to the brachial plexus resulting from shoulder positioning during latissimus dorsi flap pedicle dissection. *Br J Plast Surg* 1985;38:380.
25. Mackinnon S, Dellon L. Technical considerations of the latissimus dorsi muscle flap: a segmentally innervated muscle transfer for facial reanimation. *Microsurgery* 1988;9:36–45.
26. Maruyama Y, Nakajima H, Fossati E, Fujino T. Free latissimus dorsi myocutaneous flaps in the dynamic reconstruction of cheek defects; a preliminary report. *J Microsurg* 1979;1:231.
27. Maruyama Y, Urita Y, Ohnishi K. Rib-latissimus dorsi osteomyocutaneous flap in reconstruction of a mandibular defect. *Br J Plast Surg* 1985;38:234.
28. Mathes S, Nahai F. *Clinical Applications for Muscle and Musculocutaneous Flaps.* Toronto: CV Mosby; 1982.
29. Maves M, Panje W, Shagets F. Extended latissimus dorsi myocutaneous flap reconstruction of major head and neck defects. *Otolaryngol Head Neck Surg* 1984;92:551.
30. Maxwell G. Iginio Tansini and the origin of the latissimus dorsi musculocutaneous flap. *Plast Reconstr Surg* 1980;65:686.
31. Maxwell G, Manson P, Hoopes J. Experience with thirteen latissimus dorsi myocutaneous free flaps. *Plast Reconstr Surg* 1979;64:1.
32. Maxwell G, McGibbon B, Hoopes J. Vascular considerations in the use of a latissimus dorsi myocutaneous flap after a mastectomy with an axillary dissection. *Plast Reconstr Surg* 1979;64:771.
33. Mayou BR, Watson J, Harrison D, Wynn-Parry C. Free microvascular and microneural transfer of the extensor digitorum brevis muscle for the treatment of unilateral facial palsy. *Br J Plast Surg* 1981;34:362.
34. Olivari N. The latissimus flap. *Br J Plast Surg* 1976;29:126.
35. Olivari N. Use of thirty latissimus dorsi flaps. *Plast Reconstr Surg* 1979;64:654.
36. Pennington D, Stern H, Lee K. Free flap reconstruction of large defects of the scalp and calvarium. *Plast Reconstr Surg* 1989;83:655.
37. Quillen C. Latissimus dorsi myocutaneous flaps in head and neck reconstruction. *Plast Reconstr Surg* 1979;63:664.
38. Quillen C, Shearin J, Georgiade N. Use of the latissimus dorsi myocutaneous island flap for reconstruction in the head and neck area. *Plast Reconstr Surg* 1978;62:113.
39. Robson MC, Zachary LS, Schmidt DR, Faibisoff B, Hekmatpanah J. Reconstruction of large cranial defects in the presence of heave radiation damage and injection utilizing tissue transferred by microvascular anastomoses. *Plast Reconstr Surg* 1989;83:438–442.
40. Rowsell A, Godfrey A, Richards M. The thinned latissimus dorsi free flap: a case report. *Br J Plast Surg* 1986;39:210.
41. Rubinstein ZJ, Shafir R, Tsur H. The value of angiography prior to use of the latissimus dorsi myocutaneous flap. *Plast Reconstr Surg* 1979;63:374.
42. Russell R, Pribaz J, Zook E, Leighton W, Eriksson E, Smith C. Functional evaluation of the latissimus dorsi donor site. *Plast Reconstr Surg* 1986;78:336.
43. Schlenker J, Indresano A, Raine T, Meredith S, Robson M. A new flap in the dog containing a vascularized rib graft—the latissimus dorsi myoosteocutaneous flap. *J Surg Res* 1980;29:172–183.
44. Schmidt D, Robson M. One-stage composite reconstruction using the latissimus myoosteocutaneous free flap. *Am J Surg* 1982;144:470.
45. Schuller D. Latissimus dorsi myocutaneous flap for massive facial defects. *Arch Otolaryngol* 1982;108:414.
46. Serra J, Samayoa V, Valiente E, Kloehn G. Neurotization of the remaining latissimus dorsi muscle following muscle flap transplant. *J Reconstr Microsurg* 1988;4:415.
47. Shestak K, Schusterman M, Jones N, Johnson J. Immediate microvascular reconstruction of combined palatal and midfacial defects using soft tissue only. *Microsurgery* 1988;9:128.

48. Smith P, Morgan B, Crockard H. Immediate total scalp and skull reconstruction. *Microsurgery* 1983;4:23.
49. Stueber K, Saloman M, Spence R. The combined use of the latissimus dorsi musculocutaneous free flap and split-rib grafts for cranial vault reconstruction. *Ann Plast Surg* 1985;15:155.
50. Tansini I. Spora il mio nuovo processo di amputazione della mammaella per cancre. *Riforma Med (Palermo, Napoli)* 1896;12:3.
51. Taylor GI, Palmer J. The vascular territories (angiosomes) of the body; experimental study and clinical applications. *Br J Plast Surg* 1987;40:113.
52. Terzis J, Manktelow R. Pectoralis minor: a new concept in facial reanimation. *Plast Surg Forum* 1982;5.
53. Tobin G, Moberg A, DuBou R, Weiner L, Bland K. The split latissimus dorsi myocutaneous flap. *Ann Plast Surg* 1981;7:272–280.
54. Tobin GR, Schusterman M, Peterson GH, Nichols G, Bland KI. The intramuscular neurovascular anatomy of the latissimus dorsi muscle: the basis for splitting the flap. *Plast Reconstr Surg* 1981;67: 637–641.
55. Watson JS. The use of the latissimus dorsi island flap for intra-oral reconstruction. *Br J Plast Surg* 1982;35:408.
56. Watson JS, Craig R, Orton C. The free latissimus dorsi myocutaneous flap. *Plast Reconstr Surg* 1979;64:299.
57. Watson JS, Lendrum J. One stage pharyngeal reconstruction using a compound latissimus dorsi island flap. *Br J Plast Surg* 1979;64:654.
58. Watson JS, Robertson GA, Lendrum J, Stranc MF, Pohl MJ. Pharyngeal reconstruction using the latissimus dorsi myocutaneous flap. *Br J Plast Surg* 1982;35:401–407.
59. Whitney T, Buncke H, Alpert B, Buncke G, Lineaweaver W. The serratus anterior free muscle flap: experience with 100 consecutive cases. *Plast Reconstr Surg* 1990;86:481.
60. Zancolli E, Mitre H. Latissimus dorsi transfer to restore elbow flexion. *J Bone Joint Surg [Am]* 1973;55A:1265.

Iliac Crest Osteocutaneous and Osteomusculocutaneous

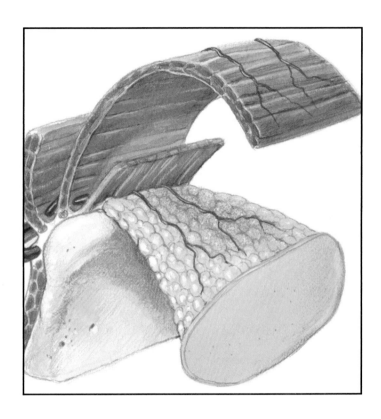

Mark L. Urken, M.D.

The search for sources of expendable bone in other parts of the skeleton for reconstruction of maxillomandibular defects has continued for several decades. Of any donor site, the ilium has arguably been placed under the greatest assault for this purpose (18) (Figures 18-1 to 18-3). It has been used as a source of nonvascularized bone blocks, corticocancellous chips, and more recently, vascularized bone through application of microvascular techniques. The amount of bone stock, and the ease of harvesting with a separate surgical team, make this an attractive donor site. Manchester (6) was one of the first to report on the similarity in shape and curvature of the anterior ilium to the native hemimandible. The era of microvascular surgery and the use of vascularized bone-containing free flaps brought multiple attempts to transfer portions of the ilium based on a variety of different vascular pedicles. The superficial circumflex iliac artery (SCIA) is the vascular supply to the groin flap, which was one of the first free flaps to be reported (12). Although the SCIA provides excellent vascularity to the overlying skin, it has a variable anatomy and a marginal nutrient flow to the bone (11). The ilium was also transferred as a compound flap with the tensor fasciae latae, which was based on the ascending branch of the lateral circumflex femoral artery (1). The superior deep branch of the superior gluteal artery has also been used as the nutrient pedicle for iliac bone transfers (3).

However, it was not until 1979, when two separate reports by Taylor et al. (16) in Australia and Sanders and Mayou (13) in England identified the deep circumflex iliac artery (DCIA) and vein (DCIV) as the most reliable and most favorable vascular pedicle for transfer of the ilium. Dye-injection studies by Taylor et al. (16) revealed both an endosteal and a periosteal supply to the entire iliac bone, extending from the

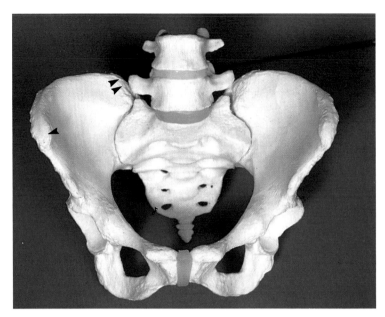

Figure 18-1. The pelvic girdle is formed by the paired coxal or innominate bones, which articulate with the sacrum. Each coxal bone is composed of three parts: the ilium, the ischium, and the pubis. The ilium provides a large amount of bone that can be transferred for reconstructive purposes in the maxillomandibular skeleton. The natural curvature of the iliac crest provides an excellent match to the contour of the hemimandible. The area of vascularized bone that can be harvested on the DCIA extends from the ASIS (*arrow*) to the posterior superior iliac spine (PSIS) (*double arrows*).

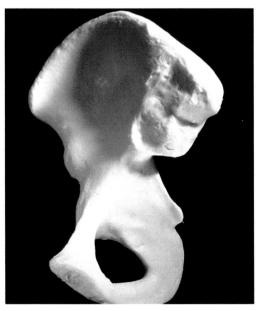

Figure 18-2. The medial aspect of the right ilium is composed largely of the iliac fossa, which is filled anteriorly by the iliacus muscle. The transversus abdominis muscle inserts on the inner aspect of the crest.

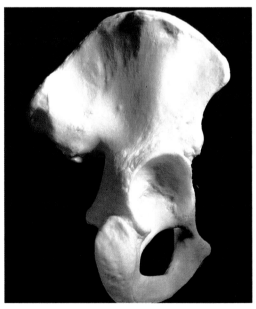

Figure 18-3. A variety of muscles insert on the lateral aspect of the ilium (right ilium shown here). Moving anteriorly to posteriorly, the sartorius, tensor fasciae latae, external oblique, internal oblique, and latissimus dorsi insert along the crest. However, the gluteus minimus, medius, and maximus muscles occupy the majority of the surface area of the lateral aspect of the ilium. The distance between the crest and the acetabulum provides a significant amount of bone height in addition to the length that can be harvested extending from the ASIS to the PSIS.

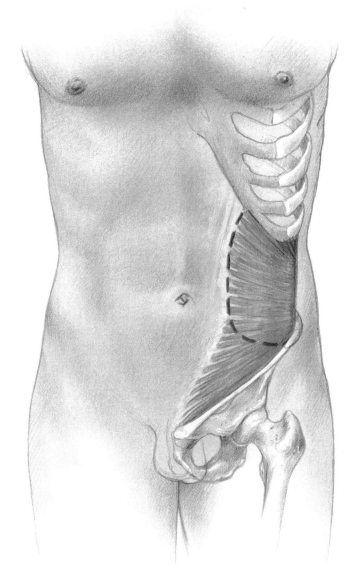

Figure 18-4. The internal oblique muscle arises from the thoracolumbar fascia, the iliac crest, and the lateral aspect of the inguinal ligament. It inserts into the linea semilunaris of the rectus sheath and the 10th through the 12th ribs.

anterosuperior iliac spine (ASIS) to the sacroiliac joint. The DCIA was also found to supply the skin overlying the ilium through an array of perforators that traverse the three muscle layers of the abdominal wall (13).

In 1984, experimental work by Ramasastry et al. (8) identified the ascending branch of the DCIA as the primary blood supply to the internal oblique muscle. It therefore became possible to transfer two separate soft tissue flaps, the skin and the internal oblique muscle, with the iliac bone based on the DCIA and DCIV. Ramasastry et al. reported the use of this composite free flap for extremity reconstruction. In the latter part of the 1980s, we became increasingly dissatisfied with the skin paddle of the iliac osteocutaneous flap because of its bulk, its limited maneuverability relative to the bone, and its tenuous blood supply. In 1989, my colleagues and I reported the adaptation of the iliac osteomusculocutaneous flap to oromandibular reconstruction (19,20). The major advantage that the inclusion of the internal oblique muscle brought to this composite flap was its increased maneuverability and decreased bulk, which enhanced is utility in intraoral reconstruction (Figure 18-4).

Additional soft tissue flaps have been transferred with the iliac bone. The antero-lateral thigh flap has been incorporated into this flap, but a second set of anastomoses is required to vascularize the skin (5). Alternatively, an iliac crest musculoperitoneal flap was used, with the blood supply to the layer of peritoneum derived from the ascending branch of the DCIA (4). However, both of these flaps have received little attention since their initial reports.

FLAP DESIGN AND UTILIZATION

Although the DCIA can be used to transfer the skin of the groin and the internal oblique muscle, these soft tissue flaps are rarely used independent of the iliac bone because of the large number of alternative soft tissue donor sites from which to choose. The design of the skin paddle usually assumes a fusiform shape to facilitate donor-site closure. There is little variability in the skin flap aside from the size and position on the abdominal wall. The size of the skin paddle must be large enough to incorporate a sufficient number of musculocutaneous perforators. Its maximum size is not clearly defined, but primary closure of the abdominal wall usually determines the upper limits of the skin that can be harvested. The relationship of the skin to the bone is somewhat fixed by the array of perforators that exit the external oblique just cephalad to the ilium. The skin flap achieves greater mobility relative to the bone when designed in a more cephalad location on the abdominal wall (21), provided that its inferior portion incorporates the zone of the cutaneous perforators (17).

The internal oblique muscle is usually harvested in its entirety pedicled inferiorly on its attachment to the inner table of the iliac crest. In 80% of cases, there is a single dominant ascending branch that allows the surgeon to isolate the entire muscle solely on its nutrient vascular supply (Figure 18-5).

The rich vascularity of the ilium allows great flexibility in the size and shape of the segment of bone that is harvested. The iliac bone is composed of a thick layer of cancellous bone that is sandwiched between two layers of cortical bone. The amount of bone, based on the cross-sectional surface area, was determined to be greater than the fibula, scapula, and radius (7). There is a wide range of bone orientations that can alter the position of the flap's pedicle, depending on the location of the recipient vessels. The natural curvature of the ilium must be accounted for in designing and planning the bone to be harvested. Height may be added to the bone by extending the osteotomies deeper into the body of the ilium. According to the principles established by Manchester (6), the ASIS can be used to fashion the angle of the neomandible, and the ramus and condyle may be formed by extending the bone cuts to the anteroinferior iliac spine (Figure 18-6). The iliac bone may be further contoured to match the curvature of the symphysis by making osteotomies. These osteotomies result in wedge-shaped openings in the bone that must be packed with corticocancellous bone chips. Alternatively, wedge-shaped segments of the ilium may be removed to collapse the bone and match virtually any defect's shape. The vascularity to the distal segments is preserved by maintaining the integrity of the inner periosteum and the DCIA–DCIV pedicle, which lies in close proximity to the inner table of bone (Figure 18-7). Finally, unicortical segments of vascularized ilium may be harvested by making a sagittal cut through the crest. By preserving the outer cortical layer of the ilium, the attachments of the upper thigh muscles remain undisturbed, which helps to reduce postoperative morbidity and to preserve normal hip contour (Figure 18-8). However, we have found it advantageous to harvest bicortical segments of ilium to achieve a more functional mandibular reconstruction that can receive endosteal osteointegrated dental implants.

The most common application of the iliac composite flap in head and neck surgery is the reconstruction of segmental mandibular defects. Up to 16 cm of bone can be harvested, which is suitable for the restoration of most ablative defects of the lower jaw. Subtotal or total mandibular reconstruction requires the use of the fibula. There

Text continues on page 269.

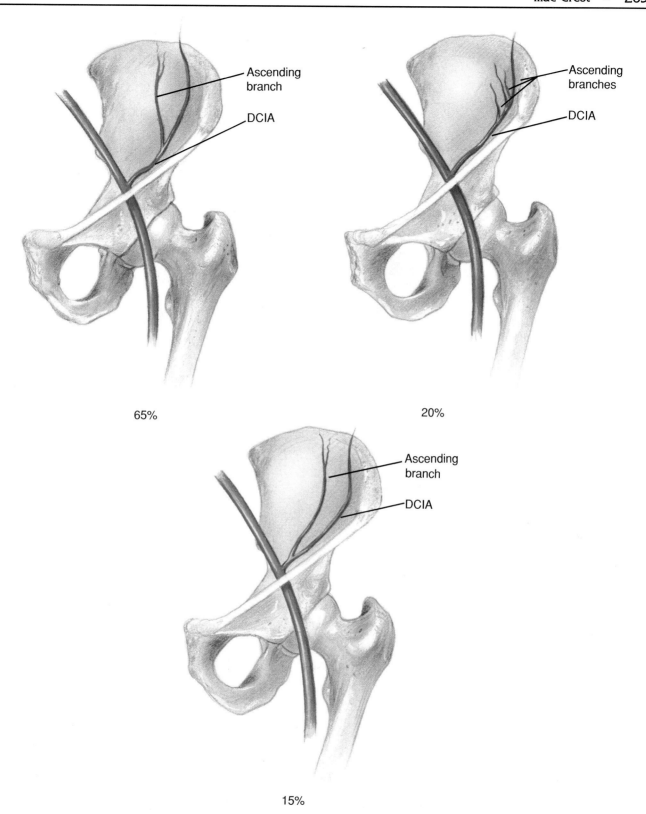

65%

20%

15%

Figure 18-5. Two separate series of cadaver dissections revealed almost identical incidence rates for the three different anatomic patterns of the ascending branch (9,17). In 65% of cases, the ascending branch originates from the DCIA within 1 cm medial to the ASIS. In 15% of cases, the ascending branch originated in a more medial location, *i.e.*, 2 to 4 cm from the ASIS. In the final group, constituting 20% of dissections, there was no single dominant ascending branch. Instead, the internal oblique muscle was supplied by a series of smaller branches arising at various points along the course of the DCIA.

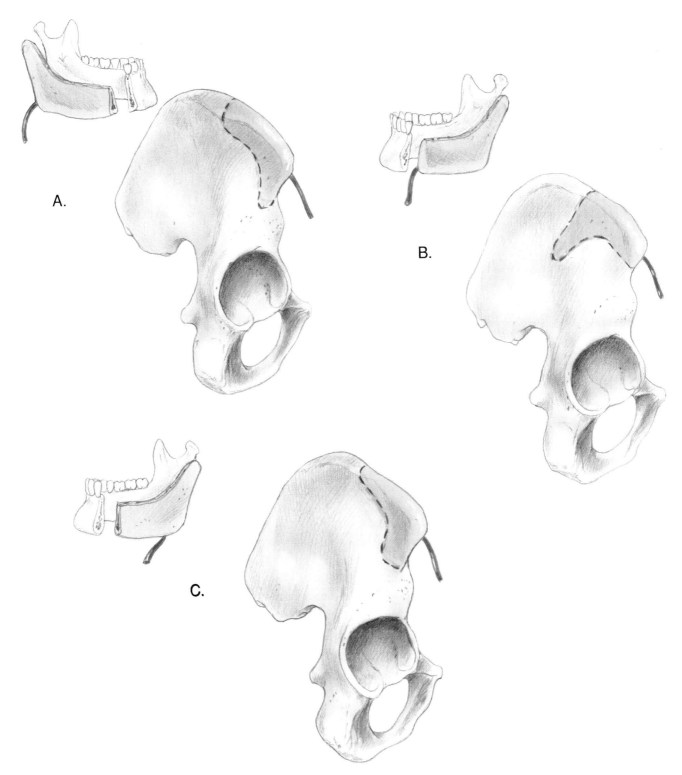

Figure 18-6. Different shapes of the iliac bone may be harvested, depending on which portion of the mandible must be reconstructed and where the recipient vessels are located. The variations become even more numerous when we consider that the bone may be oriented with the crest either along the neoridge or along the inferior border of the new mandible. There are three different bone designs that have been demonstrated in these illustrations that reflect a number of different options that are available for reconstructing the hemimandible. **A:** A hemimandible designed from the ipsilateral hip provides a neomandible of appropriate curvature and the pedicle arising at the angle. **B:** By selecting a flap from the contralateral side of the pelvis, the hemimandible can be restored with the pedicle arising near the midline. **C:** When the defect is limited to the ramus and condyle, the design can be changed so that the crest is used to achieve appropriate mandibular height.

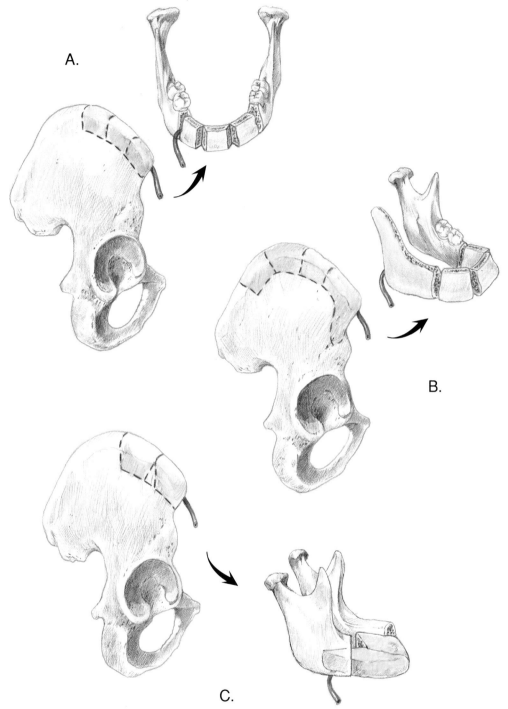

Figure 18-7. Several different orientations of the iliac bone may be harvested, based on the demands of the mandibular defect. **A:** When symphyseal defects are present, a straight piece of iliac bone is harvested that requires osteotomies to achieve a gentle curvature that matches the anterior mandible. **B:** This same principle applies when extending the defect from the ramus or condyle across the midline, in which case the length of bone to be harvested extends more posteriorly. The ramus, condyle, and body of the mandible rarely require significant contouring because of the similarity in shape of the pelvis to the hemimandible. However, distal osteotomies are needed to achieve a gentle curvature of the central mandible. **C:** The iliac bone may also be placed as a platform in a horizontal position to reconstruct the symphysis and the tongue in patients who have undergone composite resections that involve the anterior mandible and significant or total glossectomies. Placement of the bone in a horizontal position allows the skin to be supported against the effects of gravity while duplicating the gentle curvature of the symphysis. This is achieved by removing a V-shaped ostectomy of the ilium, which allows the bone to be collapsed and, therefore, produces the desired curvature.

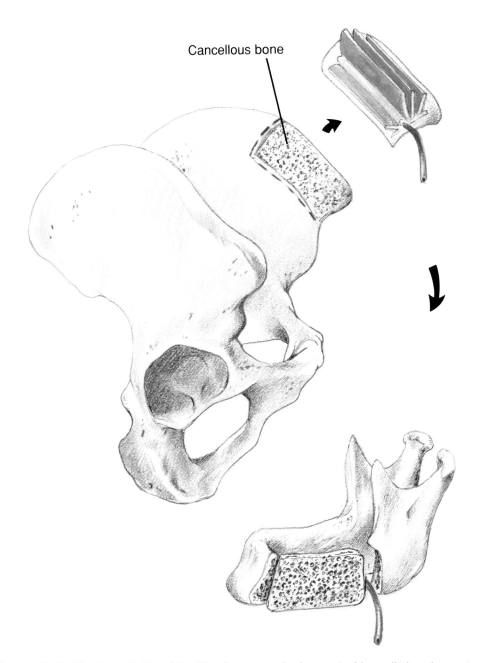

Cancellous bone

Figure 18-8. The inner table of the iliac bone may be harvested by splitting the cortex in the sagittal direction and transferring only the inner cortex of the bone with the muscle cuffs that protect the DCIA. This can then be used to reconstruct the mandible as shown. In the process of insetting the bone, the cancellous portion is oriented on the buccal aspect of the mandible. The advantage of this bone design is that it preserves the attachments of the upper thigh muscles, which facilitates the rehabilitation of the hip in the postoperative period.

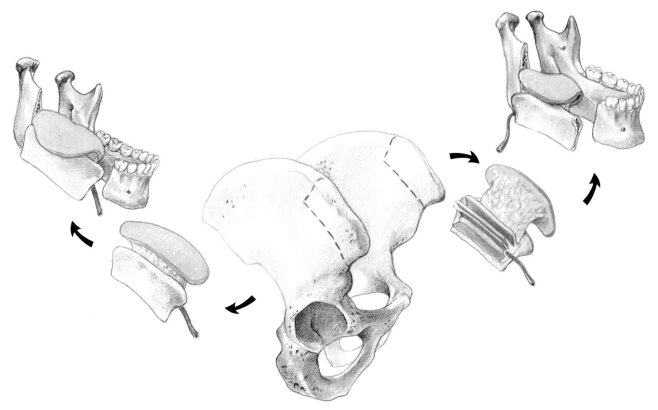

Figure 18-9. The iliac osteocutaneous flap may be inset with the crest forming the ridge of the neomandible. This orientation places the skin in its normal anatomic position relative to the bone and, therefore, avoids any torsion on the delicate musculocutaneous perforators. This flap configuration is suitable for use in patients who have very thin subcutaneous tissue overlying the inguinal region. The selection of the appropriate donor hip is determined by the location of the recipient vessels. When this osteocutaneous flap is harvested from the contralateral hip, the vessels exit at the angle of the neomandible. When the ipsilateral hip is utilized, the pedicle exits nearer the midline, in closer proximity to recipient vessels in the contralateral neck.

is a tremendous amount of versatility in the use of the soft tissue components of the iliac composite flap. The osteocutaneous flap may be placed with the crest as the neoridge and the skin situated on top of the crest in its normal anatomic relationship to the bone (Figure 18-9). Alternatively, the crest may be placed at the inferior aspect of the neomandible, leaving the cut surface of the cancellous bone to form the new alveolar ridge. In the latter orientation, the skin must be tunneled on the lingual or the buccal aspect of the neomandible. In virtually all cases, the bone is oriented with the DCIA and DCIV on the lingual aspect of the neomandible so that rigid fixation plates can be applied to the buccal cortex. In virtually all cases in which the skin of the osteocutaneous flap is placed in the oral cavity, secondary procedures are required to debulk the subcutaneous tissue or replace it with a skin graft.

The tripartite osteomusculocutaneous flap provides an added dimension for oromandibular reconstruction. The mobility of the internal oblique muscle, by virtue of its axial pattern blood supply in 80% of cases, allows the surgeon the freedom to position it in three dimensions relative to the bone (Figure 18-10). In most cases, the internal oblique is placed intraorally and wrapped around the neomandible or transposed posteriorly to resurface a portion of the pharynx. A split-thickness skin graft placed over the muscle serves as a primary vestibuloplasty to restore the sulcal anatomy and to maintain the mobility of the tongue (14). The denervated internal oblique muscle undergoes atrophy and provides a well-vascularized thin immobile tissue layer over the neomandible. In situations in which the mucosal defect is limited to the gingiva, then the internal oblique muscle can be left bare to remucosalize and,

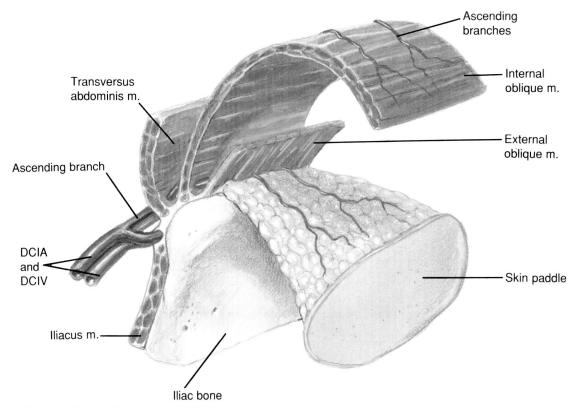

Figure 18-10. The tripartite iliac internal oblique osteomusculocutaneous flap is shown in its normal anatomic position following harvest from the left side of the pelvis. Cuffs of the iliacus, transversus abdominis, and external oblique are harvested with the internal oblique muscle to protect the perforators to the skin. When this flap is inset into the oral cavity for oromandibular reconstruction, it is usually turned 180 degrees so that the crest forms the inferior border of the neomandible.

therefore, avoid placement of a skin graft. This flap is ideal for the reconstruction of composite defects that involve mucosa, bone, and external skin. The skin of this osteomusculocutaneous flap is well positioned to resurface cutaneous defects of the neck and lower face. As it hangs from the lower border of the neomandible, the skin is in a favorable position with regard to the lack of torsion or tension on the nutrient perforators (Figure 18-11). When the cutaneous defect extends above the level of the lateral commissure, then the use of the iliac skin paddle becomes unfavorable because of the effect on its vascular supply. An alternative solution to this complex defect is to use the subscapular system of flaps, which has maximum mobility of the soft tissue components relative to the bone (20).

The reconstruction of the tongue of a patient who requires a total or subtotal glossectomy is challenging. The problem is even greater when the anterior mandible is also resected. The combination of a total glossectomy defect with a lateral mandibulectomy can be managed well with a soft tissue flap and a rigid mandibular reconstruction plate to maintain the contour of the lower jaw. However, when the bony defect involves the region of the symphysis, a vascularized bone graft should be utilized. Salibian et al. (11,12) introduced a unique design for the iliac osteocutaneous flap in which the bone was placed in the floor of the mouth in a horizontal position to act as a shelf to support the overlying soft tissue flap. The skin flap of the osteocutaneous flap was transposed into the oral cavity to reconstruct the tongue. As originally reported, both the DCIA and the SCIA were revascularized to ensure the blood supply to the skin. In our experience, it has only been necessary to anastomose the DCIA when using this flap design. This may be the result, in part, of the trapezoidal bone that was described by Salibian et al. As an alternative, we have harvested a

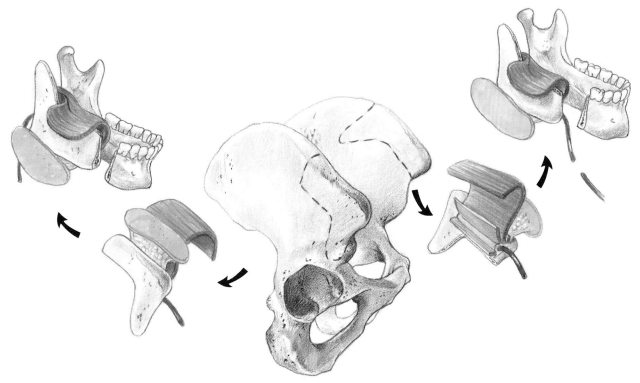

Figure 18-11. The combined iliac crest internal oblique flap transfers a skin paddle and the broad sheet of the internal oblique muscle. The selection of the appropriate hip is determined by the availability of the recipient vessels in the neck. When the recipient artery and vein are located in the contralateral neck, then harvest of the flap from the contralateral hip places the vessels at a more favorable location closer to the midline. Alternatively, when the recipient vessels are located in the ipsilateral neck, this requires a flap to be harvested from the ipsilateral hip, which allows orientation of the vessels at the angle of the mandible.

longer piece of the ilium, which is then contoured to the shape of the anterior arch and placed as a horizontal platform by removing a triangular wedge of bone that comes to a point at the crest (Figure 18-7C). The advantage of this modification is that a longer course of the DCIA and DCIV is harvested, which ensures a greater number of perforators. Long-term follow-up of patients who have undergone this type of reconstruction has shown excellent maintenance of the height of the neo-tongue because of the support provided by the bony platform.

The iliac crest has also been used for the reconstruction of hard palate defects in which the insertion of endosteal implants has allowed functional dental restoration comparable to that of the lower jaw (8). Finally, the iliac crest–internal oblique flap has been utilized in the restoration of skull base defects (10).

NEUROVASCULAR ANATOMY

The DCIA arises from the lateral aspect of the external iliac artery approximately 1 to 2 cm cephalad to the inguinal ligament. It courses toward the ASIS enclosed within a fascial envelope that consists of the fasciae of the transversalis and iliacus. In its more lateral curvilinear course, it travels along the inner table of the ilium in the groove formed by the junction of the transversus abdominis muscle and the iliacus. That groove is located from 0.4 to 2.2 cm inferior to the inner lip of the iliac crest (2). During its course, it gives off the ascending branch, which supplies the internal oblique muscle, and the periosteal and endosteal perforators to the ilium. It supplies the overlying skin through a series of branches that traverse the three layers of the abdominal wall. The DCIA terminates as a dominant skin feeder approximately 9 to 10 cm posterior to the ASIS (13) (Figure 18-12).

A series of cadaveric dissections revealed the diameter of the DCIA to be 2 to 3 mm; the DCIV ranged from 3 to 5 mm (2). The length of the free portion of the DCIA, which extends from the ASIS to its junction with the external iliac artery, is between 5 and 7 cm (2). The DCIV may be several centimeters longer because it often runs a longitudinal cephalad course prior to entering the external iliac vein. The DCIV is usually composed of two paired venae comitantes, which merge at a variable distance lateral to the external iliac vein. The DCIV receives a consistent ascending branch proximal to its junction with the external iliac vein. This branch must be transsected to achieve the maximum length of the DCIV pedicle. The DCIV may pass either superficially or deep to the external iliac artery and, therefore, diverges from the DCIA in its medial portion.

There are two important factors that the surgeon must keep in mind to ensure preservation of the blood supply to the skin. The first is related to the flap design, which must capture the three to nine perforators that exit the external oblique muscle in a zone that extends approximately 9 cm posterior to the ASIS and about 2.5 cm medial to the crest. This zone of perforators can be readily incorporated by designing a skin paddle centered along an axis drawn from the ASIS to the inferior border of the scapula. The second major technical factor is the preservation of the obligatory cuff of external oblique, internal oblique, and transversus abdominis layers through which these perforators traverse. Although the perforators can be identified on the undersurface of the skin, we usually maintain a healthy distance from the inner table of the ilium to avoid these vessels. It is this arrangement of very small perforators, located in this zone, that makes it imperative to maintain the relationship of the skin to the bone to avoid twisting or stretching these vessels.

The internal oblique muscle is a thin broad muscle that lies between the transversus abdominis and the external oblique on the anterior abdominal wall. It originates from the thoracolumbar fascia, the iliac crest, and the inguinal ligament. It inserts into the 10th through the 12th ribs and the rectus sheath (Figure 18-4). The ascending branch of the DCIA provides the dominant blood supply to the internal oblique. However, there are contributions from branches of the deep inferior epigastric artery and branches of the lower thoracic and lumbar arteries that run in the same neurovascular plane between the transversus abdominis and the internal oblique. The ascending branch is a large vessel measuring 1 to 2 mm in diameter that arises from the DCIA and courses through the transversus abdominis to reach the undersurface of the internal oblique. It is important to reiterate that the ascending branch provides no cutaneous circulation. In two independent cadaver dissections, the anatomy of the ascending branch could be categorized into three distinct groups (8,16). In

---→

Figure 18-12. The DCIA and DCIV originate from the external iliac vessels a few centimeters above the inguinal ligament. Three separate approaches to the DCIA and DCIV have been described. The first is a caudal approach that begins below the inguinal ligament by dissecting proximally along the plane of the femoral vessels underneath the inguinal ligament. The second approach is transinguinal, through the posterior wall of the inguinal canal. Finally, the third approach utilizes the ascending branch as a guide to dissect in a retrograde fashion to its takeoff from the DCIA. The DCIA and DCIV run a relatively straight course from the external iliac artery and vein to the ASIS. From the ASIS, they continue laterally in a curvilinear fashion in the groove formed by the junction of the iliacus and the transversus abdominis. In its course, the DCIA gives off the ascending branch, which runs through the transversus abdominis to supply the internal oblique muscle. It also supplies the iliac bone through endosteal and periosteal feeders. Musculocutaneous perforators are given off in an array along the inner table of the iliac crest. These perforators must traverse the three muscle layers of the abdominal wall before supplying the skin. The relationship of the femoral nerve to the external iliac artery and vein should be noted. The lateral femoral cutaneous nerve crosses medially to the ASIS, either superficially or deep to the DCIA-DCIV pedicle.

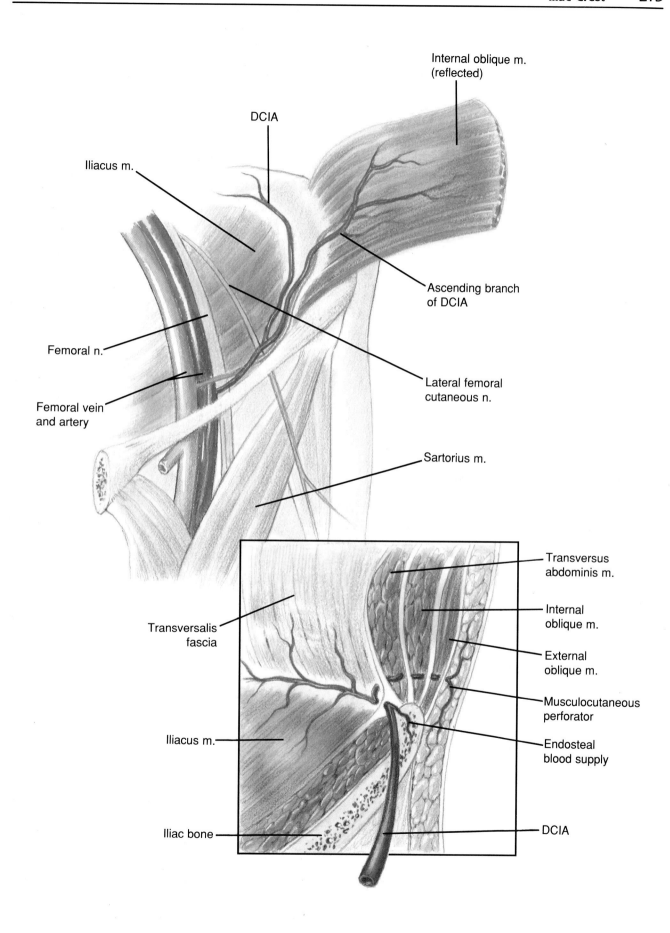

Internal oblique m. (reflected)

DCIA

Iliacus m.

Ascending branch of DCIA

Femoral n.

Lateral femoral cutaneous n.

Femoral vein and artery

Sartorius m.

Transversus abdominis m.

Transversalis fascia

Internal oblique m.

External oblique m.

Musculocutaneous perforator

Iliacus m.

Endosteal blood supply

Iliac bone

DCIA

approximately 65% of cases, the ascending branch arises from the DCIA within 1 cm of the ASIS. In 15% of dissections, the ascending branch had a more medial takeoff between 2 and 4 cm from the ASIS. In the remaining 20% of cases, there were multiple smaller branches that entered the muscle laterally to the ASIS. The important conclusion from these statistics is that approximately 80% of internal oblique muscles are supplied by a single dominant vessel arising medially to the ASIS. The surgeon therefore has the freedom to treat the internal oblique muscle as a flap with an axial pattern blood supply in these patients (7,13). In the remaining patients, the muscle must remain attached to the inner lip of the iliac crest to preserve the smaller more numerous feeders from the DCIA.

The internal oblique muscle has a segmental nerve supply from the lower thoracic (T-8 to T-12), iliohypogastric (L-1), and ilioinguinal nerves (L-1). It is therefore not a front-line muscle to reinnervate and use in a dynamic reconstruction. The lateral femoral cutaneous nerve exits from the pelvis, running a course medial to the ASIS, either superficially or deep to the DCIA and DCIV. This nerve may be preserved through meticulous dissection. However, we often harvest a portion of this nerve as a free nerve graft for bridging nerve defects in the head and neck, such as the inferior alveolar nerve. Finally, the femoral nerve runs in a deeper plane laterally to the external iliac artery and vein. Although rarely identified during the course of the dissection, its position should be noted to be certain that injury is avoided during the closure. To date, there have been no reports of restoring sensation to the skin paddle of the iliac crest composite flap.

ANATOMIC VARIATIONS

Aside from the variable position and number of branches of the ascending branch, the major anatomic variations of this donor site are few and infrequent. In the multiple series of cadaver dissections noted earlier and my own experience with more than 120 iliac crest free flaps, there have been no cases of an absent DCIA or DCIV. However, in a small number of dissections, Taylor and Daniel (15) found that the DCIA passed through the transversus abdominis medially to the ASIS, assuming a more superficial position. It is imperative that this anomalous course does not cause the surgeon to mistake the DCIA for the ascending branch.

In our experience, the ascending branch has a separate takeoff from the external iliac artery in about 5% of cases. Included in this group are the cases in which the ascending branch arises from the DCIA within 1 to 2 mm of the external iliac artery. In such cases, these two vessels must be treated as separate pedicles. We have also encountered the rare anomaly of duplication of the DCIA. In these cases, we placed a temporary microvascular clamp on each artery to determine their relative dominance before deciding which branch to anastomose in the neck. When the results of this test were inconclusive, we performed a double arterial anastomosis. Duplication of the DCIV has been encountered in only a small number of cases. However, when the two venae comitantes join within 1 to 2 mm from the external iliac vein, the ligation of that vessel often creates the necessity to perform two separate venous anastomoses.

POTENTIAL PITFALLS

There are several potential problems that may be encountered in using composite flaps from the ilium. Perhaps the greatest concern is related to the integrity of the abdominal wall. The presence of a weakness or hernia prior to surgery may suggest that an alternative donor site be used or that the surgeon should be alerted to the need for additional measures in donor-site closure. On occasion, we have utilized a synthetic mesh when the native tissues are of poor quality. As in all aspects of reconstructive microsurgery, meticulous technique and attention to detail are critical factors in producing a successful outcome. In addition to frank hernia formation, the harvest of the internal oblique muscle causes denervation of the rectus abdominis through interruption of its motor nerve supply, which runs in the neurovascular plane between the internal oblique and the transversus abdominis. These nerves are readily identified and can be preserved through careful dissection. In our experience, incisional hernias are rare as are patient complaints related to abdominal wall bulging. Attention must also be paid to vital neighboring structures, such as the femoral nerve and the intraperitoneal contents, to prevent injury during harvest or closure.

Although atherosclerotic involvement of the external iliac artery is fairly common, we have not encountered similar problems in the DCIA. There have been no cases in our experience in which this flap was abandoned intraoperatively because of atherosclerosis. There was one case in our experience in which the DCIV was too small for transfer of this flap, which was then abandoned and an alternative donor site used. The blood supply to the soft tissue components of this composite flap may be compromised by a number of factors. Prior surgery, such as an appendectomy, may lead to direct damage of the ascending branch of the internal oblique muscle. The blood supply to the skin may be at risk as a result of (a) failure of flap design to incorporate a sufficient number of perforators, (b) failure to preserve an adequate muscle cuff of the three abdominal wall muscles, and (c) altering the relationship of the skin paddle to the bone, causing tension or kinking of these perforators.

POSTOPERATIVE CARE

Postoperative care of the donor site following harvest of the iliac crest osteocutaneous or osteomusculocutaneous flaps involves progressive mobilization, which begins on the third or fourth postoperative day. Assisted ambulation usually begins by the seventh postoperative day along with passive and active range-of-motion exercises. Progressive assisted ambulation is carried out during the second postoperative week. Stair climbing does not usually begin until the third week after surgery.

Flap Harvesting Technique follows on page 276.

Flap Harvesting Technique
Internal Oblique Iliac Crest Flap

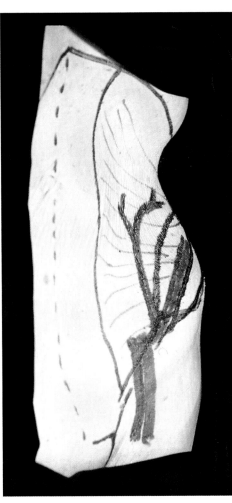

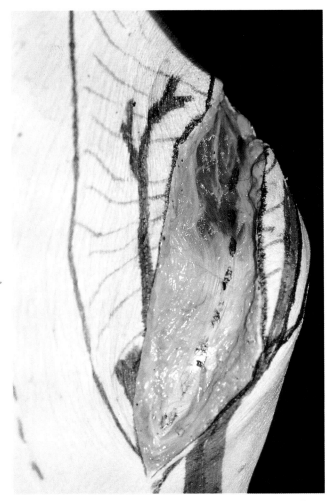

Figure 18-13. Harvest of the iliac crest internal oblique osteomusculocutaneous flap is accomplished by modification of the original technique that was described for harvesting the iliac crest osteocutaneous flap. The approach to the vascular pedicle that I use when harvesting the internal oblique muscle serves as the basis for the approach to the vascular pedicle when the osteocutaneous flap is harvested. I begin with a dissection of the internal oblique muscle.

Figure 18-14. The dissection begins by incising along the cephalad limit of the skin paddle, which is marked by drawing a fusiform skin island. This skin island is usually centered along an axis that runs from the anterior superior spine to the inferior border of the scapula. It is essential to capture the dominant musculocutaneous perforators that exit through a zone that extends from approximately 2.5 cm medially and cephalad to the crest and runs approximately 9 cm posterolaterally from the anterior superior iliac spine. The incision extends through the skin and subcutaneous tissue to expose the external oblique muscle and aponeurosis. The skin may be elevated off the external oblique muscle until approximately 2–2.5 cm from the medial aspect of the crest.

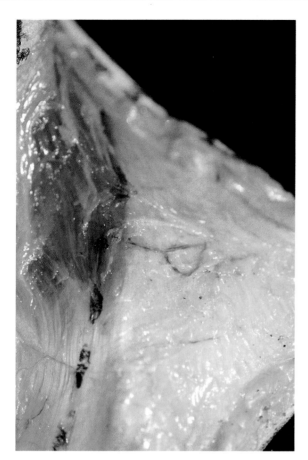

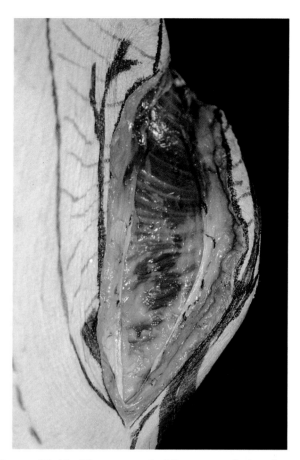

Figure 18-15. By careful dissection in this plane between the subcutaneous tissue and the external oblique muscle, the surgeon can usually identify dominant musculocutaneous perforators, as shown in this dissection. These perforators must be preserved to maintain the vascularity to the skin. A *dotted line* has been drawn in the direction of the fibers of the external oblique muscle, approximately 2.5–3 cm above the iliac crest and marks the incision that is made through the external oblique muscle and fascia.

Figure 18-16. The external oblique muscle has been incised throughout the full extent of the wound, as previously noted. This cuff of the external oblique muscle, which measures approximately 2.5 cm in width, should not be elevated in a caudal direction off the internal oblique muscle to avoid interfering with the perforators that come through the three muscle layers of the abdominal wall.

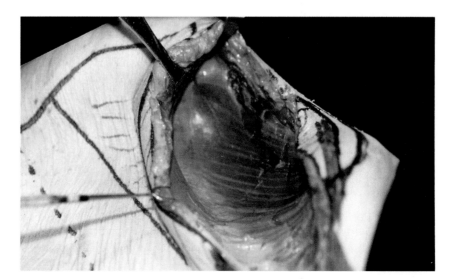

Figure 18-17. The entire internal oblique muscle is exposed by elevating the external oblique muscle up to the level of the costal margin by blunt and sharp dissection. This plane of dissection is relatively avascular.

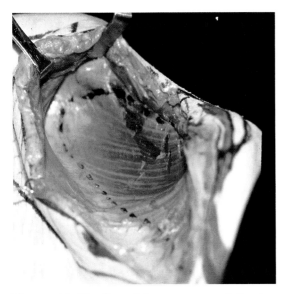

Figure 18-18. Complete exposure of the internal oblique muscle has been obtained. The 12th rib can be easily palpated. A *dotted line* has been placed along the margins of the internal oblique. Incisions are made around the perimeter of the internal oblique muscle prior to elevating it off the transversus abdominis. The inferior attachments of the muscle to the crest are left undisturbed.

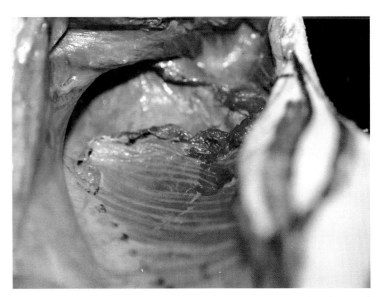

Figure 18-19. The plane of dissection between the internal oblique and the transversus abdominis is most easily identified in the region just caudal to the 12th rib. In this location, the division between the two muscle layers is the most well defined. A change in the direction of the muscle fibers signifies the correct intermuscular plane. Meticulous dissection in this plane is required to elevate the internal oblique muscle completely from cephalad to caudad.

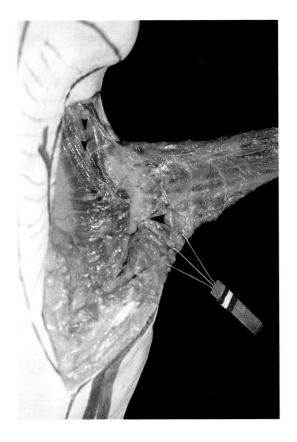

Figure 18-20. Elevation of the internal oblique muscle has been completed. In the process of elevating this muscle, the integrity of the transversus abdominis must be maintained. In addition, meticulous dissection is necessary to identify and maintain the ascending branch (*large arrow*) of the DCIA, which is the nutrient blood supply to the internal oblique muscle. Segmental neurovascular bundles traverse the abdomen laterally to medially between the internal oblique muscle and the transversus abdominis (*small arrows*). The cephalad neurovascular bundles can be maintained. However, in the more caudal locations, the terminal branches of the intercostal neurovascular bundles intertwine with the ascending branch and must be transsected. There are often interconnecting branches between the ascending branch and the segmental branches that must be carefully coagulated using bipolar cautery. Unipolar cautery should be avoided in this location.

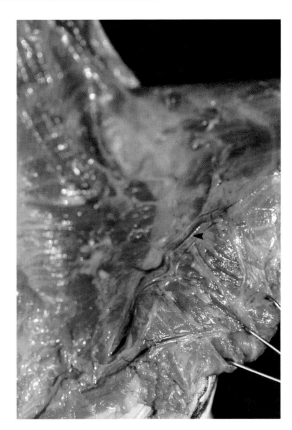

Figure 18-21. A close-up view of the undersurface of the internal oblique muscle reveals the ascending branch (*arrow*) of the DCIA. As the dissection is followed inferiorly and medially, multiple tributaries converge to the main trunk of the ascending branch which then travels through the transversus abdominis muscle layer to join with the DCIA and DCIV.

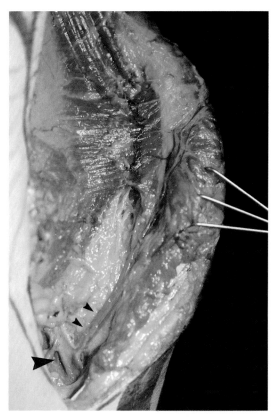

Figure 18-22. The junction of the ascending branch with the DCIA occurs most often in the region medial to the ASIS. The DCIA and DCIV (*small arrows*) are then traced to their junction with the external iliac artery and vein (*large arrow*). The preperitoneal fat must be retracted medially and cephalad to gain exposure of the iliacus.

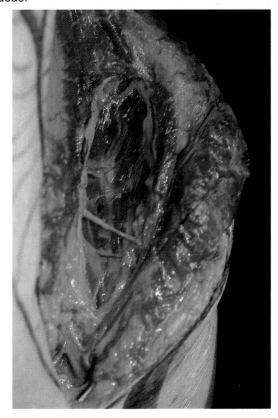

Figure 18-23. The lateral portion of the transversus abdominis is then transsected, leaving a 2-cm cuff attached to the inner table of the iliac crest. The exposure afforded by this maneuver provides access to the iliacus and to the lateral femoral cutaneous nerve (*arrow*). The DCIA and DCIV run in a fibrous tunnel created by convergence of the fasciae of the transversalis and the iliacus. The more lateral course of the DCIA and DCIV runs in the groove between the iliacus and the transversus abdominis. Although the pulse of the DCIA can be palpated in this groove, there is no reason to expose the vascular pedicle lateral to the ASIS.

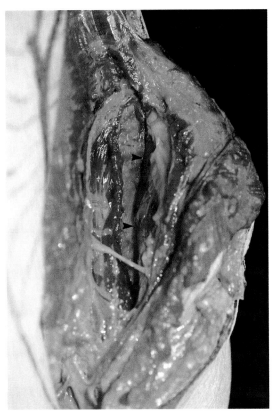

Figure 18-24. The iliacus is transsected to expose the inner table of the ilium. A 2-cm cuff of iliacus (*arrows*) is left attached to the inner table as protection for the DCIA and DCIV.

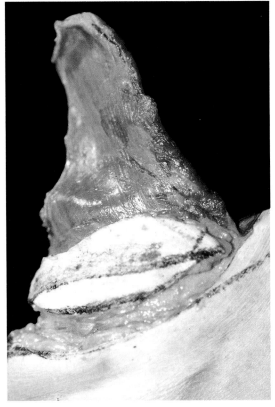

Figure 18-25. The lateral dissection now begins by incising along the inferior border of the skin paddle to the level of the tensor fasciae latae and the tendon of the gluteus medius.

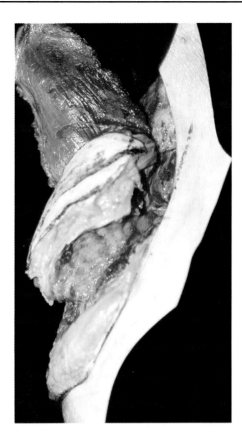

Figure 18-26. Sharp dissection along the entire lateral border of the iliac crest provides exposure to the outer table of the ilium to perform the osteotomies. A strip of tensor fasciae latae may be left attached to the outer lip of the iliac crest to help secure the bone in selected situations.

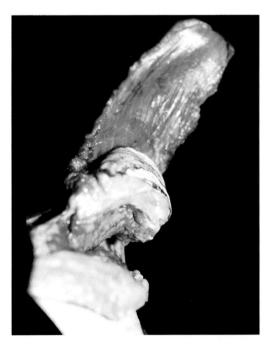

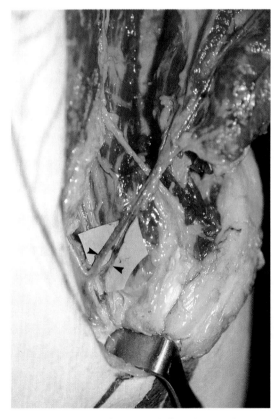

Figure 18-27. The dissection is viewed from the vantage point of the midabdomen, looking directly at the ASIS. The internal oblique muscle has been completely elevated, and the skin paddle sits in its normal anatomic position atop the iliac crest. The lateral thigh muscles have been transsected to provide exposure of the outer table of the ilium.

Figure 18-28. The DCIA and DCIV (*arrows*) must be dissected free of the surrounding soft tissues in the region between their takeoff from the external iliac artery and vein to the ASIS. Meticulous dissection around the ASIS determines whether the lateral femoral cutaneous nerve runs a course superficial or deep to the DCIA and DCIV. Careful transsection of the iliopsoas and sartorius along the medial aspect of the ilium completes the soft tissue dissection.

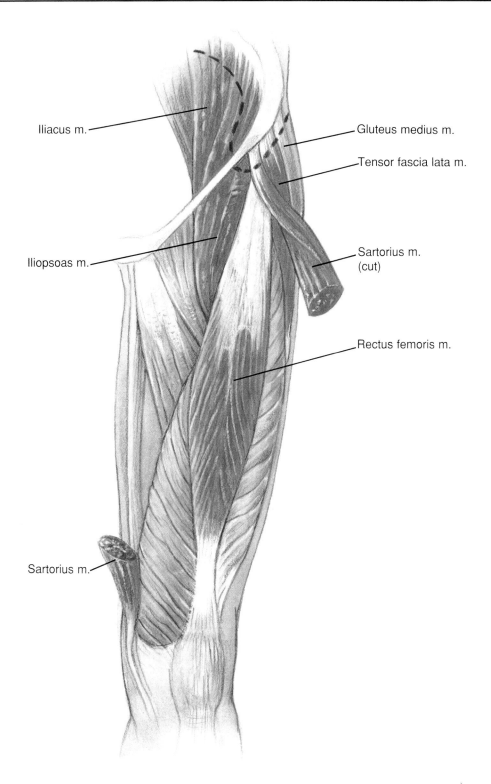

Iliacus m.

Gluteus medius m.

Tensor fascia lata m.

Iliopsoas m.

Sartorius m.
(cut)

Rectus femoris m.

Sartorius m.

Figure 18-29. The *dotted line* marks the cuts that are made to gain exposure of the iliac bone. A 2- to 3-cm cuff of iliacus is left attached to the ilium to protect the DCIA. Medial exposure of the ilium is made by cutting the iliopsoas muscle with the DCIA and DCIV completely mobilized and protected in that region. The gluteus medius, sartorius, and tensor fasciae latae are removed flush with the outer table of the ilium. Alternatively, if a unicortical bone graft is to be harvested, then the upper thigh muscles are left attached at this point in the dissection, and bone cuts are made sagittally through the crest and transversely through the inner table.

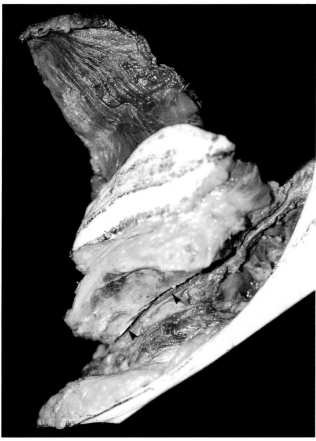

Figure 18-30. While protecting the abdominal contents by using deep retractors, osteotomies (*arrows*) are made from the lateral exposure. The protection of the DCIA and DCIV must be maintained while making the medial bone cuts.

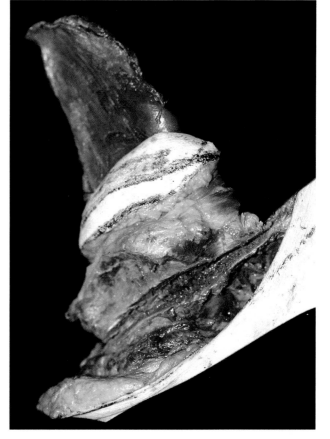

Figure 18-31. The osteotomy has been completed and the bone segment that is to be included in this composite flap is now freed.

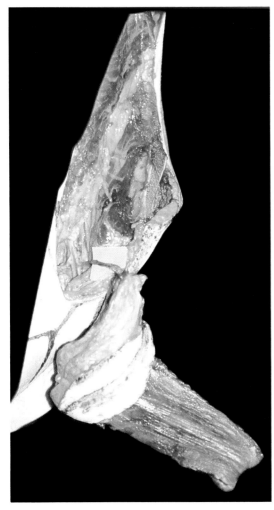

Figure 18-32. From a medial vantage point, the composite flap has been rotated 180 degrees while still attached to the external iliac artery and vein. Harvesting of this flap is completed by a double ligation of the DCIA and a single ligation of the DCIV.

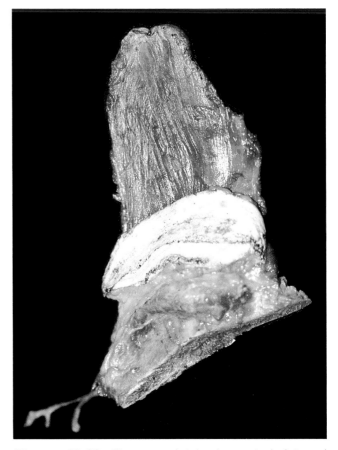

Figure 18-33. The completely harvested internal oblique iliac crest osteomusculocutaneous flap with its vascular pedicle is shown from a lateral view. A bicortical segment of bone with the upper thigh muscles completely freed from the lateral table of the crest is demonstrated.

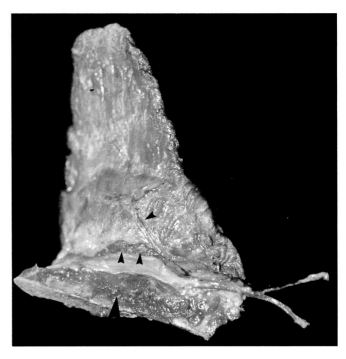

Figure 18-34. Examination of the medial aspect of this composite flap reveals the undersurface of the internal oblique muscle with the ascending branch (*small arrow*). The cuff of the transversus abdominis is demonstrated by the *double small arrows*. The cuff of the iliacus is demonstrated by the *large arrow*. The cuff of the external oblique muscle and aponeurosis, which lies superficial to the internal oblique muscle, is not visualized.

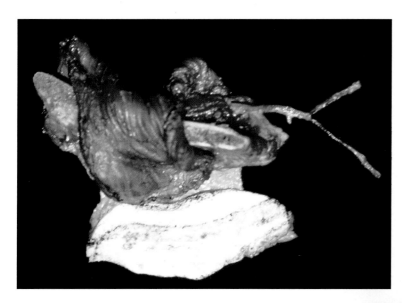

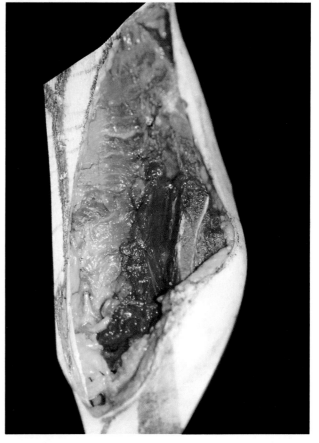

Figure 18-35. The use of the internal oblique muscle as coverage of the bone is demonstrated by wrapping the sheath of muscle over the cut margin of the iliac bone. Using this technique, the ascending branch runs on the undersurface of the muscle adjacent to the bone.

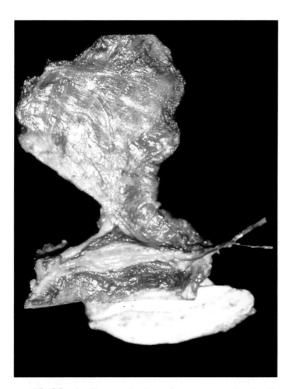

Figure 18-36. In the majority of cases, a single dominant ascending branch provides an axial blood supply to the internal oblique muscle. Further mobilization of the internal oblique muscle may be achieved by making a back cut parallel to the bone, from laterally to medially, to the ascending branch. It is imperative to maintain a 2–2.5-cm cuff of internal oblique muscle while making this back cut to protect the integrity of the musculocutaneous perforators that are traversing the three layers of the abdominal wall.

Figure 18-37. Closure of the abdominal wall must be completed in a meticulous fashion to prevent a ventral hernia. After copious irrigation and hemostasis, the first layer of closure is achieved by approximating the transversus abdominis to the iliacus. To reinforce this layer of the closure, drill holes may be placed along the cut margin of the iliac bone through which sutures are placed that traverse the iliacus and the transversus abdominis. It is essential to note the position of the femoral nerve, which lies laterally to the femoral artery. Deep sutures in this region must be avoided to prevent injury to that nerve.

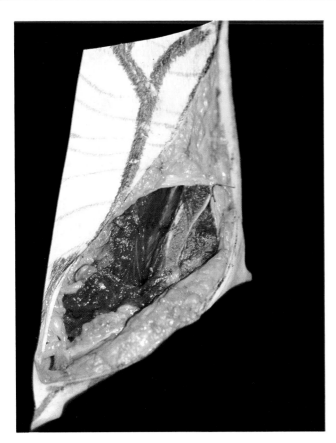

Figure 18-38. The next layer of closure approximates the external oblique muscle and aponeurosis to the tensor fasciae latae and the tendon of the gluteus medius.

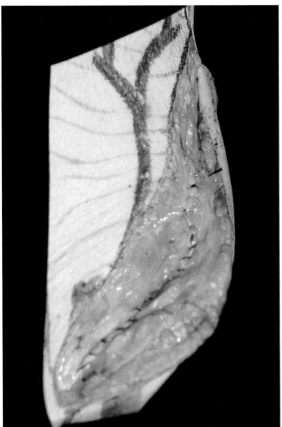

Figure 18-39. The second muscle layer closure has been completed.

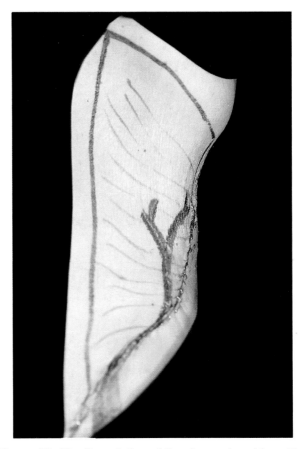

Figure 18-40. Completion of the closure is achieved by a layered approximation of the subcutaneous tissue and the skin.

Flap Harvesting Technique
The Iliac Crest Osteocutaneous Flap

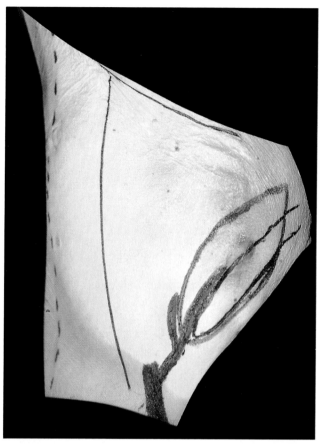

Figure 18-41. The harvest of the iliac crest osteocutaneous flap is performed by using a technique similar to that described for the osteomusculocutaneous flap. The topographical anatomy of the left hip is drawn at the outset of this dissection.

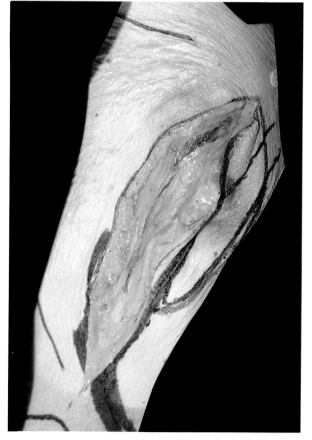

Figure 18-42. The cephalad margin of the skin paddle has been incised to the level of the external oblique muscle and fascia.

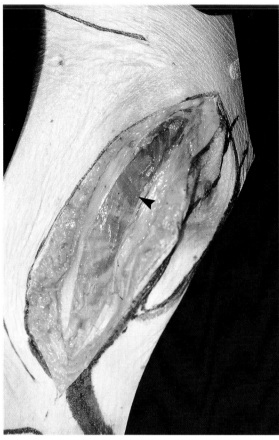

Figure 18-43. The external oblique muscle and aponeurosis have been transsected, leaving a cuff of external oblique (*arrow*), approximately 2 cm in width, attached to the inner table of the ilium.

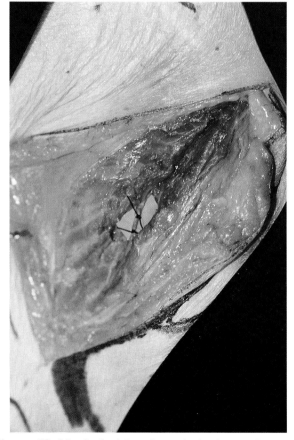

Figure 18-44. An incision through the internal oblique muscle, which leaves 2 cm attached to the ilium, provides exposure of the ascending branch, which runs on its undersurface. Ligatures are shown on the ascending branch, which is then transsected.

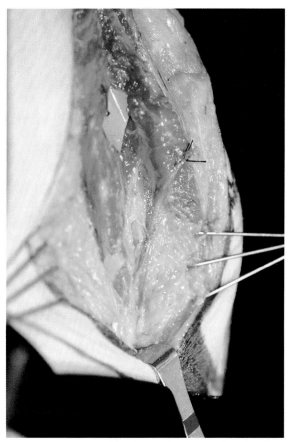

Figure 18-45. A medial view of the dissection reveals the ligated ascending branch as it courses through the transversus abdominis.

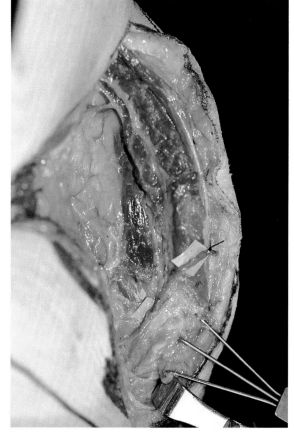

Figure 18-46. The ascending branch has been followed through the transversus abdominis, exposing the DCIA and DCIV to their junction with the external iliac vessels. The transversus abdominis has been incised laterally to expose the preperitoneal fat and the iliacus. The remainder of this dissection follows that of the description for the osteomusculocutaneous flap. The closure of this defect is modified as a result of the preservation of the internal oblique muscle, which is incorporated with the transversus abdominis for the inner layer of the abdominal wall closure.

REFERENCES

1. Baker S. Reconstruction of mandibular defects with the revascularized free tensor fascia lata osteomyocutaneous flap. *Arch Otolaryngol Head Neck Surg* 1981;107:404.
2. Fredrickson JM, Man SC, Hayden RE. Revascularized iliac bone graft for mandibular reconstruction. *Acta Otolaryngol (Stockh)* 1985;99:214.
3. Gong-Kang H, Hu R, Miao H, Yin Z, Lan T, Pan G. Microvascular free transfer of iliac bone based on the deep superior branches of the superior gluteal vessel. *Plast Reconstr Surg* 1985;75:69.
4. Karener H, Helborn B, Radner H. The osteomusculocutaneous musculoperitoneal groin flap in head and neck reconstruction. *J Reconstr Microsurg* 1989;5:31.
5. Koshina I, Fakuda H, Soeda S. Free combined anterolateral thigh flap and vascularized iliac bone graft with double vascular pedicle. *J Reconstr Microsurg* 1989;5:55.
6. Manchester W. Immediate reconstruction of the mandible and temporomandibular joint. *Br J Plast Surg* 1965;18:291.
7. Moscoso J, Keller J, Genden E, Weinberg H, Biller H, Buckbinder D, Urken ML. Vascularized bone flaps in oromandibular reconstruction: a comparative anatomic study of bone stock from various donor sites to assess suitability for enosseous dental implants. *Arch Otolaryngol Head Neck Surg* 1884;120:36.
8. Ramasastry SS, Granick MS, Futrell J. Clinical anatomy of the internal oblique muscle. *J Reconstr Microsurg* 1986;2:117.
9. Ramasastry SS, Tucker JB, Swartz WM, Hurwitz DJ. The internal oblique muscle flap: an anatomic and clinical study. *Plast Reconstr Surg* 1984;73:721.
10. Riediger D. Restoration of masticatory function by microsurgically revascularized iliac crest bone grafts using enosseous implants. *Plast Reconstr Surg* 1988;81:861.
11. Salibian A, Rappaport I, Allison G. Functional oromandibular reconstruction with the microvascular composite groin flap. *Plast Reconstr Surg* 1985;76:819.
12. Salibian A, Rappaport I, Furnas D, Achauer B. Microvascular reconstruction of the mandible. *Am J Surg* 1980;140:499.
13. Sanders R, Mayou B. A new vascularized bone graft transferred by microvascular anastomosis as a free flap. *Br J Surg* 1979;66:787.
14. Shenaq SM. Reconstruction of complex cranial and craniofacial defects utilizing iliac crest-internal oblique microsurgical free flap. *Microsurgery* 1988;9:154.
15. Taylor GI, Daniel RK. The free flap: composite tissue transfer by vascular anastomosis. *Aust N Z J Surg* 1973;43:1.
16. Taylor GI, Townsend P, Corlett R. Superiority of the deep circumflex iliac vessels as the supply for free groin flaps: experimental work. *Plast Reconstr Surg* 1979;64:595–604.
17. Taylor GI, Watson N. One-stage repair of compound leg defects with free, revascularized flaps of groin skin and iliac bone. *Plast Reconstr Surg* 1978;61:494–506.
18. Urken ML. Composite free flaps in oromandibular reconstruction. Review of the literature. *Arch Otolaryngol Head Neck Surg* 1991;118:724–732.
19. Urken ML, Vickery C, Weinberg H, Buchbinder D, Biller HF. The internal oblique-iliac crest osseomyocutaneous microvascular free flap in head and neck reconstruction. *J Reconstr Microsurg* 1989;5:203.
20. Urken ML, Vickery C, Weinberg H, Buchbinder D, Lawson W and Biller HF. The internal oblique-iliac crest osseomyocutaneous free flap in oromandibular reconstruction: report of 20 cases. *Arch Otolaryngol Head Neck Surg* 1989;115:339.
21. Urken ML, Weinberg H, Vickery C, Buchbinder D, Lawson W, Biller HF. The internal oblique-iliac crest free flap in composite defects of the oral cavity involving bone, skin and mucosa. *Laryngoscope* 1991;101:257.

19
CHAPTER

Fibular
Osteocutaneous

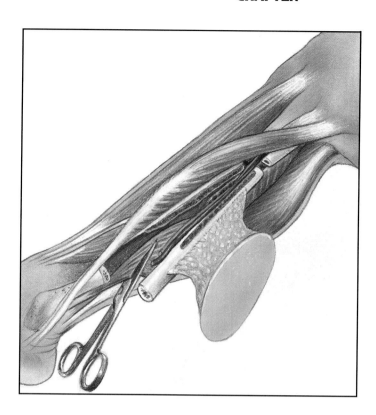

Mark L. Urken, M.D. and
Michael J. Sullivan, M.D.

Taylor et al. (28) were the first to report the successful transfer of the vascularized fibular bone flap for reconstruction of an open fracture of the lower extremity in 1975. A posterior approach to harvesting this flap was described. Gilbert (7) introduced a much simpler lateral approach to fibular flap harvest in 1979, and it is this technique that is universally applied today. Chen and Yan (4) are credited with being the first to report the transfer of a fibular osteocutaneous flap in 1983 (4). In the same year, Yoshimura et al. (33) described the transfer of the fibular bone with a "buoy" flap of skin that served as a monitor of the circulation. The primary purpose for using the fibular donor site was to reconstruct long bone defects of the extremities until Hidalgo (14) adapted this flap to the restoration of segmental mandibulectomy defects in 1989. A number of detailed anatomic dissections have helped to clarify the circulation from the peroneal artery to the skin (2–4,22,26,31). However, the variability in the vascular supply to the skin occasionally limits the use of this flap in oromandibular reconstruction in which defects of the mucosa and the skin are commonly encountered. The ease of harvest and the distance from the head and neck region have enhanced the popularity of this donor site.

The fibula is a long thin nonweight-bearing bone of the lower extremity (Figure 19-1). It has a tubular shape, with thick cortical bone around the entire circumference that renders it one of the strongest bones available for transfer (27). Approximately 22 to 25 cm of bone can be harvested while preserving 6 to 7 cm of bone both distally and proximally to maintain the integrity of the knee and ankle joints. The path of the common peroneal nerve, which wraps around the neck of the fibula, also limits proximal dissection and bone harvest. However, the ability to transfer up to 25 cm of

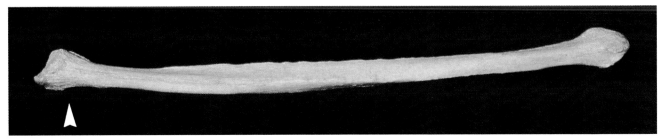

Figure 19-1. A lateral view of the fibula reveals the head at the proximal end (*arrow*) and the lateral malleolus distally. This long narrow bone is triangular on cross section. It forms a tube of dense cortical bone that surrounds the central medullary cavity and can supply up to 25 cm of vascularized bone.

bone makes this donor site unique in terms of the ability to restore total or subtotal defects of the mandible (8).

FLAP DESIGN AND UTILIZATION

The fibula can be transferred as a free osseous or as a free osteocutaneous flap. The skin of the lateral aspect of the calf is supplied by either septocutaneous or musculo-cutaneous perforators arising from the peroneal artery and vein. Variations in the location of these perforators occur along the posterior crural septum. It is therefore advisable to design a longer skin paddle that accounts for these variations (Figure 19-2). Fleming et al. (6) described a division of the skin flap for internal and external linings when multiple skin perforators were visualized. The width of the skin paddle is limited by the ability to achieve primary closure, although a skin graft can be effectively applied to the donor defect when needed.

The vascular pedicle to the fibular flap, although consistent in the location and caliber of the vessel's lumen, is often limited in length by the bifurcation of the posterior tibial artery (11). Additional length can be obtained on the vascular leash by harvesting a more distal segment of bone and skin while discarding the more proximal fibula. A subperiosteal dissection of the soft tissue surrounding the proximal bone that is to be removed effectively preserves the blood supply to the distal flap. Hidalgo (16) reported obtaining vascular pedicles as long as 12 cm by using this technique. In addition, Wei et al. (30) designed a proximal skin paddle combined with a distal bone segment to separate and increase the flexibility of the two components of this composite flap. The vascular supply of the skin was preserved by performing a subperiosteal dissection and discarding the proximal bone segment.

The peroneal artery and vein run along the entire length of the fibula without a significant change in the caliber of the vessel. This arrangement permits the use of the fibula as a "flow-through" flap to supply a second free flap anastomosed to the free ends of the distal artery and vein. Wei et al. (30) transferred two free flaps supplied by one set of donor vessels by using this technique.

The primary application of the fibular donor site in the head and neck has been in the reconstruction of segmental defects of the mandible. The strength of the cortical bone effectively withstands the powerful forces of mastication. There are certain situations in which the characteristics of the fibula are particularly conducive to a successful reconstruction. As noted previously, the length of bone that can be harvested makes it the only donor site that is suitable for the reconstruction of subtotal or total mandibular defects. In the secondary reconstruction of mandibular defects that involve the ramus and condyle, it is often possible to create only a narrow tunnel for the placement of the graft into the glenoid fossa. The creation of a larger tunnel is limited by scarring and concerns about injury to the facial nerve. The narrow fibula is much easier to pass through such a tunnel than a bulkier segment of bone, such as the ilium.

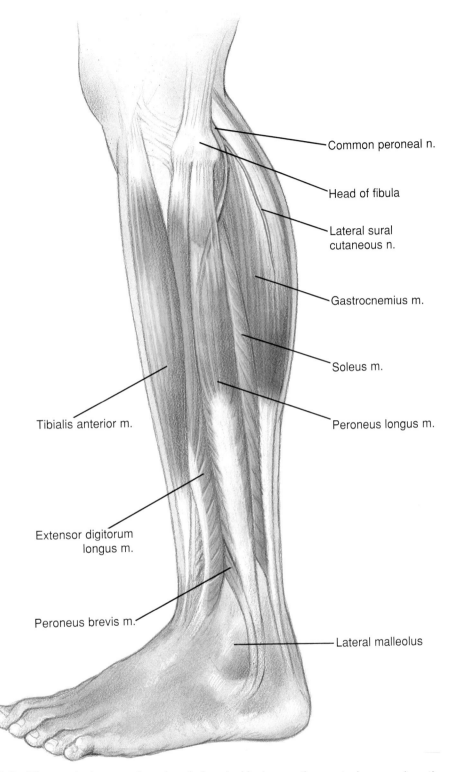

Figure 19-2. The posterior crural septum is located between the posterior muscles, the gastrocnemius and soleus, and the anterior muscles, the peroneus longus and brevis. The approximate position of the septum can be gauged by drawing a line between the head of the fibula and the lateral malleolus. The lateral sural cutaneous nerve arises from the common peroneal nerve and supplies sensation to the skin of the fibular osteocutaneous flap.

The long straight fibular bone must be contoured to match the shape of the mandible by creating wedge-shaped closing osteotomies. Hidalgo (16) described a series of techniques that allow more aesthetic contouring of the fibula to mimic the shape of the native mandible. Multiple osteotomies can be performed without compromising distal bone circulation if the periosteum is not significantly traumatized. Hidalgo advised against stripping the periosteum when performing an osteotomy by performing the bone cuts directly through the periosteum and the bone. Jones et al. (18) showed that the fibular bone could be osteotomized and folded on itself to produce a "double-barreled" vascularized bone graft. The vascularity to the distal segment was maintained through the periosteum. The double-barreled fibular flap was applied to the reconstruction of segmental defects of the femur.

This technique was advanced even further by Sadove and Powell (23) who removed a 3-cm segment of the fibula, in addition to performing osteotomies, to contour the bone to reconstruct the mandible and the maxilla in a patient with a severe post-traumatic deformity. The segment of bone was removed in a subperiosteal plane, which permitted the proximal and distal segments to be rotated and placed into two separate three-dimensional planes.

When reconstructing the mandible, the bone should be oriented so that the vascular pedicle of the fibula is located on the lingual surface of the neomandible, which places the skin paddle along the inferior border. The skin can be delivered into the oral cavity by transposing it over the buccal surface, which also provides coverage of the fixation hardware. In addition, the cuff of the flexor hallucis longus provides augmentation in the submandibular region (12).

Functional mandibular reconstruction involves the successful placement of a lower dental prosthesis to restore mastication. In patients who have residual teeth in the native mandible, a tissue-borne partial prosthesis can be effectively used. Such a prosthesis gains stability and retention through clasps that attach to the remaining teeth. However, when the patient is edentulous or there are no remaining teeth of sufficient quality to allow the use of clasps, then successful dental rehabilitation requires the use of endosteal implants that function as tooth root analogs. The thick cortical bone of the fibula appears to accept implants well (21,34). However, the smaller dimensions of the bone require the use of a shorter dental implant than can be used in the ilium. Long-term follow-up is required to determine whether marginal bone loss around the implant will lead to extrusion because, with a shorter implant, there is a greater percentage of implant exposure for the same amount of bone loss.

The introduction of the sensate fibular osteocutaneous flap by Hayden and O'Leary (12) added a new dimension to this donor site. The lateral sural cutaneous nerve can be harvested and anastomosed to a suitable recipient nerve to restore sensation to the skin component. These authors also described the harvest of the peroneal communicating branch for use as a vascularized nerve graft to bridge the gap in the inferior alveolar to mental nerve for the restoration of sensation in the lower lip. Sadove et al. (24) used the sensate fibular osteocutaneous flap to achieve a one-stage penile reconstruction. The lateral sural cutaneous nerve was anastomosed to an appropriate recipient nerve, which reportedly restored sensation to the neophallus.

NEUROVASCULAR ANATOMY

The peroneal artery and vein provide the primary blood supply to the fibular osteocutaneous flap. The popliteal artery is classically described as bifurcating into the anterior and posterior tibial arteries, and the latter vessel subsequently gives rise to the peroneal artery (Figures 19-3 to 19-4). The peroneal artery and its two venae comitantes descend in the lower leg between the flexor hallucis longus and the tibialis posterior. A discussion of the vascular supply to the fibular flap, of necessity, must include a description of the various patterns of vascular supply to the foot. Knowledge of these variations and a preoperative evaluation to determine their presence is imperative to avoid ischemic complications.

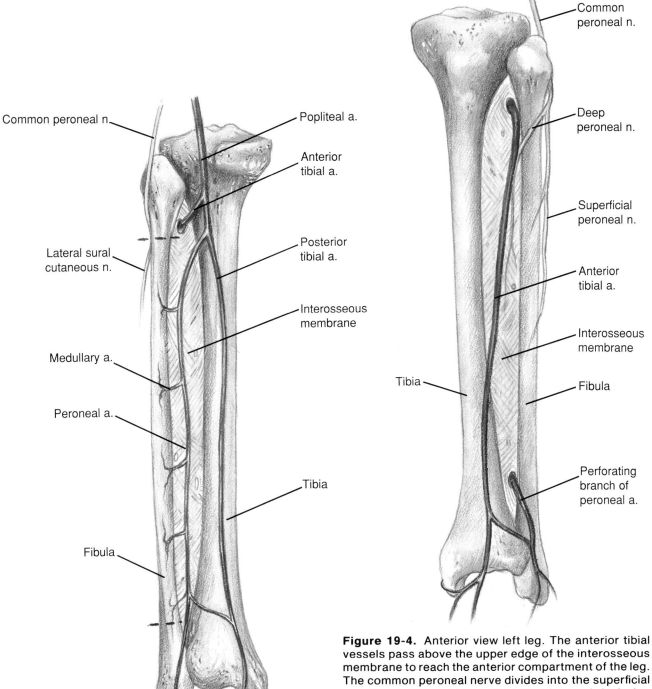

Figure 19-3. Posterior view left leg. The popliteal artery usually divides into the anterior and posterior tibial arteries. The peroneal artery arises from the posterior tibial artery within 2–3 cm of the bifurcation of the popliteal artery. The peroneal artery provides an endosteal vascular supply to the fibula through the nutrient medullary artery as well as numerous periosteal feeders. Proximal and distal segments of the fibula at the ankle and knee must be preserved (*dashed line*). The common peroneal nerve winds around the neck of the fibula where it is most susceptible to injury.

Figure 19-4. Anterior view left leg. The anterior tibial vessels pass above the upper edge of the interosseous membrane to reach the anterior compartment of the leg. The common peroneal nerve divides into the superficial and deep peroneal nerves. The latter descends in the leg in conjunction with the anterior tibial artery. The distal portion of the peroneal artery passes through a gap in the interosseous membrane to reach the anterior compartment where it joins with the lateral malleolar branch of the anterior tibial artery forming a plexus around the heel and the lateral malleolus.

In addition to supplying the nutrient artery of the fibula and musculoperiosteal vessels, the peroneal artery and vein also give rise to fasciocutaneous perforators that run in the posterior crural septum to supply the skin. There has been a considerable amount of interest and research into the location, size, course, and reliability of the blood vessels supplying the skin. This is a particularly important issue when dealing with composite defects of the head and neck in which mucosal and cutaneous defects often require soft tissue flaps in addition to the bone that is used to reconstruct the mandible. In Hidalgo's (14) initial description of the application of the fibular free flap to mandibular reconstruction, he reported 12 cases. Among these 12 patients, 4 had intraoral mucosal defects, and one had an external cutaneous defect. Only one of the five skin paddles survived entirely, and one developed a 30% necrosis. The remaining three skin paddles were excised intraoperatively because of ischemia. Hidalgo's conclusion from this experience was that the fibular donor site should not be used for reconstructing mandibular defects with large intraoral mucosal defects.

This rather pessimistic view of the fibular skin paddle is not shared by others who have successfully used this composite flap in head and neck reconstruction. It is worthwhile to review and summarize the anatomic studies that have been reported on the blood supply to the fibular skin. The blood vessels that enter the skin in the vicinity of the posterior crural septum have been classified in a variety of different ways. In 1983, Yoshimura et al. (33) described three different types of arteries: type A vessels pass through the peroneus longus in the more proximal portion of the leg; type B vessels run between the soleus and peroneus muscles, giving off muscular branches prior to supplying the skin; type C branches run a course similar to that of type B but without the muscular branches. Beppu et al. (1) adopted the same classification system in their anatomic study reported in 1992. Wei et al. (31) described two types of septocutaneous perforators: those that traverse the posterior crural septum throughout their entire course and those that travel through either the flexor hallucis longus, tibialis posterior, or soleus before entering the septum and supplying the skin. Wei et al. referred to the latter branches as musculocutaneous vessels. However, Shusterman et al. (26) classified the vessels that have a muscular course before traveling through the septum to the skin as septomuscular perforators to distinguish them from the musculocutaneous branches that exit the surface of the muscle before ramifying in the subcutaneous layer. It is important to recognize the course of the septomuscular branches to include a protective cuff of muscle around the bone (Figure 19-5).

A number of cadaveric dissection studies have addressed the quantity and the geography of these different vessels to help in flap planning and harvest. Carriquiry et al. (3) reported that the diameter of the perforators ranged from 0.4 to 1.3 mm, with the largest perforators located at either end of the fibula. The proximal large perforator crosses in close proximity to the common peroneal nerve and has been referred to as the "circumflex peroneal" artery. However, this vessel commonly arises from the posterior tibial artery instead of the peroneal. Chen and Yan (4) observed that there were four to five cutaneous branches that exited the soleus muscle in a segmental distribution along the length of the calf. Yoshimura et al. (32) reported an average of 4.8 cutaneous branches from the peroneal artery, each with a minimum diameter of 0.3 mm. The posterior tibial artery contributed 5.7% of the cutaneous branches to the lateral calf skin; the popliteal artery gave rise to 3.5% and the anterior tibial artery, to only 0.4%. The cutaneous branches arising from the arteries other than the peroneal were primarily noted in the proximal portion of the leg. Yoshimura et al. divided the length of the fibula into ten zones and quantified the perforators arising in each zone. The greatest density of peroneal cutaneous branches was concentrated in the zone that was eight tenths of the way along the fibula. The authors also noted that 71% of the cutaneous perforators were musculocutaneous and 29% were septocutaneous.

Beppu et al. (1) similarly studied the distribution of cutaneous branches to the lateral calf and found that one perforator was consistently located at the midpoint between the head of the fibula and the lateral malleolus. In 21 of 23 dissections, a cutaneous branch was identified within 2 cm of that point. The proximal third of the calf was inconsistently supplied by the peroneal artery. In 5 of 23 dissections, there

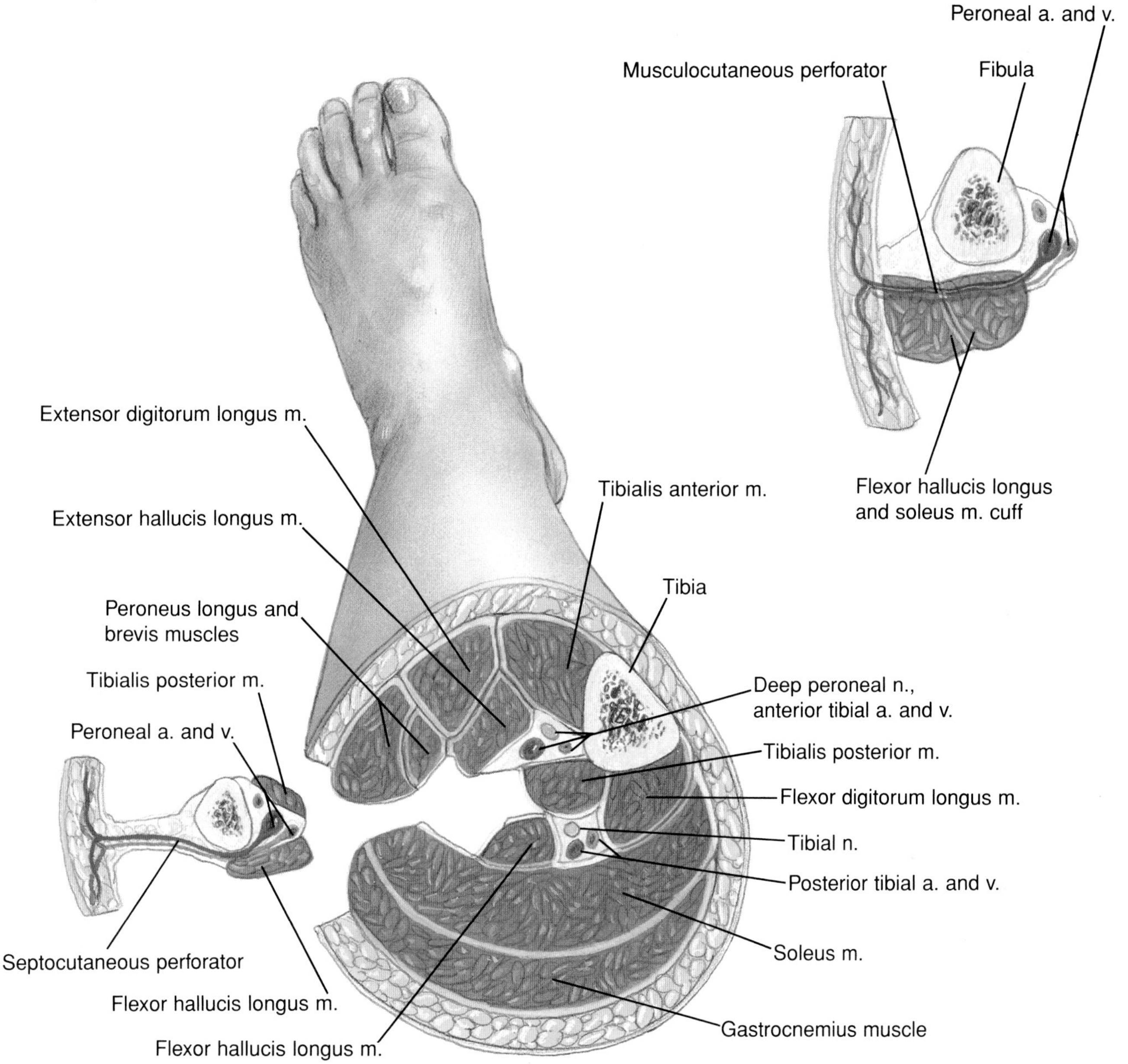

Peroneal a. and v.

Musculocutaneous perforator

Fibula

Flexor hallucis longus
and soleus m. cuff

Extensor digitorum longus m.

Tibialis anterior m.

Extensor hallucis longus m.

Tibia

Peroneus longus and
brevis muscles

Deep peroneal n.,
anterior tibial a. and v.

Tibialis posterior m.

Tibialis posterior m.

Peroneal a. and v.

Flexor digitorum longus m.

Tibial n.

Posterior tibial a. and v.

Septocutaneous perforator

Soleus m.

Flexor hallucis longus m.

Gastrocnemius muscle

Flexor hallucis longus m.

Figure 19-5. The cross-sectional anatomy of the lower leg reveals the path of the septocutaneous perforators, which may run entirely through the septum or, in part, through the flexor hallucis longus before entering the lateral aspect of the septum. A cuff of the flexor hallucis longus is harvested to protect these perforators. The musculocutaneous perforators (inset) run their entire course through the posterior muscle group, necessitating a cuff of both the soleus and flexor hallucis longus.

were no branches from the peroneal artery to the proximal calf skin. Beppu et al. reported that at least one septocutaneous vessel was noted in the middle third of the calf in all 23 dissections. Wei et al. (31) reported their findings in 35 dissections in which they found four to seven cutaneous branches arising from the peroneal artery, they also noted one to four septocutaneous arteries, except in one leg, in which there were none. By contrast, Shusterman et al. (26) reported that 20% of the 80 cadaver leg dissections showed no septocutaneous perforators and 6.25% also showed no muscular or septomuscular vessels. The septal vessels tended to be located more distal in the leg in contrast to the muscular or septomuscular branches. It was unclear from this report whether there were any dissections that showed a total absence of both septal and muscular perforators, leading to an absolute skin paddle reliability in the range of 93% to 94%.

Despite the controversy regarding the skin paddle, Wei et al. (30) reported a 100% success rate with the skin paddle of the fibular osteoseptocutaneous flap in 80 cases of extremity reconstruction and 27 cases of mandibular reconstruction. In the latter group, there was 1 case of total flap failure, but no partial or total skin loss among the remaining 26 cases. The authors centered the skin paddle at the junction of the middle and lower third of the fibula. They warned that the posterior crural septum had to be included with the flap and that excess traction during harvest or closure was detrimental to the skin's blood supply. Despite their success with the skin paddle, Wei et al. used a second soft tissue free flap in 14 of their 26 mandibular reconstructions. In a discussion of this article, Hidalgo (16) reported that, from his experience and that of others, the skin paddle of the osteoseptocutaneous flap was reliable in only 91.5% of cases overall. He also stated that, in his experience, the skin island often survives even in the absence of any visible perforators in the septum. Despite this claim, most surgeons use the approach described by Fleming et al. (6) to harvest the skin paddle of the fibular flap from an anterior direction in a subfascial plane. A long flap is usually designed to allow for variations in the location of perforators that occur along the length of the septum. If no septal perforators are visualized, then musculocutaneous branches must be identified to supply the skin. The absence of musculocutaneous vessels that can be traced back to the peroneal system usually indicates the need for an alternative soft tissue flap (29). A cuff of flexor hallucis longus and soleus should be included, even in those cases in which a septal branch is identified, because of the possibility that it may diverge from the septum to run through the muscle as it courses toward the peroneal vessels (Figure 19-5). In his discussion of the article by Shusterman et al. (26), Hidalgo (15) questioned the validity of harvesting a large cuff of soleus muscle. In his experience, he noted that many of the large muscular perforators did not take their origins from the peroneal vessels and that large cuffs of soleus muscle are often devascularized and must be excised.

Dye-injection studies of the peroneal artery stained a skin territory that averaged 9.9 cm in width and 21.4 cm in length. Fleming et al. (6) successfully split the skin paddle by incising to, but not through, the level of the fascia. They also advised mapping cutaneous perforators preoperatively with Doppler ultrasonography.

As noted previously, the sensory supply to the skin of the lateral calf is derived from the lateral sural cutaneous nerve (Figure 19-2). This branch arises from the common peroneal nerve within or above the popliteal fossa. However, this nerve is variable, as described by Huelke (17), who reported it to be absent in 22% of cases. Kosinski (19) reported only a 1.7% incidence of this nerve being absent but also noted that, in an additional 9.4% of cases there were no cutaneous branches before the lateral sural nerve joined the medial sural cutaneous nerve. The peroneal communicating nerve is a second superficial nerve that traverses the territory of the fibular flap. It also arises from the common peroneal nerve and joins with the medial sural cutaneous nerve to form the sural nerve. That junction may occur at virtually any location from the popliteal fossa to the lateral malleolus. This nerve was absent in 50% of dissections reported by Kosinski (19) and 20% of those reported by Huelke (17). As noted above, Hayden and O'Leary (12) described using the peroneal communicating branch as a vascularized nerve graft.

ANATOMIC VARIATIONS

The fibula is the most common long bone in the body to be absent or markedly diminished in size to the extent that it is replaced by a fibrous band. The anomaly of an absent fibula is usually associated with a shortened leg and an abnormal tibia, which is bowed forward, findings that would be readily apparent on preoperative radiographs of the donor limb.

Variations in the arterial supply to the foot are the greatest concern in sacrificing the peroneal artery. According to Senior (25), there have been no reports of the absence of the peroneal vessels, and the same holds true for the anterior tibial artery. The latter, however, may be significantly diminished in size. In roughly 10% to 20% of cases, either the anterior tibial or the posterior tibial artery may become attenuated during their course in the lower leg. When this happens, a communicating branch from the peroneal artery supplies the missing or diminutive vessel's territory in the distal extremity. It is evident that, under such circumstances, the sacrifice of the peroneal artery would result in ischemia of the foot.

POTENTIAL PITFALLS

The most serious consequence of fibula flap transfer is the lack of collateral circulation to the foot, leading to ischemia following interruption of the peroneal artery. Preoperative assessment helps to avoid this potential problem.

There are a variety of donor-site complaints that have been reported, including cold intolerance and edema. Functional deficits include weakness in dorsiflexion of the great toe, related either to injury to branches of the peroneal nerve or scarring of the muscles, in particular, the flexor hallucis longus (9). Patients have reported pain and weakness on ambulation for several months after surgery. Muscle weakness is believed to be caused by the disruption of the muscular origins that attach to the fibula and the interosseous membrane. Detailed gait analysis revealed abnormalities in stride, joint angles, and "ground reaction forces," which were thought to be attributable to muscle weakness and altered load transmission (20).

Injury to the common peroneal nerve may occur as a result of traction or errant dissection, leaving the patient with an equinovarus deformity and anesthesia along the anterior and lateral sides of the leg and dorsum of the foot. This complication can be avoided by identifying this nerve early in the dissection. A 6- to 7-cm segment of bone should be left attached to the knee as an additional protection. A similar quantity of bone should be preserved distally to maintain the integrity of the ankle joint. Hematomas were reported in 25% of 20 patients in whom the fibula was used for long-bone reconstruction. This complication was attributed, in part, to oozing from the exposed medullary surfaces of the bone's ends (5).

There continues to be some uncertainty in the blood supply to the skin of the fibular osteocutaneous flap. The surgeon cannot be assured of the skin's vascularity until after harvest. Because of the loss of the skin paddle that has been reported in 5% to 10% of cases, a backup plan should be formulated prior to surgery. The patient should be informed of the potential need for a second soft tissue flap. This is especially true in those patients with defects that require significant soft tissue reconstruction. An alternative flap, such as the scapula, or a separate soft tissue flap combined with the fibula should be anticipated.

The width of the fibular skin paddle is usually limited by the ability to achieve primary wound closure. Excess tension must be avoided to prevent a compartment syndrome. A skin graft may be applied to the defect on the lateral calf and then subsequently removed by serial excision. Alternatively, a tissue expander may be placed primarily through the defect to expand the dorsal skin of the calf. Secondary closure with a linear scar may then be achieved (10).

PREOPERATIVE ASSESSMENT

The possible absence or diminished size of the anterior or posterior tibial arteries and the prevalence of atherosclerosis in the lower extremities requires that a preoperative evaluation be performed prior to fibula transfer. Angiography is the conventional method to perform such an evaluation. Magnetic resonance angiography has also been shown to provide at least comparable if not improved definition of the vascular anatomy of the lower extremities. This noninvasive technique provides valuable information that guides the selection of the appropriate leg to use for flap harvest or whether to select an alternative donor site (13).

Flap Harvesting Technique

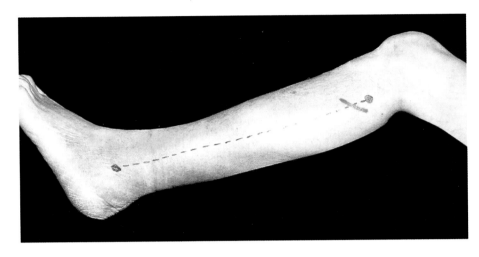

Figure 19-6. The topographical anatomy is outlined on the lateral aspect of the left leg. The landmarks to the intermuscular septum are the fibular head superiorly and the lateral epicondyle of the ankle inferiorly. A *dashed line* connecting these points identifies the location of the intermuscular septum. The peroneal nerve, which passes 1–2 cm below the fibular head, is marked in red.

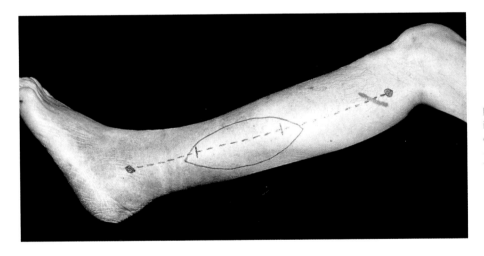

Figure 19-7. The cutaneous flap is designed with a fusiform shape centered on the intermuscular septum. The dominant septocutaneous perforators are usually located more distally in the leg, and therefore, the skin paddles are usually centered over the junction of the middle and distal thirds.

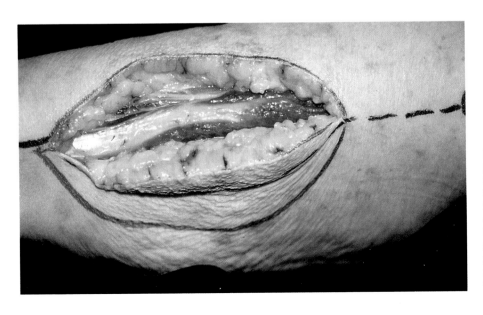

Figure 19-8. The dissection is performed with a thigh tourniquet inflated to 350 mmHg. The skin paddle is incised anteriorly through the skin and subcutaneous tissue. The fascia overlying the peroneus longus and brevis is also incised, and the dissection proceeds from anterior to posterior in a subfascial plane toward the intermuscular septum.

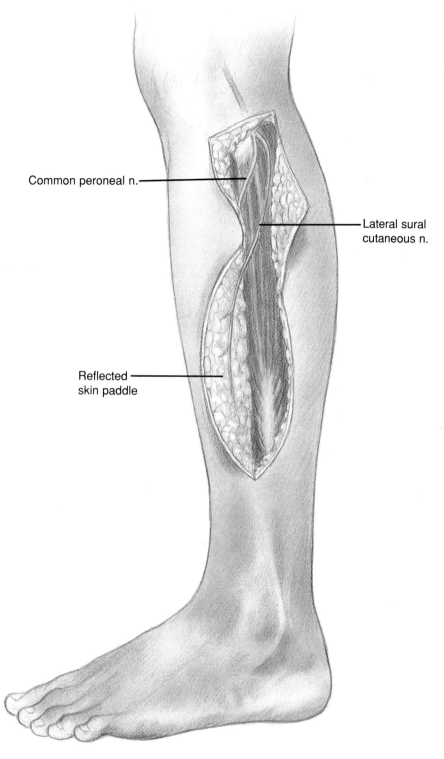

Common peroneal n.

Lateral sural
cutaneous n.

Reflected
skin paddle

Figure 19-9. When harvesting a sensate fibular osteocutaneous flap, the technique is slightly altered. The lateral sural cutaneous nerve is found by tracing the common peroneal nerve in a proximal direction into the popliteal fossa. The lateral sural cutaneous nerve arises at any point along the course of that dissection. Once identified, the lateral sural nerve can be traced caudally to the cutaneous paddle, which has been reflected anteriorly. The peroneal communicating branch also arises from the common peroneal nerve in this location and travels through the soft tissue of the flap but does not supply sensation to the flap skin. The peroneal communicating branch may be included in the flap and used as a vascularized nerve graft.

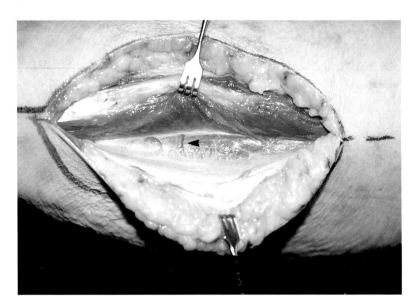

Figure 19-10. The skin paddle has been reflected to reveal the posterior crural septum. The peroneus longus is retracted. A septocutaneous perforator is identified coursing out to the skin (*arrow*).

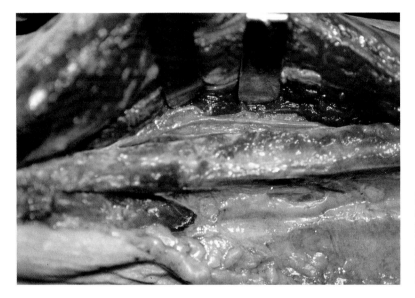

Figure 19-11. Dissection along the anterior aspect of the fibula requires elevation of the peroneus longus, peroneus brevis, and extensor hallucis longus. The deep peroneal nerve, anterior tibial artery, and anterior tibial vein are identified in the anterior compartment.

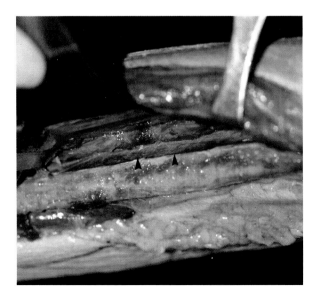

Figure 19-12. Further dissection along the medial aspect of the fibula reveals the interosseous membrane (*arrows*).

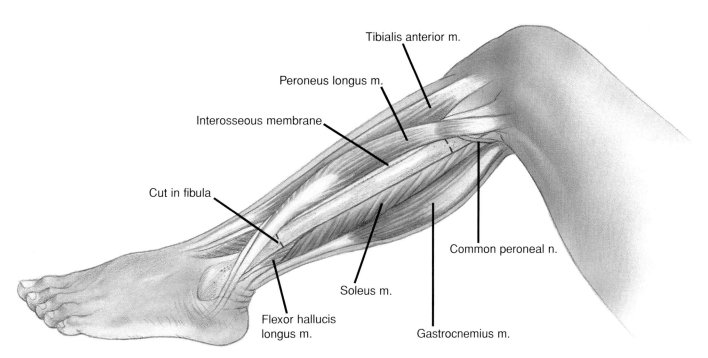

Tibialis anterior m.

Peroneus longus m.

Interosseous membrane

Cut in fibula

Common peroneal n.

Soleus m.

Flexor hallucis
longus m.

Gastrocnemius m.

Figure 19-13. At this juncture in the dissection, bone cuts are made in the proximal and distal fibula. A segment of fibula must be preserved both proximally and distally, as shown. Distraction of the fibula is needed to proceed with the remainder of the dissection.

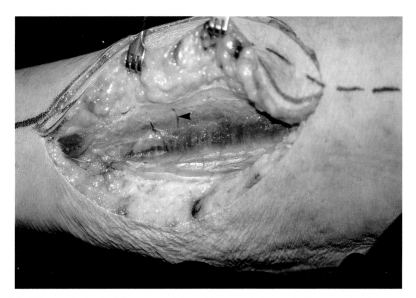

Figure 19-14. The posterior incision around the skin paddle is made down to the fascia overlying the gastrocnemius and soleus. In this particular dissection, a septocutaneous perforator (*arrow*) has been identified, and therefore, a septocutaneous, rather than a musculocutaneous flap, will be harvested.

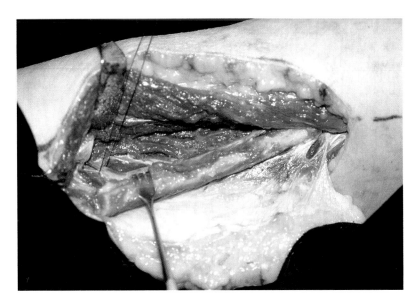

Figure 19-15. The distal portion of the peroneal artery and vein are identified after distraction of the fibula. The distal pedicle is ligated and transsected.

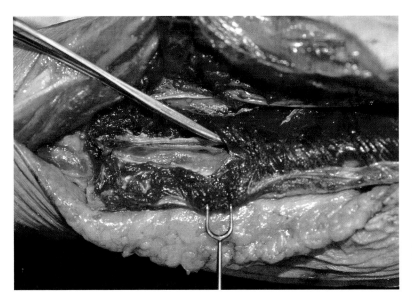

Figure 19-16. After cutting the interosseous membrane, the chevron-oriented muscle fibers of the tibialis posterior are visualized and transsected to follow the peroneal artery and vein proximally in the calf.

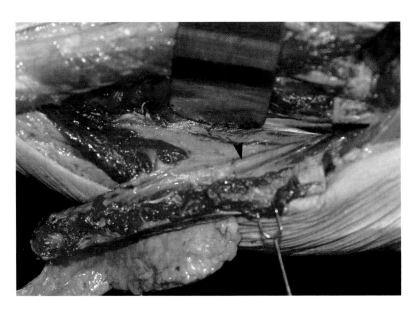

Figure 19-17. The entire length of the peroneal vascular system (*arrow*) has been dissected to the bifurcation of the posterior tibial vessels.

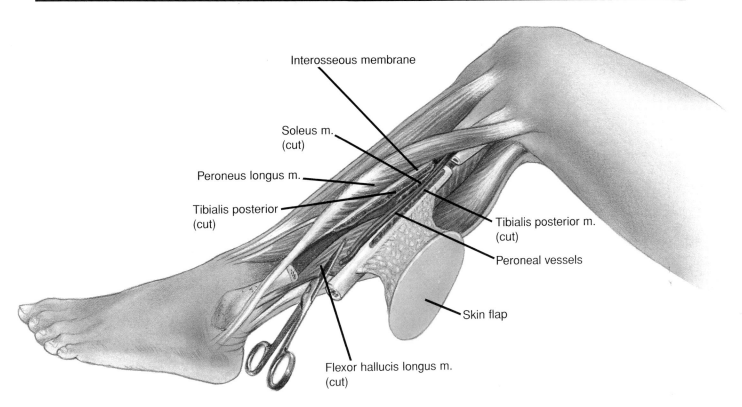

Interosseous membrane

Soleus m.
(cut)

Peroneus longus m.

Tibialis posterior
(cut)

Tibialis posterior m.
(cut)

Peroneal vessels

Skin flap

Flexor hallucis longus m.
(cut)

Figure 19-18. Prior to ligation of the pedicle, the flexor hallucis longus is transsected, leaving a cuff attached to the composite flap.

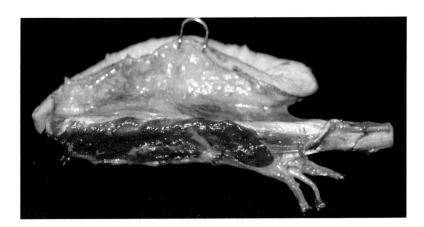

Figure 19-19. The fibular osteocutaneous flap has been harvested with a cuff of flexor hallucis longus and tibialis posterior. The vascular pedicle consisting of the peroneal artery and two venae comitantes, can be lengthened by performing a subperiosteal dissection and removing the proximal bone but preserving the intervening periosteum and muscles.

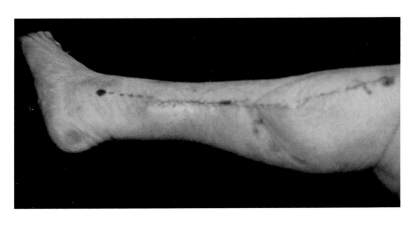

Figure 19-20. Primary closure of the leg has been accomplished. If necessary, a skin graft can be applied to this defect. Following closure, a posterior splint is fashioned for the lower leg and foot.

REFERENCES

1. Beppu M, Hanel D, Johnston G, Carmo J, Tsai T. The osteocutaneous fibula flap: an anatomic study. *J Reconstr Microsurg* 1992;8:215–223.
2. Carr A, MacDonald D, Waterhouse A. The blood supply of the osteocutaneous free fibular graft. *J Bone Joint Surg [Br]* 1988;70B:319–321.
3. Carriquiry C, Costa A, Vasconez L. An anatomic study of the septocutaneous vessels of the leg. *Plast Reconstr Surg* 1985;76:354–361.
4. Chen Z, Yan W. The study and clinical application of the osteocutaneous flap of fibula. *Microsurgery* 1983;4:11–16.
5. Coghlan B, Townsend P. The morbidity of the free vascularized fibula flap. *Br J Plast Surg* 1993;46: 466.
6. Fleming A, Brough M, Evans N, Grant H, Harris M, James J, Lawlor M, Laws I. Mandibular reconstruction using vascularized fibula. *Br J Plast Surg* 1990;43:403–409.
7. Gilbert A. Vascularized transfer of fibula shaft. *Int J Microsurg* 1979;1:100.
8. Gilbert R, Dovion D. Near total mandibular reconstruction: the free vascularized fibular transfer. *Oper Tech Otolaryngol Head Neck Surg* 1993;4:145.
9. Goodacre TE, Walker CJ, Jawad AS, Jackson AM, Brough MD. Donor site morbidity following osteocutaneous free fibula transfer. *Br J Plast Surg* 1990;43:410–412.
10. Hallock G. Refinement of the fibular osteocutaneous flap using tissue expansion. *J Reconstr Microsurg* 1989;5:317–322.
11. Harrison DH. The osteocutaneous free fibular graft. *J Bone Joint Surg [Br]* 1986;68B:804–807.
12. Hayden R, O'Leary M. A neurosensory fibula flap: anatomical description and clinical applications. Presented at the 94th Annual Meeting of the American Laryngological, Rhinological and Otological Society Meeting in Hyatt Regency Waikoloa, Big Island of Hawaii, Hawaii, May 8, 1991.
13. Hayden RE, Carpenter J, Thaler E. Magnetic resonance angiography: noninvasive evaluation of potential free flaps. Presented at the Annual Meeting of the American Academy of Facial Plastic and Reconstructive Surgery in Minneapolis, Minnesota, on October 1, 1993.
14. Hidalgo D. Fibula free flap: a new method of mandible reconstruction. *Plast Reconstr Surg* 1989;84: 71.
15. Hidalgo D. Discussion of "The osteocutaneous free fibula flap: Is the skin paddle reliable?" by Schusterman et al. *Plast Reconstr Surg* 1992;90:797.
16. Hidalgo D. Discussion of "Fibula osteoseptocutaneous flap for reconstruction of composite mandibular defects" by Wei F, Seah C, Tsai Y, Liu S, Tseu M. *Plast Reconstr Surg* 1994;93:305.
17. Huelke DF. The origin of the peroneal communicating nerve in adult man. *Anat Record* 1958;131:81.
18. Jones N, Swartz W, Mears D, Jupiter J, Grossman A. The "double-barrel" free vascularized fibular bone graft. *Plast Reconstr Surg* 1988;81:378.
19. Kosinski C. The course, mutual relations and distribution of the cutaneous nerves of the metazonal region of leg and foot. *J Anat* 1926;60:274.
20. Lee EH, Goh JC, Helm R, Pho RW. Donor site morbidity following resection of the fibula. *J Bone Joint Surg [Br]* 1990;72:129–131.
21. Lyberg T, Olstad O. The vascularized fibular flap for mandibular reconstruction. *J Craniomaxillofac Surg* 1991;19:113.
22. Onishi K, Maruyama Y, Iwahira Y. Cutaneous and fascial vasculature of the leg: an anatomic study of fasciocutaneous vessels. *J Reconstr Microsurg* 1986;2:181.
23. Sadove R, Powell L. Simultaneous maxillary and mandibular reconstruction with one free osteocutaneous flap. *Plast Reconstr Surg* 1993;92:141.
24. Sadove R, Sengenzer M, McRoberts J, Wells M. One stage total penile reconstruction with a free sensate osteocutaneous fibula flap. *Plast Reconstr Surg* 1993;92:1314.
25. Senior HD. An interpretation of the recorded arterial anomalies of the human leg and foot. *J Anat* 1919;53:130.
26. Shusterman MA, Reece GP, Miller MJ, Harris S. The osteocutaneous free fibula flap: is the skin paddle reliable? *Plast Reconstr Surg* 1992;90:787–793.
27. Serra A, Paloma V. Mesa F, Ballesteros A. The vascularized fibula graft in mandibular reconstruction. *J Oral Maxillofac Surg* 1991;49:244–250.
28. Taylor GI, Miller DH, Ham FJ. The free vascularized bone graft: a clinical extension of microvascular techniques. *Plast Reconstr Surg* 1975;55:533.
29. Von Twisk R, Pavlov P, Sonneveld J. Reconstruction of bone and soft tissue defects with free fibula transfer. *Ann Plast Surg* 1988;21:555–558.
30. Wei F, Seah C, Tsai Y, Liu S, Tsai M. Fibula osteoseptocutaneous flap for reconstruction of composite mandibular defects. *Plast Reconstr Surg* 1994;93:294.
31. Wei FC, Chen HC, Chuang CC, Noordhoff MS. Fibular osteoseptocutaneous flap: anatomic study and clinical application. *Plast Reconstr Surg* 1986;78:191–199.
32. Yoshimura M, Shimada T, Hosokawa M. The vasculature of the peroneal tissue transfer. *Plast Reconstr Surg* 1990;85:917–921.
33. Yoshimura M, Shimamura K, Iwai Y, Yamauchi S, Ueno T. Free vascularized fibular transplant. *J Bone Joint Surg [Am]* 1983;65A:1295–1301.
34. Zlotolow I, Huryn J, Piro J, Lenchewski E, Hidalgo D. Osseointegrated implants and functional prosthetic rehabilitation in microvascular fibular free flap reconstructed mandibles. *Am J Surg* 1992;165: 677–681.

Free Jejunal Autograft

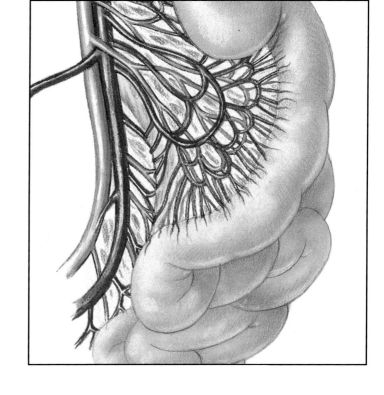

Michael J. Sullivan, M.D. and
Mark L. Urken, M.D.

Free jejunal autografts (FJA) have a unique place in the history of microvascular surgery because this was the first tissue to be transplanted in humans. Seidenberg et al. (49) conducted a number of canine experiments involving FJA transfers to the head and neck to replace the pharyngoesophagus. In 1959, they reported their experience in one patient, who underwent a pharyngoesophagectomy for recurrent cancer. The patient survived for 5 days until a cerebrovascular accident caused his death. However, the findings at autopsy revealed a viable jejunal transplant. This procedure was performed without the benefit of a microscope. The arterial anastomosis was sutured, and the venous anastomosis was performed by using a tantalum ring prosthesis (28).

Although 1959 marks the beginning of the era of human free tissue transfer, the concept of moving tissue around the body and reestablishing its circulation was introduced in the writings of Alexis Carrel (9). In 1907, he reported his experimental work in an animal model with organ transfers, including the successful autotransplantation of a segment of jejunum to the neck. He described the resumption of peristaltic activity after completing the microvascular anastomoses.

The first successful transfer of a FJA in which a patient was able to resume swallowing was described by Roberts and Douglas (46) in 1961. After the introduction of the operating microscope for performing microvascular anastomoses, this technology was rapidly applied, both clinically and experimentally. In 1966, Green and Som (17) performed a number of animal experiments involving the transfer of FJAs with the help of the microscope. In addition, they introduced the concept of the split jejunal patch graft, which was created by incising the jejunum along its antimesenteric border to change it from a mucosa-lined tube to a flat mucosal patch. The split jejunal autograft has since been used to reconstruct various noncircumferential defects of the upper aerodigestive tract.

In addition to being the first reported free tissue transfer, the FJA has perhaps been written about the most of any reconstructive free flap in the head and neck. Various issues related to the technique, perioperative management, and postoperative function are addressed in this chapter.

FLAP DESIGN AND UTILIZATION

Prior to its use in humans as a free flap, the jejunum was introduced as a pedicled intestinal transfer to reconstruct the thoracic esophagus. Wiillstein (59) reported this technique in 1904. Pedicled segments of jejunum were transferred by cutting the first two vascular arcades and basing the segment on the vascular supply through the third and fourth arcade. However, ischemic necrosis of the most cephalad portion of the jejunum was common, and this technique was restricted to esophageal defects that did not extend above the inferior pulmonary vein (18). The concept of "turbocharging" the pedicled jejunum was introduced by Chang et al. (10) in 1985. To circumvent the problem of ischemia in the most cephalad portion of the pedicled jejunum, they described the reestablishment of flow through the first or second arcade by anastomoses to recipient vessels in the neck. This partially attached and partially free segment of jejunum provided an effective conduit for the replacement of the entire thoracic and cervical esophagus.

Currently, the jejunum is primarily transferred as a microvascular autograft. It is most commonly used as a mucosal tube or a mucosal patch, depending on the configuration of the defect. A reliable and functional reconstruction of pharyngoesophageal defects has been pursued by head and neck surgeons for many decades. Pedicled cervical flaps were popularized by Wookey (60) in the early 1940s, but this technique was criticized because of the necessity for multiple staged procedures. The use of a skin graft over a stent was also advocated but was soon superseded by pedicled regional flaps, the most important of which was the tubed, deltopectoral flap which was introduced for pharyngoesophageal reconstruction by Bakamjian (2) in 1965. This last technique was a significant advance. However, it was still limited by the necessity for a two-staged procedure. Other regional flaps most importantly the pectoralis major musculocutaneous flap, were applied to this problem by fashioning them into an epithelial conduit. However, these flaps were often too bulky to form into a tube and, therefore, were unreliable for circumferential defects. The problem of bulk was corrected in part by the use of free cutaneous flaps, which could be more readily formed into a tube in a one-stage procedure (22).

The transfer of pedicled visceral flaps such as the stomach and colon, has been used extensively to replace the thoracic and cervical esophagus. However, both of these mucosal flaps require extensive abdominal and thoracic dissections, which are fraught with complications and are not warranted when the defect is confined to the cervical region. The gastric pull-up (GPU) procedure is also problematic because of its limited reach when used to resurface defects that extend more cephalad into the oropharynx. When a GPU is used in heavily radiated tissues, its weight and the effect of the gravitational pull on it has also led to problems with wound healing. The colonic interposition is useful for thoracic esophageal replacement, but its limited reach has restricted its use when the defect extends into the cervical region. The bacterial flora of the colon can also lead to infectious problems in the abdomen and chest.

The FJA was therefore introduced and popularized as a solution for reconstructing circumferential defects that were limited to the neck (3,34). Vascularized segments of ileum have also been used (21). Unrestricted by a vascular pedicle based in the abdomen, the FJA can easily be used for defects that extend more cephalad into the oro-

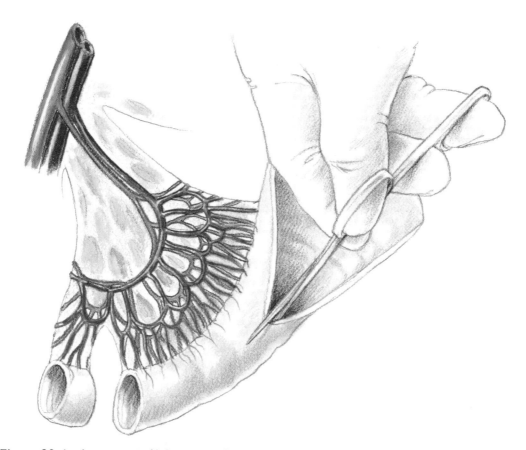

Figure 20-1. A segment of jejunum can be partially or completely divided in a longitudinal fashion along its antimesenteric border. By so doing, we can create either a completely flat mucosal patch or a partially tube-shaped and partially flat segment of mucosa.

and nasopharynx. Partially split and partially circumferential segments of jejunum can readily satisfy the need for a circumferential mucosal tube to replace the pharyngoesophagus and a flat piece of mucosa to replace the posterior pharyngeal wall all the way up to the base of the skull. This partially tube-shaped and partially split design can also be used for reconstructing the cervical esophagus and hypopharynx when the larynx is not involved, the function of which can be preserved (Figure 20-1).

The caliber of the lumen of the FJA matches the esophagus fairly well in most individuals. However, in a pharyngoesophageal reconstruction, the pharyngeal opening may be considerably larger. The cephalad portion of the FJA can be opened along its antimesenteric border to achieve a caliber that is more suitable for anastomosis. When the defect extends to the oral cavity following glossectomy and requires reconstruction of the entire floor of the mouth along the inner table of the mandible, the necessity to enlarge the lumen is even greater. Jones et al. (25) proposed a design for the FJA that involved folding the "split jejunum" on itself to effectively double the size of the lumen. The ability to achieve a tension-free closure of the oral cavity seemingly offsets the considerably longer suture line when the FJA is sutured to itself.

When considering the three major options for one-stage reconstruction of cervical esophageal or pharyngoesophageal defects, there are a number of points to be made. The GPU and colonic interposition are the only methods that allow resection and replacement of the thoracic esophagus. However, this is done at the expense of significant abdominal and thoracic dissections. In addition, the limited cephalad reach has been noted. Swallowing after a GPU is also problematic because of early satiety and reflux of food into the oropharynx and oral cavity. The use of tube-shaped cutaneous free flaps offers tremendous flexibility in design and little potential morbidity compared with that of a laparotomy. However, when the inferior cervical esophageal margin is very low, leaving a proximal thoracic esophageal stump that is tucked into the close confines behind the tracheal remnant, it is often difficult to perform an anastomosis between the tube-shaped skin flap and the esophagus. This can be done effectively by using a FJA with an enteric stapling device that produces a safe and reliable anastomosis without the requisite exposure that is needed for the placement of circumferential sutures. Jejunoesophageal anastomoses that are located in the upper mediastinum carry an additional risk if an anastomotic leak occurs. The recognition of such a leak and the ability to manage it effectively are compromised. Finally, the occurrence of a stricture in this location is also far more difficult to manage than one that is located in the neck (44). In our experience, the "short proximal esophagus" represents a clear indication for the harvest of a FJA and provides an alternative solution to the GPU when the thoracic esophagus itself is not involved by cancer.

The FJA has also been successfully used for reconstructing the pharyngoesophagus in benign conditions, such as strictures caused by prior surgery, radiation therapy, or gastroesophageal reflux and fistulas that have not responded to conservative treatment. This may be accomplished with either a patch graft or a circumferential tube, depending on the status of the native mucosa (7,23,26,37,43).

Reconstruction of mucosal defects of the oral cavity evolved tremendously during the 1960s and 1970s. Early in the 1960s, the primary emphasis was placed on restoring a watertight seal and avoiding a multistaged procedure through the creation of an orostoma. With the introduction of new techniques, primarily the safe and reliable transfer of free flaps, the emphasis changed so that restoration of function became the primary consideration. With this in mind, the quality of the tissue that is used to replace the oral mucosal lining has taken on paramount importance. Thin pliable tissue is required when a partial glossectomy is performed and the maintenance of tongue mobility is desired. This can be readily accomplished with thin cutaneous free flaps, such as the radial forearm and dorsalis pedis flaps, with the added advantage of also restoring sensation to that tissue. However, the introduction of cutaneous flaps into the oral cavity is not an exact duplication of the native oral lining. The advantage of using a split FJA in this setting is that it transfers a moist mucosal lining (8). This may be particularly advantageous in patients with severe xerostomia caused by prior radiotherapy. Experimental studies in animals showed that the FJA conforms well to the three-dimensional contour of the oral cavity, and the serosa adheres to the denuded or partially cut mandible (51). Another application for jejunum in the oral cavity was reported by Black et al. (6) who transferred a FJA to reconstruct a total palatal defect. The mucosal surface was used on the oral side, and the serosal surface was placed on the nasal side of the defect. This provided a functional separation of the oral and nasal cavities, which permitted the patient to resume oral nutrition.

The FJA has also been used in experimental settings to investigate its potential use as a replacement for the trachea in patients who have developed symptomatic tracheal stenosis. Jones et al. (27) introduced the idea of using a FJA for this purpose and reported their successful replacement of one half of the circumference of the trachea over a length of four rings using a vascularized mucosal patch. Letang et al. (31) replaced entire segments of the cervical trachea in dogs with a jejunal tube. A silicone tube was placed as an intraluminal stent for 2 weeks. The authors reported favorable results in 12 dogs that were followed for a maximum of 60 days after surgery. From this investigation, it was concluded that the FJA was a promising substitute for the trachea and that the potential problem of excess secretions in the airway was not realized. Constantino et al. (13) reported similar findings in a group of eight dogs that underwent circumferential replacement of the trachea. Although mucus production was not problematic, the authors did note a period of intermittent peristalsis in the FJA, which caused airway obstruction. This occurred despite placement of both a temporary intraluminal stent and a permanent rigid mesh tube on the outside of the FJA to which it was sutured. They raised concerns about the reliance on the FJA to attach to the surrounding tissues in the neck by fibrosis to achieve a stable airway when a rigid framework was not added. Somatostatin was used to reduce the peristaltic activity of the FJA.

As an extension of this application of the FJA, Zeismann et al. (61) described the use of a segment of jejunum to produce speech following laryngopharyngectomy. A portion of the bowel was used to replace the gullet, and a segment was sutured to the end of the trachea to create a shunt for air to pass into the neopharynx. The midpoint of the loop of jejunum was sutured to the floor of mouth so that the tracheal limb rose to a higher level than the pharyngojejunal anastomosis did. By so doing, aspiration was prevented. In three patients who were treated in this manner, fluent speech was achieved in two, and none of the patients had significant aspiration.

NEUROVASCULAR ANATOMY

The small intestine extends from the pylorus to the ileocecal valve and is divided into three segments: the duodenum, the jejunum, and the ileum. The duodenum and the jejunum are demarcated by the ligament of Treitz. The jejunum and ileum are attached to the posterior abdominal wall by the mesentery and are arranged in a series of loops. This fan-shaped mesentery contains the jejunum and ileum, branches of the superior mesenteric artery and vein, together with the autonomic nerves, lymph nodes, lymphatic channels, and a variable amount of fat (Figure 20-2).

The superior mesenteric artery is the second ventral unpaired branch of the abdominal aorta. The jejunal arteries (range, 12 to 15) arise from the left side of the superior mesenteric artery. They run nearly parallel to one another, and each vessel divides into two arteries that unite with the adjacent branches to form a series of convex arches within the mesentery. A second and third series of arches may arise, particularly in the more distal segment. Each successive arch has a smaller caliber as the jejunum is approached. Eventually, small straight vessels (vasa recta) arise, which pass alternately to one or the other side of the small intestine. The veins that supply the jejunum and ileum accompany the arteries and drain into the superior mesenteric vein. There are often two venae comitantes for each mesenteric artery.

PREOPERATIVE ASSESSMENT

A thorough history and physical examination must be carried out during the initial evaluation to determine whether there are any contraindications to performing a FJA. The two major factors in the recipient site that argue against FJA transfer are the absence of suitable recipient vessels and the extension of disease into the thoracic esophagus (4). The presence of either of these problems represents absolute indication for the use of a GPU or colonic interposition.

There are a number of donor-site factors that should point the surgeon toward an alternative method of reconstruction. The presence of ascites is considered a contraindication to harvesting a FJA. Likewise, chronic intestinal diseases, such as Crohn's disease, should alter a surgeon's plan to harvest a jejunal segment. Relative contraindications to performing a FJA are a history of extensive prior abdominal surgery or intraperitoneal sepsis, both of which predispose to the development of adhesions. Patients with compromised pulmonary reserve are at increased risk of postoperative complications when a laparotomy is performed, and this factor should be considered when an alternative form of reconstruction is available. The development of safe laparoscopic techniques for the harvest of FJAs will probably greatly reduce the morbidity of an open laparotomy.

SURGICAL TECHNIQUE

As with all large head and neck procedures in which the upper aerodigestive tract is violated, perioperative antibiotics are administered. However, because of the violation of the lower intestinal tract, additional antimicrobial precautions, such as the

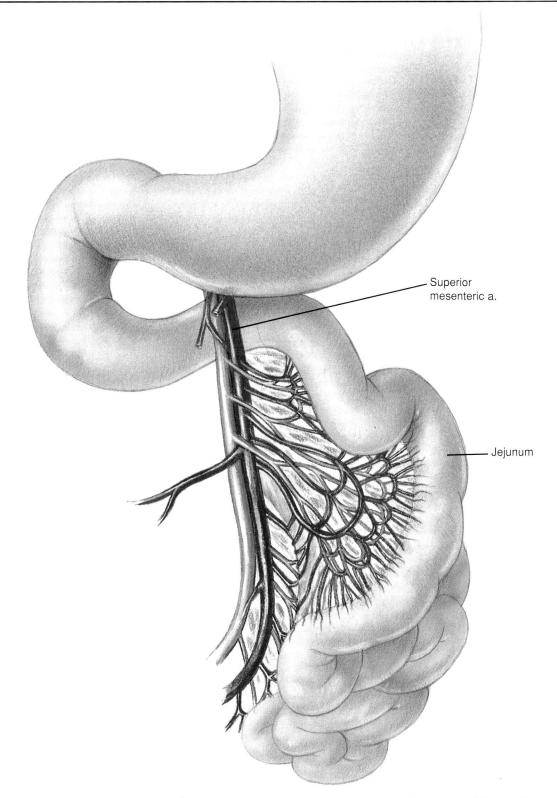

Superior
mesenteric a.

Jejunum

Figure 20-2. The transition from duodenum to jejunum occurs at the ligament of Treitz. The jejunum and ileum are arranged in a series of loops. The vascular supply to the small bowel runs in the mesentery along with the lymphatic and neural channels. A segment of jejunum to be used as a FJA can be harvested from virtually any location.

use of a bowel preparation, have been discussed but remain controversial. As early as 1959, experimental studies by Lillehei et al. (32) did not demonstrate any increase in survival in dogs that had undergone bowel sterilization prior to clamping of the superior mesenteric artery for a 5-hour period. Additional experiments in dogs by McGill et al. (35) in 1979 showed no decrease in the extent of mucosal injury when intraluminal antisepsis was instituted before rendering a segment of jejunum ischemic for 90 minutes. Although preoperative bowel preparation has been advocated by a few authors, most do not consider it to be essential for free jejunal transfers (12,15,16).

A two- and sometimes three-team approach is usually instituted when using a FJA to reconstruct a head and neck defect. The general surgical service that harvests the jejunal segment must be attuned to the needs of the microsurgeon, and therefore, preoperative and intraoperative communication is essential for a successful outcome. The same holds true when the reconstructive team differs from the ablative team and the fate of potential recipient vessels is at stake.

The size of the FJA is determined by the dimensions of the defect. The particular segment must be supplied by a single vascular arcade with nutrient vessels of sufficient size for microsurgical transfer. The selection of a suitable segment may be facilitated by transilluminating the mesentery, which highlights the vascular arcades (12,14). There is some controversy in the literature regarding the ideal location of the jejunum that is to be harvested. Some authors have proposed harvesting from just beyond the ligament of Treitz; others have advocated segments that are 100 to 150 cm distal to this structure (36,41,52). Virtually every location between these extremes has also been proposed (3,30,42,52,58).

The FJA is left attached to its nutrient supply in the abdomen until the head and neck defect is prepared. It is imperative that the orientation of the FJA be marked with a suture so that isoperistaltic reconstruction of the pharyngoesophagus can be achieved. The preparation of the vessels before harvest is usually performed with loupe magnification. Particular attention must be given to handling the mesenteric vein, which is fragile and easily injured.

There has been considerable controversy in the literature regarding the necessity for improving the FJA tolerance to ischemia through the use of pharmacotherapy or hypothermia. Fisher et al. (15) advocated using a hyperosmolar perfusate infused into the mesenteric artery to stabilize the endothelium and prolong the ischemic tolerance. Heparinized saline has been instilled through the FJA to exsanguinate the vascular system (41,58). However, McKee and Peters (36) reported no difference in outcome between a group of FJA transfers in which a heparin perfusate was used and a second group in which there was no perfusion.

There is general agreement that the ischemic tolerance of a FJA can be increased by instituting hypothermia during the transfer period prior to reestablishing the flap's circulation. Lillehei et al. (32) demonstrated that FJAs that were cooled to 5°C could survive an ischemic period of 5 hours. McGill et al. (35) reported a significant improvement in the extent of mural injury following 90 minutes of ischemia when a FJA was cooled to between 6°C and 12°C. Elaborate methods to achieve cooling have been proposed, such as a system of glass rods placed in the lumen through which water at 10°C was continuously instilled (52).

In most situations in which ischemia time is kept to a minimum, pharmacotherapy and hypothermia are not believed to be necessary. Lillehei et al. (32) and Mullens and Pezacki (38) reported successful FJA transfers in an animal model following 2 hours of euthermic ischemia. Reuther et al. (45) also reported that some therapeutic value was achieved by a 2-hour period of warm ischemia, leading to a decrease in the amount of mucus production from the FJA. There are two situations in which ischemic tolerance may be an issue and warrant the consideration of instituting hypothermia during the ischemic period. Walkinshaw et al. (57) reported a lesser tolerance to ischemia for distal jejunal segments compared with those harvested from the region close to the ligament of Treitz. When prior abdominal surgery limits the selection of jejunum to this region, then the surgeon should be concerned about the length of the ischemic period. The other circumstance in which improving ischemic tolerance should be entertained is during salvage procedures for a failing FJA. Under conditions in which the exact length of secondary bowel ischemia cannot be determined, it may be helpful to use a perfusate and hypothermia to enhance the chances for successful salvage.

As noted previously, the circulation to the FJA should not be interrupted until the head and neck defect is prepared and the recipient vessels are isolated and examined under the microscope. Insetting of the FJA should be performed before the microvascular anastomoses for a variety of reasons. The length and geometry of the vascular pedicle can be more precisely gauged when the enteric anastomoses have been completed, thereby establishing the exact position of the FJA (55). The enteric anastomoses, in particular that of the esophagus to the jejunum, may be technically difficult to perform, especially when the proximal esophageal stump is low in the thoracic inlet. This anastomosis is made even more difficult when performed on a revascularized bowel because of the bleeding end, the postischemic engorgement, and the limited mobility of the FJA for fear of disrupting the microvascular anastomoses. As noted previously, the size mismatch between the jejunum and the pharynx, following laryngopharyngoesophagectomy, often requires opening of the antimesenteric border of the FJA. The FJA should be inset in an isoperistaltic direction when it is used as a tubular conduit. In addition, it is important to have the FJA under a slight amount of stretch during insetting of the ischemic bowel to account for the elongation that occurs after revascularization and to avoid the problem of a redundant conduit.

The use of an enteric stapling device to perform the jejunoesophageal anastomosis was mentioned earlier. This technique is reserved for those specific cases in which the circumferential sutures cannot be placed or are placed only with difficulty and compromised precision. Schusterman et al. (53) reported a 33% incidence of stenosis for stapled anastomoses compared with a 17% incidence for anastomoses that were sewn. Green and Som (17) cautioned against the use of a running suture, which led to a higher incidence of stenosis in their experience. The use of the stapler for the proximal pharyngojejunal repair is rarely feasible because of the mismatch in luminal size. Following inset of the FJA and completion of the revascularization, any redundant mesentery should be used to cover the enteric anastomoses if it does not lead to a distortion of the vascular pedicle.

After the reconstruction is completed, the wounds are closed and drained with either passive or suction drains. Decompression of the bowel is usually performed with a nasogastric tube. Enteric feedings may be effectively carried out with a jejunostomy tube. Because of the postoperative ileus that usually results from FJA harvest and jejunojejunostomy repair, feedings are usually withheld until the third or fourth day after surgery.

POSTOPERATIVE MANAGEMENT

Aside from the routine postoperative care following a major head and neck procedure, the problem of monitoring the circulation to the FJA must be addressed. Different techniques have been proposed. However, few satisfy the criteria for the ideal monitor, which include (a) continuous, (b) rapid determination of either arterial or venous compromise, (c) noninvasive, (d) reliable, (e) objective, and (f) easy to perform (56). Some authors have reported monitoring the circulation with implantable devices, such as probes for Doppler sonography, which register the flow of blood across the anastomoses. Temperature probes have also been used to monitor changes in the temperature recorded from the intraluminal mucosal surface (53). The problem with all implantable devices is that any changes that occur raise the question of whether the circulation has changed or the probe has become dislodged.

Direct graft observation can easily be performed when the defect extends into the oral cavity or oropharynx where the color, bleeding to needle stick, and peristalsis to manual stimulation can be observed. The problem arises when the FJA is not accessible unless a laryngoscope or a fiberoptic nasopharyngoscope is passed (52,54). Both of these techniques are problematic because of limited exposure, patient discomfort, and the fact that they are not continuous and must be performed by experienced personnel.

The most reliable method of FJA monitoring is to observe a portion of the flap directly. This was initially done by exteriorizing a portion of the serosal surface through a "window" in the skin that was either covered with Silastic or a skin graft (24). The most direct method, however, was introduced by Katsaros et al. (29) in 1985. They described exteriorizing a small segment of jejunum that was completely isolated from the "primary" segment of jejunum, except for its vascular connections to the main vascular pedicle through a common mesentery. We adopted this technique and found it to be effective. To avoid potential soilage of the neck, the two ends of the jejunal segment are stapled, and then the serosa is sutured to the opening in the neck skin through which it is passed. A small opening into this blind loop must be created to allow an egress for the enteric secretions. An ostomy bag may be placed around the monitor to help prevent a wound infection. The exteriorized jejunum can be excised under local anesthesia and the mesentery ligated 5 to 7 days after surgery (Figure 20-3).

A barium swallow is usually performed 7 to 12 days after surgery, depending on whether prior radiation therapy was administered to the neck. The jejunostomy tube can be removed when the patient's oral nutrition is satisfactory. In those patients who are to undergo postoperative adjuvant radiotherapy, we routinely leave the feeding tube in place until after that treatment is completed.

It is well established that postoperative adjuvant radiotherapy can be administered without a significant risk of complications. Several studies have demonstrated that doses of 6,000 cGy produce few, if any, adverse sequelae (5,15,54). McCaffrey and Fisher (33) reported an increased incidence of graft failure in a small number of FJAs placed into previously irradiated defects. However, the group of patients that were reconstructed with FJAs and treated with postoperative radiotherapy had an equal incidence of complications compared with a similar group of FJA recipients who were not treated with radiotherapy. Mustoe et al. (39) confirmed the tolerance of FJAs to radiation in a dog model. Despite a submucosal inflammatory response and flattening of jejunal folds, they did not find an increased incidence of mucosal slough or stricture formation. Gullane et al. (19) described a functional benefit derived from postoperative radiotherapy, which resulted from decreased mucus production and decreased intrinsic motility. The latter finding was believed to produce improved deglutition by producing a more passive conduit.

POTENTIAL PITFALLS

The outcome of FJA transfers to the head and neck depends in part on the defect to which they are applied. Most series report experience with FJAs used for circumferential pharyngoesophageal defects. Early outcome measures for this type of defect include the success of flap transfer, avoidance of salivary fistulas, and avoidance of stricture formation. The long-term measures of success include the functional parameters of swallowing and speech.

Transfer of a FJA is a relatively safe and reliable method of reconstruction. Shangold et al. (50) compiled a review of 633 reported cases in the literature in which there was a 4.4% incidence of perioperative death. Successful FJA transfer was reported to occur in 91.1% of cases. Fistulas occurred in approximately 18% of cases in which FJAs were used to reconstruct the pharyngoesophagus. In those patients who devel-

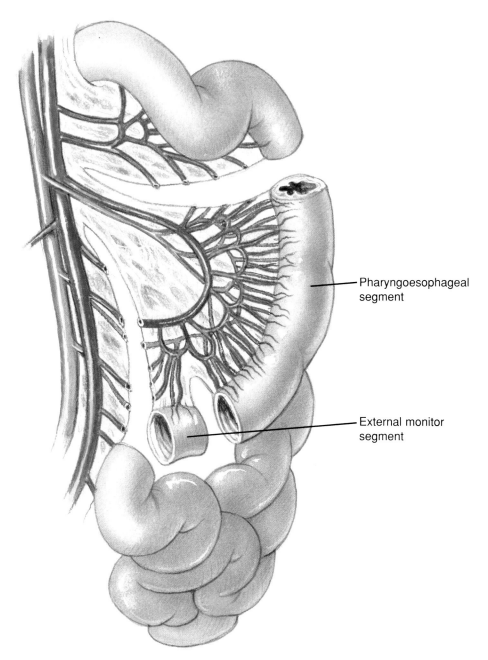

Figure 20-3. A small segment of jejunum can be transferred with the FJA to serve as a monitor of the circulation. The vascular supply to the monitor is derived from the primary mesenteric vessels that supply the main portion of the jejunum used in the reconstruction.

oped salivary fistulas, most had these defects at the proximal anastomosis between the jejunum and pharynx. In two thirds of cases, the fistulas resolved without additional surgery.

The most important functional parameter following the reestablishment of continuity between the pharynx and the esophagus is the resumption of oral intake. Swallowing can be assessed on many different levels, of which the most basic is the ability of the patient to satisfy all nutritional requirements by oral intake to maintain normal body weight. However, swallowing may be more critically assessed based on the type of food that the patient is able to eat and also the time that it takes for the completion of an average meal. Both of these latter factors may have a significant impact on a patient's ability or willingness to eat meals with family members and to dine in public restaurants.

More detailed data were not available in most published articles on FJAs. However, in the review by Shangold et al. (50), 81.8% of 402 patients were able to maintain their nutrition entirely by oral intake. Most series reported some degree of dysphagia in all patients in whom the reconstruction was done with a FJA. However, it is important to recognize that the extent of the defect in a pharyngoesophageal reconstruction may vary considerably. Patients who have also lost portions of their tongues would be expected to experience greater swallowing problems, regardless of the method used to restore the pharyngoesophageal segment (48).

The actual function of the FJA during the act of swallowing is somewhat controversial. Although some investigators maintain that the FJA plays a role in propelling a food bolus into the esophagus by coordinated peristalsis, there is considerable evidence to the contrary (27,40,46). Manometric and electrical tests demonstrated a variable amount of contractile activity in the FJA but did not show that the contractions occurred in a coordinated fashion (30,46). Nakamura et al. (41) stated that the motility of a FJA diminishes over time. The diminution in peristaltic activity leading to the development of a more passive conduit may help to explain why swallowing tends to improve with time following FJA reconstruction. In an attempt to eliminate the factor of early FJA contraction, Harashina et al. (20) described a technique whereby a FJA was harvested at a length that was twice the size of the defect. The FJA was opened on its antimesenteric border and then sutured to itself to achieve twice the diameter of the fabricated gullet. This not only doubled the lumen but also disrupted the muscular ring of the FJA. Swallowing was thought to be improved by using this technique.

The reports on alaryngeal speech rehabilitation in patients who have undergone FJA reconstructions are limited. This may be a reflection of the difficulties that these patients encounter in the restoration of this function. Bafitis et al. (1), however, reported that all six patients in their series were able to achieve a voice using a duckbill prosthesis placed through a tracheojejunal shunt. There are additional reports of patients with FJA reconstructions who were able to gain functional neoesophageal speech (50).

There is a range of abdominal complications that have been reported following the harvest of a segment of jejunum. They were reported to occur with a frequency of 5.8%. The most common reported abdominal complications were abdominal wound dehiscence, bowel obstruction, gastrointestinal hemorrhage, G-tube leakage, and prolonged ileus (50).

The FJA is unique among all the free flaps used in head and neck reconstruction because of its serosal surface, which is believed to be the reason why the FJA does not undergo neovascularization and remains dependent on its vascular pedicle. Late graft necrosis, occurring up to 18 months after surgery, has been reported as a result of transsection of the vascular pedicle (47,54).

Various other potential problems have been reported. Redundancy of the pharyngoesophageal reconstruction has been described, which is caused by an underestimation of the true length of the FJA when inset in its ischemic state (11). Unlike the rugae of the gastric mucosa, which disappear over time, the plicae circularis of the jejunum tend to persist. These mucosal folds often trap food particles and lead to halitosis (37).

The transfer of FJAs is a highly reliable and safe method of restoring defects of the upper aerodigestive tract with vascularized mucosa. However, the success of this procedure depends on the successful completion of five anastomoses: two microvascular anastomoses to restore circulation and three enteric anastomoses to restore continuity of the gullet and the small intestine. The failure of any one of these anastomoses may result in a significant complication requiring further surgery, prolonged hospitalization, and untoward long-term sequelae that may have a severe detrimental effect on the patient's function and quality of life.

REFERENCES

1. Bafitis H, Stallings JO, Ban J: A reliable method for monitoring the microvascular patency of free jejunal transfers in reconstructing the pharynx and cervical esophagus. *Plast Reconstr Surg* 1989;83: 896–898.
2. Bakamjian VY: A two-stage method for pharyngoesophageal reconstruction with a primary pectoral skin flap. *Plast Reconstr Surg* 1965;36:173.
3. Berger A, Tizian C, Hausamen J, Schulz-Coulon H, Lohlein D: Free jejunal graft for reconstruction of oral, oropharyngeal, and pharyngoesophageal defects. *J Reconstr Microsurg* 1984;1:83.
4. Biel MA, Maisel RH: Free jejunal autograft reconstruction of the pharyngoesophagus: review of a 10-year experience. *Otolaryngol Head Neck Surg* 1984;97:369.
5. Biel MA, Maisel RH: Postoperative radiation-associated changes in free jejunal autografts. *Arch Otolaryngol Head Neck Surg* 1992;118:1037.
6. Black P, Bevin G, Arnold P: One-stage palate reconstruction with a free neovascularized jejunal graft. *Plast Reconstr Surg* 1971;47:316.
7. Brain RHF: The place for jejunal transplantation in the treatment of simple strictures of the esophagus. *Ann R Coll Surg* 1967;40:100.
8. Buckspan GS, Newton ED, Franklin JD, Lynch JB: Split jejunal free-tissue transfer in oral pharyngo-esophageal reconstruction. *Plast Reconstr Surg* 1986;77:717–728.
9. Carrel A: The surgery of blood vessels, etc. *Johns Hopkins Hosp Bull* 1907;190:18.
10. Chang T, Wang W, Huang O: One-stage reconstruction of esophageal defect by free transfer of jejunum: treatment and complications. *Ann Plast Surg* 1985;51:492.
11. Coleman JJ, Searles JM Jr, Hester TR, Nahai F, Zubowicz V, McConnel FM, Jurkiewicz MJ: Ten years experience with free jejunal autograft. *Am J Surg* 1987;154:394–398.
12. Coleman JJ 3rd, Tan KC, Searles JM, Hester TR, Nahai F: Jejunal free autograft: analysis of complications and their resolution: *Plast Reconstr Surg* 1989;84:589–595.
13. Constantino P, Nuss D, Snyderman C, Johnson J, Friedman G, Narayanan K, Houston G: Experimental tracheal replacement using a revascularized jejunal autograft with an implantable macron mesh tube. *Ann Otol Rhinol Laryngol* 1992;101:807.
14. Deane LM, Gilbert DA, Schecter GL, Baker JW: Free jejunal transfer for the reconstruction of pharyngeal and cervical esophageal defects. *Ann Plast Surg* 1987;19:499.
15. Fisher SR, Cole TB, Meyers WC, Seigler HF: Pharyngoesophageal reconstruction using free jejunal interposition grafts. *Arch Otolaryngol Head Neck Surg* 1985;111:747–752.
16. Flynn MB, Acland R: Free intestinal autografts for reconstruction following pharyngolaryngoesophagectomy. *Surg Gynecol Obstet* 1979;749:858.
17. Green GE, Som ML: Free grafting and revascularization of intestine. I. Replacement of the cervical esophagus. *Surgery* 1966;60:1012.
18. Grimes OF: Surgical reconstruction of the diseased esophagus. Part I: Interposition of the jejunum. *Surgery* 1967;61:325.
19. Gullane P, Havas T, Patterson A, Todd T, Boyd B: Pharyngeal reconstruction: current controversies. *J Otolaryngol* 1987;16:169–173.
20. Harashina T, Inoue T, Andoh T, Sugimoto C, Fujino T: Reconstruction of cervical oesophagus with free double-folded intestinal graft. *Br J Plast Surg* 1985;38:483–487.
21. Harashina T, Kakegawa T, Imai T, Suguro Y: Secondary reconstruction of oesophagus with free re-vascularized ileal transfer. *Br J Plast Surg* 1981;34:17.
22. Harii K, Ebihara S, Ono I, Saito H, Terui S, Takato T: Pharyngoesophageal reconstruction using a fabricated forearm free flap. *Plast Reconstr Surg* 1985;75:463–476.
23. Hester TR, McConnel F, Nahai F, Cunningham SJ, Jurkiewicz MJ: Pharyngoesophageal stricture and fistula. *Ann Surg* 1984;199:762–769.
24. Hester TR, McConnel FM, Nahai F, Jurkiewicz MJ, Brown RG: Reconstruction of cervical esophagus, hypopharynx and oral cavity using free jejunal transfer. *Am J Surg* 1980;140:487–491.
25. Jones NF, Eadie P, Myers E: Double lumen-free jejunal transfer for reconstruction of the entire floor of mouth, pharynx, and cervical esophagus. *Br J Plast Surg* 1991;44:44.
26. Jones B, Gustavson E: Free jejunal transfer for reconstruction of the cervical oesophagus in children. A report of two cases. *Br J Plast Surg* 1983;36:162.
27. Jones R, Morgan R, Marcella K, Mills S, Kron I: Tracheal reconstruction with autogenous jejunal microsurgical transfer. *Ann Thorac Surg* 1986;41:636.
28. Jurkiewicz MJ: Vascularized intestinal graft for reconstruction of the cervical esophagus and pharynx. *Plast Reconstr Surg* 1965;36:509.
29. Katsaros J, Banis JC, Acland RD, Tan E: Monitoring free vascularized jejunum grafts. *Br J Plast Surg* 1985;38:22.
30. Kerlin P, McCafferty GJ, Robinson DW, Theile D: Function of a free jejunal "conduit" graft in the cervical esophagus. *Gastroenterology* 1986;90:1956–1963.
31. Letang E, Sanchez-Lloret J, Gimferrer J, Ramirez J, Vicens A: Experimental reconstruction of the canine trachea with a free vascularized bowel graft. *Ann Thorac Surg* 1990;49:955.
32. Lillehei RC, Goott B, Miller FA: The physiological response of the small bowel of the dog to ischemia including prolonged in-vitro preservation of the bowel with successful replacement and survival. *Ann Surg* 1959;150:543.
33. McCaffrey TV, Fisher J: Effects of radiotherapy on the outcome of pharyngeal reconstruction using free jejunal transfer. *Ann Otol Rhinol Laryngol* 1987;96:22.
34. McDonough JJ, Gluckman JL: Microvascular reconstruction of the pharyngoesophagus with free jejunal graft. *Microsurgery* 1988;9:116.
35. McGill CW, Taylor BH, Flynn MB, Acland RD, Flint LM: Effects of cooling and intraluminally

administered antiseptics on surgically induced ischemia of the intestine in dogs. *Surg Gynecol Obstet* 1979;149:377–379.

36. McKee DM, Peters CR: Reconstruction of the hypopharynx and cervical esophagus with microvascular jejunal transplant. *Clin Plast Surg* 1978;5:305.

37. McLear P, Hayden R, Muntz H, Fredrickson J: Free flap reconstruction of recalcitrant hypopharyngeal stricture. *Am J Otolaryngol* 1991;12:76.

38. Mullens JE, Pezacki EJ: Reconstruction of the cervical esophagus by revascularized autografts of intestine: an experimental study using the Inokuchi stapler and reporting the use of revascularized intestine to construct an artificial human larynx. *Int Surg* 1971;55:157.

39. Mustoe T, Fried M, Horowitz Z, Botnick LE, Strome M: Reconstruction de l'oesophage cervical par transplant libre d'anse jejunale. Etude experimentale chez la chien. *Ann Otolaryngol Chir Cevicofac (Paris)* 1986;102:227–233.

40. Meyers WC, Seigler HF, Hanks JB, Thompson WM, Postlethwart R, Jones RS, Akwai OK, Cole TB: Postoperative function of "free" jejunal transplants for replacement of the cervical esophagus. *Ann Surg* 1980;192:439–450.

41. Nakamura T, Inokuchi K, Sugimuchi K: Use of revascularized jejunum as a free graft for cervical esophagus. *Jpn J Surg* 1975;5:92.

42. Nozaki M, Huang TT, Hayashi M, Endo M, Hirayama T: Reconstruction of the pharyngoesophagus following pharyngoesophagectomy and irradiation therapy: *Plast Reconstr Surg* 1985;76:386–394.

43. Pash AR, Putnam T: Jejunal interposition for recurrent gastroesophageal reflux in children. *Am J Surg* 1985;150:248.

44. Peters CR, McKee DM, Berry BE: Pharyngoesophageal reconstruction with revascularized jejunal transplant. *Am J Surg* 1971;121:675.

45. Reuther JF, Steinaw H, Wagner R: Reconstruction of large defects in the oropharynx with a revascularized intestinal graft: an experimental and clinical report. *Plast Reconstr Surg* 1984;73:345.

46. Roberts RE, Douglas FM: Replacement of the cervical esophagus and hypopharynx by a revascularized free jejunal autograft: report of a case successfully treated. *N Engl J Med* 1961;264:342.

47. Salamoun W, Swartz WM, Johnson JT, Jones NF, Myers EN, Schramm VL Jr, Wagner RL: Free jejunal transfer for reconstruction of the laryngopharynx. *Otolaryngol Head Neck Surg* 1987;96:149–150.

48. Schecter GL, Baker JW, Gilbert DA: Functional evaluation of pharyngoesophageal reconstruction techniques. *Arch Otolaryngol Head Neck Surg* 1987;112:40.

49. Seidenberg B, Rosznak SS, Hurwittes, et al: Immediate reconstruction of the cervical esophagus by a revascularized isolated jejunal segment. *Ann Surg* 1959;149:162.

50. Shangold LM, Urken ML, Lawson W: Jejunal transplantation for pharyngoesophageal reconstruction. *Otolaryngol Clin North Am* 1991;24:1321.

51. Sheen R, Mitchell M, Macleod A, O'Brien B: Intraoral mucosal reconstruction with microvascular free jejunal autografts: an experimental study. *Br J Plast Surg* 1988;41:521.

52. Shumrick DA, Savoury LW: Recent advances in laryngopharyngoesophageal reconstruction. *Acta Otolaryngol Suppl (Stockh)* 1988;458:190.

53. Schusterman MA, Shestak K, de Vries EJ, Swartz W, Jones N, Johnson J, Myers E, Reilly J Jr: Reconstruction of the cervical esophagus: free jejunal transfer versus gastric pull-up. *Plast Reconstr Surg* 1990;85:16–21.

54. Theile DE, Robinson DW, McCafferty GJ: Pharyngolaryngectomy reconstruction by revascularized free jejunal graft. *Aust N Z J Surg* 1986;56:849.

55. Urken ML, Vickery C, Weinberg H, Buckbinder D, Biller HF: Geometry of the vascular pedicle in free tissue transfers to the head and neck. *Arch Otolaryngol Head Neck Surg* 1989;115:954–960.

56. Urken ML, Weinberg H, Vickery C, Buckbinder D, Biller HF: Free flap design in head and neck reconstruction to achieve an external segment for monitoring. *Arch Otolaryngol Head Neck Surg* 1989;115:1447–1453.

57. Walkinshaw M, Downey D, Gottlieb JR: Ischemic injury to enteric free flaps: an experimental study in the dog. *Plast Reconstr Surg* 1988;81:939.

58. Wang ID, Sun YE, Chen Y: Free jejunal grafts for reconstruction of the pharynx and cervical esophagus. *Ann Otol Rhinol Laryngol* 1986;95:348.

59. Wiillskin L: Ueber antethorakale Oesophago-jejunostomie und Operationen nach gleichem Prinzipo. *Dtsch Med Wochenschr* 1904;31:734.

60. Wookey H: Surgical treatment of carcinoma of the pharynx and upper esophagus. *Surg Gynecol Obstet* 1942;75:499.

61. Zeismann M, Boyd B, Manktelow R, Rosen I: Speaking jejunum after laryngopharyngectomy with neoglottic and neopharyngeal reconstruction. *Am J Surg* 1989;158:321.

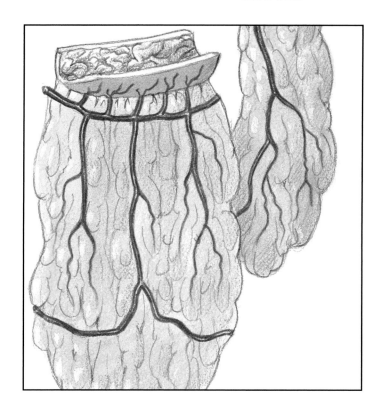

Free Omentum and Gastro-Omentum

Mark L. Urken, M.D. and
Mack L. Cheney, M.D.

The function of the omentum in the abdomen has captured the imagination of physicians and philosophers for centuries. Morison (23) referred to the greater omentum as the "abdominal policeman." Wilkie (37) reported other early opinions as to the function of the omentum, noting that Aristotle ascribed a protective role in preventing cold from reaching the viscera. He also reported that Verhagen viewed the omentum as a protector of the viscera against sudden jars and friction. Hansen believed that the omentum helped to pull the stomach downward when it was full to assist the downward excursion of the diaphragm in respiration. At times, the omentum has been given an almost mystical intelligence and motility that allowed it to seek areas of injury and disease.

Many of these qualities have been refuted through animal experiments which have shown that the omentum does not possess a higher intelligence or a separate motility. It travels about the abdomen by way of intestinal peristalsis and the movement of the diaphragm. The omentum has the ability to form adhesions that help to wall off inflammatory processes and toxic substances within the abdomen. The omentum is also endowed with a rich vascular and lymphatic network that allows it to absorb large quantities of fluid (30).

Buncke (5) is credited with being the first to investigate the potential transfer of the greater omentum in an experimental setting. McLean and Buncke (20) were the first to use the greater omentum as a free flap clinically when they reconstructed a large scalp defect with omentum which was covered with a skin graft. This was soon followed by a report by Harii and Ohmori (15) in 1973 where the greater omentum was used in two cases. They successfully transferred the omental flap to resurface the scalp in one patient and the forehead in another. In addition, these authors reported the use of the gastroepiploic pedicle as recipient vessels to supply a free flap used for chest wall reconstruction. Kiricuta and Goldstein (19) described other uses of the omentum in reconstructive surgery.

For many years, the stomach has been viewed as a reservoir of mucosa to reconstruct the upper alimentary tract. A variety of different procedures, including the gastric pull up and the reversed gastric tube, have been used in certain situations to reconstruct the thoracic and cervical esophagus (17,39). In 1959, Siedenberg et al. (32) reported the first successful transfer of tissue from a distant site to the head and neck in humans, using microvascular techniques. They used a segment of jejunum to reconstruct the pharyngoesophagus following laryngopharyngectomy. In 1961, Heibert and Cummings (16) reported the first successful transfer of a segment of the gastric antrum to reconstruct the cervical esophagus and pharynx. They described the microvascular aspect of this procedure as "Lilliputian surgery" and relegated the technique to those situations in which a gastric pull-up or colon interposition could not be performed.

Interest in the stomach as a potential donor site waned in the 1960s and 1970s, in large part due to the enthusiasm of surgeons and researchers for the experimental and clinical work using free jejunal transfers. Renewed interest in the use of the free gastric mucosal flap began with the experimental work of Papachristou's group. In 1977, these investigators described the use of a pedicled gastric island flap that was based on the left gastroepiploic vessels, which was passed through a subcutaneous tunnel along with the greater omentum to reach the head and neck (28). In a subsequent article published in 1979, Papachristou et al. (29) reported their experimental work in canines with free gastric mucosal flaps to resurface portions of the pharynx and cervical esophagus. These flaps were based on the left gastroepiploic artery and vein. Although this technique was successful in the 16 animals who were able to eat 1 week following surgery, the experience in one animal that died was instructive. In that particular case, a flap was obtained from the acid-secreting part of the stomach. The animal's demise was attributed to the development of a perforated ulcer in the esophageal wall opposite to the flap. From this experience, the authors cautioned against the harvest of antral mucosal flaps from acid-secreting portions of the stomach.

The first successful transfer of a composite flap of greater omentum and stomach was reported by Baudet (3) in 1979. This flap was used for the secondary closure of a pharyngostome. The right gastroepiploic pedicle was selected along with a more proximal portion of the greater curvature of the stomach for the harvest of the mucosa. This provided a vascular pedicle that was 30 cm in length and allowed the microvascular anastomoses to be performed to the subscapular artery and vein in the axilla. The greater omentum was draped over the anterior neck and then covered with a split-thickness skin graft. The patient resumed an oral diet on the 17th day after surgery. In addition, pH measurements of 5 were obtained from the reconstructed region.

The gastro-omental free flap was subsequently popularized by Panje et al. (25) in 1987 when they reported its successful transfer in five of seven patients with defects of the oral cavity and pharynx. The right gastroepiploic vessels were used as the vascular pedicle, and the authors described the successful application of a stapling device for flap harvest and simultaneous closure of the stomach. The authors delineated the attributes of the gastric mucosa, which are that it is nonhair-bearing tissue, pliable, and readily fashioned to restore complex three-dimensional defects of the upper aerodigestive tract. The smooth mucosal surface of the stomach was considered to be a better replacement for the digestive tract than was skin or jejunum, both of which tend to trap food. The persistence of circular folds of the jejunum are less desirable than the rugae of the stomach that tend to flatten within a few days after transfer. As with free jejunal grafts, the early excessive mucus production of the gastric mucosa may be problematic. The quantity of mucus usually subsides over time but is sufficient to provide relief of xerostomia in the postradiation patient. Panje et al. (25) also noted the use of the greater omentum to provide coverage of the carotid artery, soft tissue augmentation, and a bed for a split-thickness skin graft. They reported a 50% atrophy in the volume of the omental flap during the first 6 months. The extensive lymphatic channels within the omentum provided grounds for speculation that it might be advantageous in reducing facial edema following radical neck dissection and in forming an immunologic barrier to the spread of cancer.

Moran et al. (22) investigated a number of questions related to the gastro-omental flap in an animal model in which a patch of gastric mucosa was transferred to the floor of mouth and the omentum was placed in the neck following lymphadenectomy. A pH probe recorded measurements in the range of 6.4 to 6.9 from the oral secretions up to 5 months following surgery. The histologic evaluation of the gastric mucosa revealed atrophy and fibrosis, which may partially explain the diminished acid secretions. In addition, interstitial lymphoscintigraphy was performed following injection of technetium-99m antimony sulfide colloid into the gastric mucosal flap. The post-injection images showed uptake in two to three nodes in the omentum, which was interpreted as preliminary evidence that the omentum may provide drainage to help decrease edema and possible oncologic benefits through immunosurveillance.

FLAP DESIGN AND UTILIZATION

The greater omentum is a double layer of peritoneum that hangs like a sheet from its major attachments to the greater curvature of the stomach and the transverse colon (Figure 21-1). The blood supply to this structure arises from the right and left gastroepiploic vessels, which run in the cephalad edge of the omentum where it attaches to the stomach. Numerous epiploic branches are given off from these primary vessels, which descend toward the free edge of the greater omentum. The interconnecting arcade of vessels within the omentum permits dividing and lengthening the omental apron while still maintaining its viability (1,7). The omentum has been used as a pedicled flap in a variety of different reconstructive tasks, ranging from the head and neck and thorax to the perineum (11–13,19).

There is a considerable variation in the length and width of the greater omentum found in the virgin abdomen. In an extensive study of 200 cadavers and 100 laparotomies, Das (7) reported a rough correlation between the size of the omentum and the patient's height and weight. However, he warned that the ability to predict the length and width of the omentum in any individual situation based on these parameters is limited. Prior abdominal surgery or peritonitis causes significant scarring and contraction of the omentum, which usually makes it unsuitable for use in reconstructive procedures.

The application of the greater omentum to a variety of different reconstructive problems is a direct outgrowth of our understanding of its range of function within the abdomen. In 1911, Rubin (30) dispelled the belief that the omentum was capable of independent motility, chemotaxis, and intelligence, which assist in its protective functions. Rubin also refuted the ability of the omentum to repair visceral perforations spontaneously or to restore vascularity to nonviable tissues. Attributes of this unusual organ that continue to be upheld are its ability to form adhesions to tissues that are ischemic, inflamed, or contaminated so that they become excluded from the remainder of the abdomen. It achieves this through fibroblast and capillary ingrowth. Although unable to revascularize and restore viability to necrotic tissue, the omentum is capable of surrounding and encapsulating such tissues. The omentum also appears to have the ability to promote hemostasis when applied to raw surfaces through the activation of prothrombin and the conversion of fibrinogen to fibrin. Although unable to restore vitality to nonvital tissues, the omentum appears to be able to provide neovascularization to ischemic tissues through capillary ingrowth. Yonekawa and Yasargil (38) investigated the ability of the omentum to revascularize

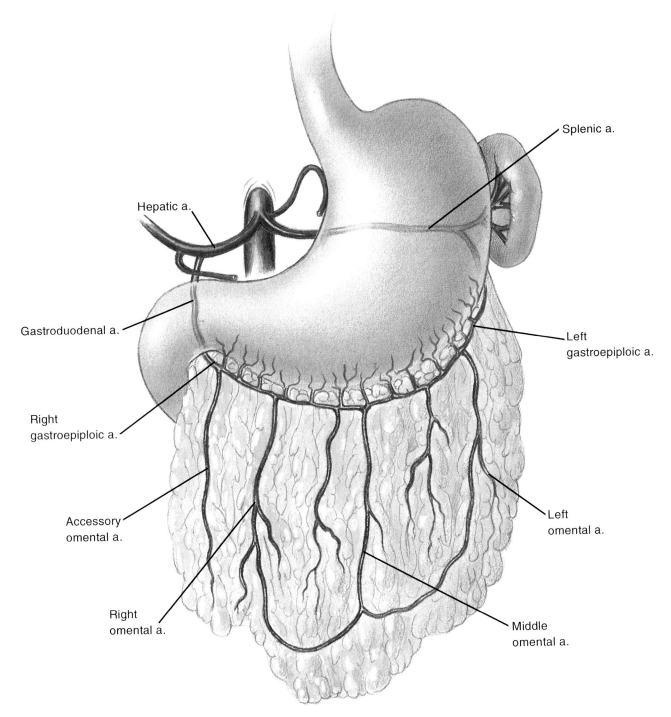

Figure 21-1. The blood supply to the greater curvature of the stomach and to the greater omentum is derived from the right and left gastroepiploic artery and vein. Both of these vessels most commonly arise from the celiac axis. The four major omental arteries are shown, but the patterns of branching and anastomoses within the omentum are variable.

an ischemic brain when applied to its denuded surface. Through animal studies, these authors found that the ingrowth of vessels after the removal of the arachnoid layer provided protection against cerebral infarction when the middle cerebral artery was ligated. Vineberg (35) reported his experience with using omentum to revascularize the ischemic heart. His technique entailed removal of the epicardium and revascularization of the myocardium by implantation of the internal mammary artery into the myocardium of the left ventricle. In addition, a free nonvascularized omental graft was placed over the myocardium to serve as a conduit for the ingrowth of mediastinal vessels. Vineberg's study was purported to demonstrate that the omentum was a critical avenue for vessel ingrowth and the prevention of extensive myocardial infarction.

The final quality that has been attributed to the omentum is the absorption of fluid through its extensive lymphatic channels. The omentum reportedly absorbs one third of the fluid that is removed from the peritoneal cavity. This absorptive function and rich lymphatic network led to speculation that the omentum may be valuable in relieving chronic lymphedema of the extremities. Harii (14) reported no reduction in swelling when omental transfers were applied clinically to this problem. There has been continued speculation about the potential role of the omentum in relieving facial edema following radical neck dissection (25).

The omentum has been used for protection in a variety of surgical procedures, such as to wrap a prosthetic vascular graft following radical resection of an inguinal tumor (11). Goldsmith et al. (13) transferred pedicled omentum through an opening in the diaphragm to reinforce an anastomotic suture line in the thoracic esophagus. Goldsmith and Beattie (12) also described a technique of transferring omentum through a subcutaneous tunnel to protect the carotid artery against salivary contamination or exposure following the breakdown of cervical skin flaps. As an extension of this technique, Freeman et al. (10) reported favorable results of using omentum to protect the carotid artery following a gastric pull-up or colon interposition for the reconstruction of pharyngolaryngoesophagectomy defects.

Since the initial publication of McLean and Buncke (20) on the use of omentum to cover a large scalp defect, there have been a number of additional reports describing the use of omentum for the same purpose (15,18). Brown et al. (4) reported their experience in reconstructing an extensive midface defect by using a free omental flap to cover a nonvascularized framework composed of split rib grafts. Panje et al. (27) expanded the range of defects in the head and neck that were reconstructed with an omental free flap. These defects included a stomal recurrence and osteoradionecrosis of the mandible and maxilla.

The greater omentum has been used in treating osteomyelitis of the extremities and the head and neck (2). Sanger et al. (31) reported a case of chronic osteomyelitis of the skull that was successfully treated by aggressive débridement followed by coverage with a vascularized omental transfer and long-term antibiotics. The authors favored the omentum to achieve coverage because of its pliability, its predictable vascularity, and its ability to provide increased vascularity to the bone for improved antibiotic delivery. Moran and Panje (21) reported the use of free omentum to achieve coverage following sequestrectomy of the mandible affected by osteoradionecrosis. The rich vascularity of the omentum and its pliability, allow it to conform to the spaces of resected tissues. These two important attributes were cited by the authors to explain the application of this technique to this clinical problem.

The final application of the free omental flap in head and neck reconstruction is to augment soft tissue defects to restore facial contour. Wallace et al. (36) were the first to describe the use of this flap to treat hemifacial microsomia. They noted that the omentum is well suited for this problem because of the ability to compartmentalize the flap and the natural feel that omentum creates in the augmented side of the face. Upton et al. (33) reported on a more extensive series using omental free flaps to correct the facial deformity of hemifacial atrophy and microsomia. Emphasis was placed on creating three subcutaneous pockets and compartmentalizing the omen-

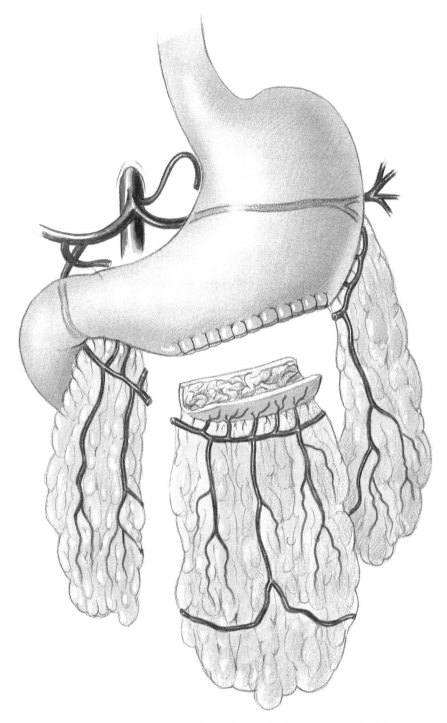

Figure 21-2. A gastro-omental flap has been harvested, and the defect in the stomach has been closed. This can be effectively performed with a stapling device. The right gastroepiploic artery is a more favorable choice for supplying this flap. It is imperative not to harvest gastric mucosa in the vicinity of the pylorus to avoid causing a gastric outlet obstruction. A longer pedicle may be achieved by more proximal dissection and by harvesting the mucosal flap at a greater distance from the pylorus. A portion of or the entire greater omentum may be harvested.

tum in these pockets to avoid migration caused by gravity. In addition, the three segments of omentum were sutured to the fascial layer in the temporal and midface regions.

Das et al. (8) studied the long-term effects of using nonvascularized omental grafts to achieve soft tissue augmentation. In a rabbit model, it was found that the peripheral zones of the omentum survived through neovascularization but the central zones underwent necrosis, which was proportional to the size of the graft. Three months after surgery, some of the larger flaps weighed only 37% of their original weight. However, with longer periods, the weight of the omental grafts increased in proportion to the increase in the body weight of the animal.

As noted previously, Hiebert and Cummings (16) performed the first successful gastric mucosal free flap in the early 1960s. They used a segment of gastric mucosa that was shaped into a tube for replacement of a circumferential defect of the pharyngoesophagus. The rich vascularity of the stomach permits a large segment of mucosa to be transferred to complete the reconstruction of virtually any mucosal defect in the head and neck. Baudet (3) described the transfer of a composite gastro-omental free flap (Figure 21-2). The omentum may be used for virtually all the indications outlined previously. In addition, a piece of the omentum may be exteriorized in a suture line to serve as a monitor of the vascularity of the entire flap (34). Calteux et al. (6) described the use of the gastro-omental flap to reconstruct the oral cavity following total glossectomy. The omentum was wrapped around the mandible and also placed beneath the mucosal graft to provide bulk. These authors reported that a segment of mucosa, measuring 15 × 10 cm, may be harvested from the greater curvature and body of the stomach. Six weeks after surgery, acid secretion from the transplanted gastric mucosa was measured after pentagastrin stimulation and found to be 25 times less than in the normal stomach. The pH of the oral secretions was 7. They reported no intraoral or esophageal ulceration. Panje and Moran (26) reported that the secretions from gastric mucosal grafts were alkaline and attributed this to the histologic finding of progressive atrophy of the gastric glands. An added factor determining the nature of the secretions from the transplanted gastric mucosa is the fact that it is also denervated and no longer under vagal control. Following truncal vagotomy, there is an average 85% reduction in basal acid secretion and a 50% reduction in maximal acid output. The denervated parietal cell has a markedly reduced sensitivity to circulating gastrin, which is probably also true of the parietal cells in the transplanted mucosa.

There are two major factors that determine the position along the greater curvature for mucosal harvest. The first is concern for narrowing the region near the pylorus, which could lead to gastric outlet obstruction. The second consideration is related to the length of the vascular pedicle. Increased lengths of the right gastroepiploic artery and vein can be obtained by harvesting mucosa from the more proximal portion of the greater curvature.

NEUROVASCULAR ANATOMY

The stomach has a rich vascular supply making it possible to perform such procedures as the gastric pull-up. The dominant blood supply to the greater curvature is derived from the right and left gastroepiploic artery and vein. Both of these arteries are terminal branches of the celiac axis. The right gastroepiploic artery arises from the gastroduodenal artery, which is a branch of the common hepatic artery. There is considerable variability in the branching pattern of the celiac axis with the gastroduodenal artery arising from a variety of different sources, including the superior mesenteric artery or directly from the aorta. The anterior and posterior superior pancreaticoduodenal arteries are usually given off prior to the point at which the right gastroepiploic artery assumes a course along the greater curvature. The left gastroepiploic artery is a branch of the splenic artery that arises at a variable distance proximal to the hilum of the spleen (Figure 21-1). Both arterial systems give rise to a series of corporeal branches that supply the stomach. The right and left gastroepiploic systems anastomose with each other to a variable extent and on a variety of different anatomic levels. These anastomoses occur along the greater curvature, in the submucosal layer of the stomach through the gastric branches, and in the omentum by the epiploic branches (9).

The right gastroepiploic artery is usually dominant when compared with the left in terms of its size and the distance that it courses along the greater curvature. The diameter of the right gastroepiploic artery ranges from 1.5 to 3.0 mm; the left gastroepiploic artery has a diameter of 1.2 to 2.9 mm. The pattern of branching of the main omental arteries is variable. However, there are usually right, left, and middle omental arteries with an accessory omental artery arising proximally from the right gastroepiploic artery (Figure 21-1). The branching pattern of the omental vessels has been divided into five different types. The presence of these patterns in a given patient is important from a surgical perspective if there is a need to lengthen or divide the greater omentum (1,33).

POTENTIAL PITFALLS

Microvascular surgery has greatly expanded the available donor sites and the range of tissue from which to choose for the reconstruction of a given defect in the head and neck. The desirability of restoring mucosal defects of the upper aerodigestive tract with mucosal flaps from the gastrointestinal tract is self-evident. However, the necessity for a laparotomy should not be taken lightly. The surgeon must ask the critical question of whether the tissue that is to be harvested from the abdominal cavity offers a distinct functional or aesthetic advantage that justifies the risks of the abdominal procedure.

A wide range of intra-abdominal complications may occur following gastro-omental flap harvest including gastric leak with peritonitis and intra-abdominal abscess formation. Upton et al. (33) advised the placement of sutures between the greater curvature of the stomach and the transverse colon to help avoid the formation of a volvulus. Gastric outlet obstruction is another potential problem that may occur if the mucosal flap is too large and harvested too close to the pylorus. A careful history and physical examination should be obtained preoperatively to avoid doing a laparotomy in patients who have had prior abdominal surgery or infection. A history of gastric outlet obstruction or peptic ulcer disease is a contraindication to using a gastroomental flap.

Excess mucus production should be anticipated during the postoperative period, and protection of the airway is essential. The extent to which the volume of the transferred omentum will diminish is somewhat controversial. Ohtsuka and Shioya (24) reported no loss of volume following an extended follow-up. However, Panje and Moran (26) noted omental atrophy in the range of 20% to 50% within the first 3 months.

REFERENCES

1. Alday E, Goldsmith H. Surgical technique for omental lengthening based on arterial anatomy. *Surg Gynecol Obstet* 1971;135:103–107.
2. Azuma H, Kondo T, Mikami M, Harii K. Treatment of chronic osteomyelitis by transplantation of autogenous omentum with microvascular anastomosis. *Acta Orthop Scand* 1976;47:271.
3. Baudet J. Reconstruction of the pharyngeal wall by free transfer of the greater omentum and stomach. *Int J Microsurg* 1979;1:53.
4. Brown R, Nahai F, Silverton J. The omentum in facial reconstruction. *Br J Plast Surg* 1978;31:58–62.
5. Buncke HJ. Early experimental omental transplantation by microvascular anastomosis. In: *Transactions of the Sixth International Congress of Plastic and Reconstructive Surgery.* Paris: Masson; 1976:58.

6. Calteux N, Hamoir M, van den Eeckhaut J, Vanioijck R. Reconstruction of the floor of the mouth after total glossectomy by free transfer of a gastro-omental flap. *Head Neck* 1988;10:512–516.
7. Das S. The size of the human omentum and methods of lengthening it for transplantation. *Br J Plast Surg* 1976;29;170–174.
8. Das S, Cragun J, Wheeler E, Goshgarian G, Miller T. Free grafting of the omentum for soft tissue augmentation: a preliminary study. *Plast Reconstr Surg* 1981;68:556–560.
9. El-Eishi H, Ayoub S, Abd-el-Khalek, M. The arterial supply of the human stomach. *Acta Anat* 1973;86:565–580.
10. Freeman J, Brondbo K, Osborne M, Noyek A, Shaw H, Rubin A, Chapnik J. Greater omentum used for carotid cover after pharyngolaryngoesophagectomy and gastric "pull-up" or colonic "swing." *Arch Otolaryngol Head Neck Surg* 1982;108:685–687.
11. Goldsmith H, Beattie E. Protection of vascular prostheses following radical inguinal excisions. *Surg Clin North Am* 1969;49:413–419.
12. Goldsmith H, Beattie E. Carotid artery protection by pedicled omental wrapping. *Surg Gynecol Obstet* 1970;130:57–60.
13. Goldsmith H, Kiely A, Randall H. Protection of intrathoracic esophageal anastomoses by omentum. *Surgery* 1968;63:464–466.
14. Harii K. Clinical application of free omental transfer. *Clin Plast Surg* 1978;5:273–281.
15. Harii K, Ohmori S. Use of the gastroepiploic vessels as recipient or donor vessels in the free transfer of composite flaps by microvascular anastomoses. *Plast Reconstr Surg* 1973;52:541–548.
16. Hiebert CA, Cummings GO Jr. Successful replacement of the cervical esophagus by transplantation and revascularization of a free graft of gastric antrum. *Ann Surg* 1961;154:103–106.
17. Heimlich H. Use of a gastric tube to replace esophagus as performed by Dr. Dan Gauriliu of Bucharest. *Surgery* 1957;42:693–699.
18. Ikuta Y. Autotransplant of omentum to cover large denudation of the scalp. *Plast Reconstr Surg* 1975;55:490–493.
19. Kiricuta I, Goldstein A. The repair of extensive vesicovaginal fistulas with pedicled omentum: a review of 27 cases. *J Urol* 1972;108:724–727.
20. McLean D, Buncke H. Autotransplant of omentum to a large scalp defect, with microsurgical revascularization. *Plast Reconstr Surg* 1972;49:268–274.
21. Moran W, Panje W. The free greater omental flap for treatment of mandibular osteoradionecrosis. *Arch Otolaryngol Head Neck Surg* 1987;13:425–427.
22. Moran W, Soriano A, Little A, Montag A, Ryan J, Panje W. Free gastro-omental flap for head and neck reconstruction: assessment in an animal model. *Am J Otolaryngol* 1989;10:55.
23. Morison R. Functions of the omentum. *BMJ* 1906;1:3.
24. Ohtsuka H, Shioya N. The fate of free omental transfers. *Br J Plast Surg* 1985;38:478–482.
25. Panje WR, Little AG, Moran WJ, Ferguson M, Scher N. Immediate free gastro-omental flap reconstruction of the mouth and throat. *Ann Otol Rhinol Laryngol* 1987;95:15–21.
26. Panje W, Moran W. Gastric mucosal and omental grafts. In: Baker S, ed. *Microsurgical Reconstruction of the Head and Neck*. New York: Churchill Livingstone; 1989:261.
27. Panje W, Pitcock J, Vargish T. Free omental flap reconstruction of complicated head and neck wounds. *Otolaryngol Head Neck Surg* 1989;100:588–593.
28. Papachristou DN, Fortner J. Experimental use of a gastric flap on an omental pedicle to close defects in the trachea, pharynx or cervical esophagus. *Plast Reconstr Surg* 1977;59:382–385.
29. Papachristou DN, Trichillis E, Forner JG. Experimental use of free gastric flaps for the repair of pharyngoesophageal defects. *Plast Reconstr Surg* 1979;64:336–339.
30. Rubin IC. The functions of the great omentum. A pathological and experimental study. *Surg Gynecol Obstet* 1911;12:117–131.
31. Sanger J, Maiman D, Matloub H, Benzel E, Gingrass R. Management of chronic osteomyelitis of the skull using vascularized omental transfer. *Surg Neurol* 1982;18:267–270.
32. Seidenberg B, Rosenak S, Hurwitt E, Som M. Immediate reconstruction of the cervical esophagus by a revascularized isolated jejunal segment. *Ann Surg* 1959;149:162.
33. Upton J, Mulliken J, Hicks P, Murray J. Restoration of facial contour using free vascularized omental transfer. *Plast Reconstr Surg* 1980;66:560.
34. Urken ML, Weinberg H, Vickery C, Buchbinder D, Biller HF. Free flap design in head and neck reconstruction to achieve an external monitoring segment. *Arch Otolaryngol Head Neck Surg* 1989;115:1447.
35. Vineberg A. Revascularization of the right and left coronary arterial systems: internal mammary artery implantation, epicardiectomy, and free omental graft operation. *Am J Cardiol* 1967;19:344–353.
36. Wallace J, Schneider W, Brown R, Nahai F. Reconstruction of hemifacial atrophy with a free flap of omentum. *Br J Plast Surg* 1979;32:15–18.
37. Wilkie D. Some functions and surgical uses of the omentum. *BMJ* 1911;2:1103.
38. Yonekawa Y, Yasargil M. Brain vascularization by transplanted omentum: a possible treatment of cerebral ischemia. *Neurosurgery* 1977;1:256–259.
39. Yudin S. The surgical construction of 80 cases of artificial esophagus. *Surg Gynecol Obstet* 1944;78:561–583.

22

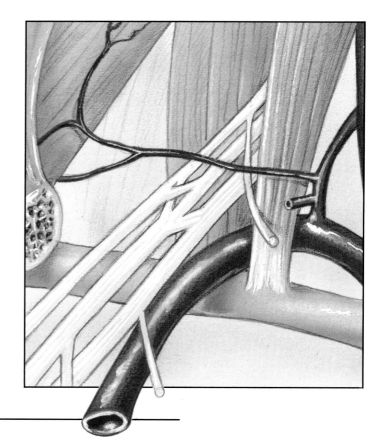

Recipient Vessel Selection in Free Tissue Transfer to the Head and Neck

Mark L. Urken, M.D.

The success of free tissue transfers to the head and neck depends on many factors. On the most basic level, the territory of tissue that is harvested must be supplied by the donor artery and vein. The design and/or the dimensions of a flap may exceed such territory, leading to areas of regional ischemia within an otherwise well-vascularized flap.

The delivery of blood into and out of the flap depends on meticulous harvesting of the nutrient pedicle, careful preparation of the recipient artery and vein in the head and neck, and technically perfect microvascular anastomoses. Careful attention must also be paid to the geometry of the vascular pedicle to prevent tension and/or kinking caused by the mobility of the head and neck (8). In this respect, free flap transfers to the head and neck differ markedly from the free flaps used in extremity reconstruction in which immobilization is readily achieved. In addition, it is absolutely essential to prevent infection in the region of the microvascular pedicle, which is far less tolerant than a regional flap of exposure to a bacterial insult. Meticulous technique must be utilized in the insetting process to help avoid a salivary fistula (9). The orientation of a flap is also important to ensure that the most well-vascularized portion of the tissue is used to complete a watertight seal of the gullet. Careful attention to proper drainage of the neck helps to ensure that accumulated blood or chyle does not lead to secondary infection. Finally, in heavily irradiated wounds, in which the problem of poor wound healing places the patient at greater risk for the formation of salivary fistulas, additional measures may be helpful. We routinely create a control pharyngostome in patients who undergo carotid artery replacement in which the pharynx is violated. In such patients, the most important life-threatening problem is protection of the bypass graft from salivary contamination. Likewise, the microvascular pedicle should also be protected in a similar fashion when there is a high likelihood of a salivary fistula. In selected patients, we advocate coverage of the pedicle by well-vascularized tissue, which may include the transfer of an additional segment of healthy tissue to cover the nutrient pedicle in the neck. This may involve the incorporation of a segment of the latissimus dorsi muscle with a scapular free flap. On occasion, we have used the pectoralis major muscle for coverage in the neck. We described a modification of the radial forearm flap that includes a segment of fascia and subcutaneous tissue to protect the microvascular pedicle in the event of a salivary leak (7).

GENERAL CONSIDERATIONS

Recipient vessel selection is one of the most critical steps in ensuring a successful outcome in microvascular surgery of the head and neck. The plethora of vessels in this region provides a wide array of choices. However, atherosclerosis or prior radiation or surgery may greatly diminish those options. Careful intraoperative selection of the recipient vessels greatly facilitates the process of revascularization and reduces the period of ischemia.

It is my practice to select and isolate the recipient vessels prior to flap harvest. When possible, I try to have multiple arteries and veins from which to choose. I also routinely do a second venous anastomosis for insurance when an additional donor vein is available. In virtually all situations, I complete the majority of flap insetting prior to beginning the anastomoses. This is vitally important for a number of reasons as follows: (a) the insetting of the flap into defects of the pharynx and oral cavity must be accomplished with maximum exposure, which may be limited when the surgeon is concerned about disruption of the completed anastomoses; (b) the insetting is also facilitated by working with an ischemic flap, which frees the surgeon from the troublesome bleeding and engorgement that occur after revascularization; and (c) the position of the donor vessels becomes fixed after insetting, which eliminates the guesswork of setting the tension on the vascular pedicle.

Despite the meticulous planning, it is often difficult to be completely certain about where the donor vessels will lie after insetting. The availability of multiple recipient arteries and veins leaves open many options to allow for variations in the positions of donor vessels. The preparation of recipient vessels prior to flap harvest affords the surgeon the freedom and the confidence to spend the time during the ischemic period to inset the flap in a meticulous fashion.

There are a variety of factors, aside from availability, that must be considered when selecting the recipient vessels. The location of the defect has a great impact on the decision-making process. Reconstruction of the skull base is much different from reconstruction of the oral cavity, with regard to recipient vessel proximity. The position of the segmental defect in the mandible also has an impact on recipient vessel selection. Reconstruction of the angle of the mandible in a patient with a high-riding carotid bifurcation may make it impossible to perform a technically perfect microvascular anastomosis to a branch of the external carotid artery. This is not the case when the segmental defect is limited to the region anterior to the midbody.

The particular flap that is selected has intrinsic restrictions in regard to the caliber and length of the donor vessels. Although insufficient length of the donor vessels is the more common problem, the surgeon may be limited in how much the donor vessels can be shortened to achieve a more favorable geometry. This is particularly true in a flap such as the iliac crest, in which the venae comitantes are often unsuitable for anastomosis until they have joined to produce a vein of sufficient caliber. The presence of a prior ipsilateral radical neck dissection severely limits the availability of recipient vessels. Advanced age and prior radiation therapy may lead to atherosclerosis, which also limits their availability. Finally, direct tumor extension from the primary tumor or a regional metastasis may also limit the surgeon's options.

An axiom of microvascular surgery is that the best microsurgical technique can be applied when the surgeon is comfortable and has maximum visualization of the microscopic field. In free tissue transfers of the head and neck, this factor should be taken into account when selecting recipient vessels. The head position must also be accounted for prior to trimming the donor and recipient vessels. Ablative procedures in the head and neck are frequently performed with the neck extended by placing a roll of towels under the shoulders. Performing the microvascular anastomoses with the neck in the extended position often exaggerates the distance between the recipient defect and the recipient vessels. In most situations, particularly when the vein is running in the long access of the neck, we advocate removal of the shoulder roll to achieve a more normal postoperative relationship.

RECIPIENT ARTERY SELECTION

The two major sources of recipient arteries in the neck are the branches of the external carotid artery and the branches of the thyrocervical trunk. Because of their availability and proximity to most head and neck defects, the lower branches of the external carotid artery are often most suitable. The superior thyroid artery, owing to its more caudal position, is usually the most accessible branch. The superior thyroid artery must be dissected to its takeoff from the carotid to permit adequate mobilization. The caliber of this vessel is usually suitable for several centimeters until it bifurcates. When cephalad branches are inaccessible and the superior thyroid artery is a poor size match, then end-to-side anastomosis to the external carotid artery can be used. It is imperative that the arteriotomy is performed at least 2 to 3 cm cephalad to the carotid bifurcation to help reduce the risk of temporary occlusion and the potential morbidity should hemorrhage from the anastomosis occur. The availability of the external carotid artery or its branches may be limited by age, radiation-induced atherosclerosis and by direct tumor invasion by the primary or a nodal metastasis. The concern for using radiated recipient vessels in the neck is more of historical interest as an issue that delayed the use of free flaps in previously irradiated patients. In my experience, this factor does not have a significant impact on the success of free flap transfers. Mulholland et al. (5) compared the success rate of free flap transfers in irradiated patients to that in nonirradiated patients. The failure rate of 3.5% in the irradiated group was not significantly different from the 2.9% reported in the nonirradiated group. They found that only two factors had an impact on free flap failure: postoperative infection in the recipient bed and the length of time between radiation and the free flap surgery. Both the reason for and the significance of the latter finding are unclear.

The branches of the thyrocervical trunk, and in particular, the transverse cervical artery (TCA), can usually be preserved following neck dissection and, in many ways, serve as a better recipient artery. The TCA can be traced for a significant distance along its course underneath the trapezius muscle. The caliber of the lumen usually remains adequate for microvascular anastomosis, despite giving off branches in the posterior triangle. Distal ligation and transsection of this vessel allows it to be transposed to a position in the midportion of the neck where it can be readily used as a recipient artery. In our experience, this vessel is far less prone to atherosclerosis than are branches of the external carotid, but it is more susceptible to vasospasm. In addition, when performing microsurgery in the previously irradiated patient, the TCA is usually outside the area of the most intense radiation. The positioning of the end of this artery in the midportion of the neck permits a comfortable microsurgical procedure with excellent exposure. An additional benefit of using the TCA is that the full length of the donor artery can be utilized without trimming back to a smaller caliber vessel. The proximity of the external carotid artery branches to the recipient defect often forces the surgeon to trim the donor artery to prevent redundancy of the pedicle. Use of the TCA allows the full length and the greatest caliber of the donor artery to be used. Trimming of the TCA, to prevent redundancy, takes it closer to its source and, therefore, usually leads to a larger lumen.

The availability of the TCA is rarely limited because of involvement by cancer. Rather, the two most common reasons why it may not be available are ligation during a neck dissection and an anatomic variation in its course. Cadaver dissections have shown that as many as 20% of TCAs arise directly from the subclavian artery and may run a circuitous course through the brachial plexus, which severely limits its suitability to be transposed. If the TCA is not identified in its normal position in the inferomedial aspect of the neck, the surgeon should explore the area lateral to the brachial plexus.

RECIPIENT VEIN SELECTION

There are three primary recipient veins in the neck that should be used in most free tissue transfers. The external jugular and the transverse cervical veins can usually be saved in a radical neck dissection. The internal jugular vein serves as an excellent outflow for a free flap when preserved following modified neck dissection.

It is often tempting to use the anterior jugular veins. However, because the majority of patients undergoing free flap reconstruction will require a tracheotomy, the caudal portions of these veins are at risk. Iatrogenic injury to the anterior jugular veins while performing a tracheotomy, or the peristomal inflammation that invariably occurs, makes the anterior jugular veins a poor choice.

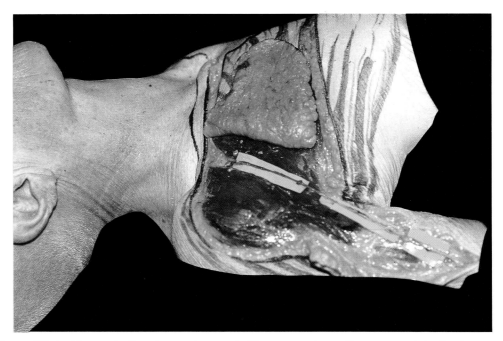

Figure 22-1. The cephalic vein may be used either as a vein graft or as a recipient vein, usually in situations in which a previous radical neck dissection has been performed. Exposure of the cephalic vein can be accomplished in a number of different ways. However, to avoid eliminating any potential reconstructive options, I routinely elevate the distal end of a deltopectoral flap. This serves not only to gain exposure, but also to delay the deltopectoral flap in the event that its use becomes necessary. The cephalic vein may be traced distally in the arm as far as necessary. The length should be measured using a free suture with the fulcrum located just inferior to the clavicle to be certain that an adequate amount of length has been obtained. It is imperative that the path of the vein into the concavity of the supraclavicular fossa be accounted for when determining a suitable length. Distal exposure of the cephalic vein may be accomplished through a linear incision or through serial transverse stair-step incisions.

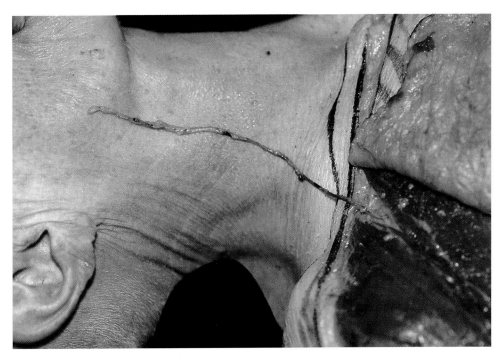

Figure 22-2. Ligation and transsection of the cephalic vein is then performed. The cephalic vein is transposed over the clavicle into position for anastomosis to the donor vein. It is essential that particular attention is paid to the turn of the cephalic vein over the clavicle. This is the most critical point at which kinking or compression may occur, leading to venous obstruction.

The cephalic veins may be used as a source for vein grafts or as recipient veins. My decision to use the cephalic vein is made only when the other options are not available and when there is a good recipient artery in the ipsilateral neck. If the recipient artery is located in the contralateral neck, then it is our preference to run the venous pedicle to that side also. We have most often used the cephalic vein in situations of flap salvage when a new recipient vein is necessary. The technique for harvesting this vein is demonstrated in Figures 22-1 and 22-2. The deltopectoral groove is exposed through elevation of the distal end of a deltopectoral flap, which serves as a delay procedure for that flap should it be needed. Particular attention must be paid to the fulcrum point of the transposed cephalic vein, which lies just below the clavicle where it enters the subclavian vein. The prevention of kinking or compression in this region is vital to the success of this procedure. On occasion, we have created a small depression in the superficial surface of the clavicle to help prevent movement and compression of the cephalic vein.

In secondary reconstructions, the paucity of recipient veins makes it tempting to consider the use of retrograde venous drainage. For example, the distal end of the superior thyroid vein may be used to provide drainage through the thyroid gland, or the distal end of the superficial temporal vein may be used to achieve drainage over the top of the scalp (5). The use of a long vein graft to the opposite neck or a transposed cephalic vein is considered a far better option than reliance on retrograde flow.

SPECIAL CONSIDERATIONS

Under certain situations, it is necessary to use interposition vein grafts to achieve a tension-free vascular pedicle that will accommodate the full range of motion of the head and neck (2). In most reconstructions, careful selection of recipient vessels, the type of free flap and the orientation of the flap during insetting help avoid the need for vein grafts.

Skull base reconstruction presents the most common situation requiring interposition vein grafts because of the distance between the defect and recipient neck vessels. In some patients, the superficial temporal artery and vein may be utilized. However, in my experience, the superficial temporal vein, in particular, is often unsuitable as a reliable recipient vessel.

Vein grafts are occasionally required in head and neck microsurgery. The potential need for them should be anticipated in "problem" reconstructions in which recipient vessels are likely to be lacking. The surgeon should anticipate the necessity for a vein graft when embarking on an emergent procedure to salvage a failing flap. Vein grafts from virtually any location can be harvested. The cephalic vein is often readily available in the surgical field. However, we have most often resorted to the greater or lesser saphenous veins. Lower extremity vein grafts can be easily harvested under tourniquet control. After harvest, the proximal end should be temporarily occluded with a microvascular clamp or a tie while a heparinized solution is perfused into the distal end. This maneuver helps to identify any side branches that require ligation. Gentle perfusion pressure also helps to dilate the vein graft so that it can be inset without underestimating its length.

There have been reports of creating arteriovenous shunts prior to flap transfer in the lower extremity to help ensure the patency of at least two anastomoses. Delayed free tissue transfer was performed several days later. When vein grafts are placed at the time of the free flap transfer, the microsurgeon has the choice of initially performing the anastomoses of the vein graft to the recipient or to the donor vessels. The arguments in favor of creating a temporary arteriovenous shunt to the recipient vessels are that it reduces the warm ischemia time and permits the proximal anastomoses to be tested (3,4,6). However, Acland (1) warned that this technique predisposes to the formation of a "high flow thrombus" at the arterial end of the graft. Alternatively, a blind vein graft loop can be created by anastomosing the vein to the flap vessels at the outset. This set of anastomoses can be comfortably performed on a side table under "laboratory-like" conditions. It is imperative that the vein loop is oriented properly to account for the directional valves. Following flap inset, the vein loop can be cut at an appropriate location for anastomoses to the recipient artery and vein.

The use of vein grafts is a necessary part of head and neck microsurgery. The anticipated requirement to perform them should not make the surgeon decide not to use a free tissue transfer. Careful planning and meticulous technique should allow the use of vein grafts without an unfavorable impact on the rate of success.

The tunneling of the vascular pedicle from the central skull base to the neck can be done through either a subcutaneous tunnel under the central cheek or through a subcutaneous tunnel created anterior to the auricle. The first approach, although more direct, is done blind and introduces uncertainty in regard to the exact orientation of the vascular pedicle in the tunnel. This may be particularly problematic when vein grafts are used and the set of anastomoses between the vein graft and the flap vessels are buried. There is no way to assess this set of anastomoses after flow has been established, following completion of the anastomoses of the vein grafts to the recipient vessels in the neck. This may be problematic if there is poor flow in the flap or if oozing from the tunnel is observed.

A preferable approach to the tunneling of the vessels is to elevate a subcutaneous cheek flap through a preauricular incision. Although a less direct course, the exposure afforded by this approach eliminates the problems outlined earlier. In either situation, the route of the vascular pedicle must be drained with a passive drainage system.

Careful attention to recipient vessel selection, pedicle geometry, and the minute details of microvascular surgery helps to eliminate some of the guesswork of this technique and to avoid some of the potential complications that may occur. Although every surgeon's skills must progress along an experience curve, adherence to the principles and suggestions outlined earlier will hasten the arrival of success rates approaching 100%.

REFERENCES

1. Acland RD: Refinements in lower extremity free flap surgery. *Clin Plast Surg* 1990;17:733–744.
2. Biemer E: Vein grafts in microvascular surgery. *Br J Plast Surg* 1977;30:197–199.
3. Gronga T, Yetman R: Temporary arteriovenous shunt prior to free myo-osseous flap transfer. *Microsurgery* 1987;8:2–4.
4. Hallock G: The interposition arteriovenous loop revisited. *J Reconstr Microsurg* 1988;4:155–159.
5. Mulholland S, Boyd J, McCabe S, Gullane P, Rotstein L, Brown D, Yoo J: Recipient vessels in head and neck microsurgery: radiation effect and vessel access. *Plast Reconstr Surg* 1993;92:628.
6. Threlfall G, Little J, Cummerie J: Free flap transfer—preliminary establishment of an arteriovenous fistula: a case report. *Aust N Z J Surg* 1982;52:182–184.
7. Urken ML, Futran N, Moscoso J, Biller HF: A modified design of the buried radial forearm free flap for use in oral cavity and pharyngeal reconstruction. Presented at the annual meeting of the American Society for Head and Neck Surgery, Los Angeles, California, April 1993. *Arch Otolaryngol Head Neck Surg* [*in press*].
8. Urken ML, Vickery C, Weinberg H, Buchbinder D, Biller HF: Geometry of the vascular pedicle in free tissue transfers to the head and neck. *Arch Otolaryngol Head Neck Surg* 1989;115:954–960.
9. Urken ML, Weinberg H, Buchbinder D, Moscoso JF, Lawson W, Catalano PJ, Biller HF: Microvascular free flaps in head and neck reconstruction: report of 200 cases and review of complications. *Arch Otolaryngol Head Neck Surg* 1994;120:633–640.

III
PART

Nerve Graft Donor Sites

Medial Antebrachial Cutaneous Nerve Graft

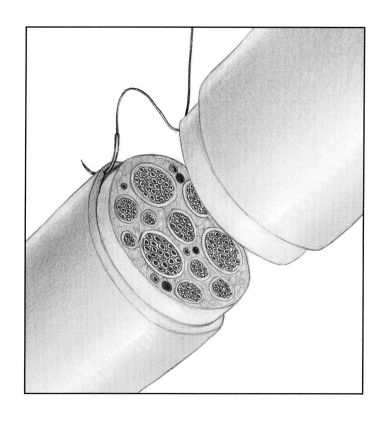

Mack L. Cheney, M.D.

During the last two decades we have gained a better understanding of the internal anatomy of peripheral nerves and the factors which influence the recovery of function. The greater understanding, coupled with advances in microsurgery, have resulted in more predictable functional results in nerve repair. The use of autogenous nerve grafts for the repair of cranial nerve defects following ablative surgery in the head and neck has become a well-recognized technique (1–5). Traditionally, the greater auricular and the sural nerves have been the primary sources of neural donor tissue. However, more recently, a branch of the median nerve, the medial antebrachial cutaneous nerve (MACN), has been introduced as an additional option for the repair of cranial and sensory nerve gaps (6–10). The sensory distribution of this nerve includes the anterior antecubital fossa and the ventral forearm (Figure 23-1). The donor site and anatomic features of the nerve offer a number of advantages for the reconstruction of peripheral nerve gaps, which may make it a useful surgical choice.

FLAP DESIGN AND UTILIZATION

The MACN offers the surgeon several advantages when faced with a branching peripheral nerve gap. The length of nerve that can be harvested ranges from 20 to 25 cm. An additional advantage of the MACN is that the cross-sectional diameter (1.5 to 2.0 mm) is consistent with the diameter of most of the cranial nerves (V, VII, X, XI, and XII), which are commonly affected in head and neck surgery. In addition, the proximal MACN, as it exits from the medial cord of the brachial plexus, is similar

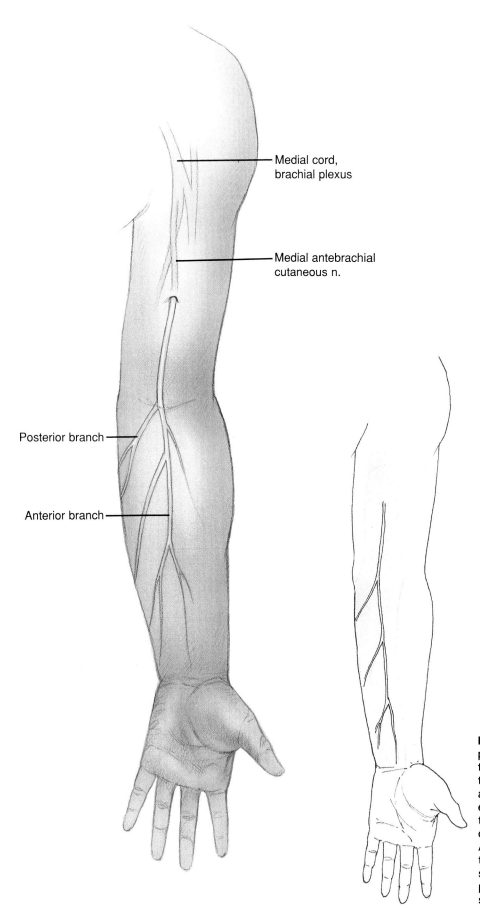

Medial cord, brachial plexus

Medial antebrachial cutaneous n.

Posterior branch

Anterior branch

Figure 23-1. The MACN arises primarily from the medial cord of the brachial plexus with contributions from the ventral rami of C-8 and the first thoracic nerve. As it enters the arm, it lies superficial to the brachial artery and runs in close proximity to the basilic vein. At the elbow, it divides into posterior and anterior branches that supply sensation to the ulnar aspect of both the flexor and extensor surfaces of the forearm.

in diameter to the facial nerve as it runs through the fallopian canal, making it useful for grafting within the temporal bone. As the nerve is traced distally, it tapers and exhibits a branching pattern, which closely resembles the peripheral arrangement of the distal facial nerve. For this reason, the nerve is well suited when a match between the main body of the facial nerve and the peripheral system is required.

In addition, the donor site has the advantage that the incision is well concealed on the medial aspect of the arm. The sensory deficit over the forearm is normally limited to a 6 × 6-cm area of the forearm and predictably diminishes in size over a 6- to 12-month period. The fact that the donor area can be accessed by a second surgical team at the time of surgical ablation expedites the procedure.

NEUROVASCULAR ANATOMY

The MACN arises from the medial cord of the brachial plexus, adjacent to the ulnar nerve, and carries fibers from the eighth cervical and first thoracic nerves (11–13). It lies medial to the axillary artery and, more distal, anterior and medial to the brachial artery. At the junction of the middle and lower thirds of the arm, it pierces the brachial fascia medially and lies in close association with the basilic vein. It is at this point that it divides into anterior and posterior (ulnar) branches (11).

The anterior branch of the MACN may pass superficial or deep to the medial cubital vein and then divides into several branches that supply the anterior medial surface of the forearm extending to the wrist. The smaller ulnar, or posterior branch, passes posteriorly to the medial epicondyle of the humerus. It then branches to supply the skin on the posterior medial aspect of the forearm.

ANATOMIC VARIATIONS

Masear et al. (7) performed 50 cadaveric dissections and found that the nerve arose from the medial cord in 78% of specimens and from the lower trunk in 22% of specimens. In 54% of the dissections, there was a common origin of the MACN and the medial brachial cutaneous nerve (T-1) from either the medial cord or the lower trunk. When this was the case, the two nerves divided an average of 6 cm distal to the common origin. Twenty-six nerves had a second medial cutaneous nerve branch from the medial antebrachial cutaneous nerve (14).

Masear et al. (7) found that the distal nerve divided into anterior and posterior branches an average of 14.5 cm proximal to the medial humeral epicondyle. The branches traveled together with the basilic vein until the posterior branch turned in an ulnar direction. The anterior branch divided into two to five branches, usually in a zone between 6 cm proximal and 5 cm distal to the elbow. It was also noted that, in 35% of specimens, there were articulating branches to the elbow (14).

The sensory distribution of the nerve includes the skin of the distal arm, the anteromedial aspect of the antecubital fossa, the posterior olecranon, and the medial aspect of the forearm from the midline ventrally to the midline dorsally.

POTENTIAL PITFALLS

The use of the MACN graft is relatively free of morbidity; however, during the dissection process, the major concern is inadvertent injury to the median nerve in the midportion of the arm (15). This can be avoided by using the basilic vein as a landmark for the identification of the MACN. In addition to this potential problem, extensive proximal dissection of the nerve may result in brachial plexus injury.

Inadvertent vascular injury is uncommon; however, the basilic vein and the brachial artery are closely associated with the course of the MACN. Therefore, these structures must be identified and avoided during the harvest of this nerve graft.

PREOPERATIVE ASSESSMENT

The preoperative assessment of candidates for MACN transfer should include a careful inspection of the upper arm. Patients who have extensive subcutaneous tissue in this area may be less favorable candidates for the use of this donor nerve because of the difficulty in harvesting. In addition to this, the upper arm and axilla should be examined for any scars because previous surgery or trauma in this area is a relative contraindication for the use of this nerve as a donor graft. The patient should be educated preoperatively in regard to the sensory field deficit that will result from the use of this nerve graft.

POSTOPERATIVE WOUND CARE

After harvesting of the nerve graft, hemostasis is obtained with a bipolar cautery. The subcutaneous tissues are closed in two layers. The wound is not routinely drained; however, a compressive dressing is applied over the donor site and is left in place for 48 hours. Elevation of the donor arm minimizes extremity edema.

Flap Harvesting Technique

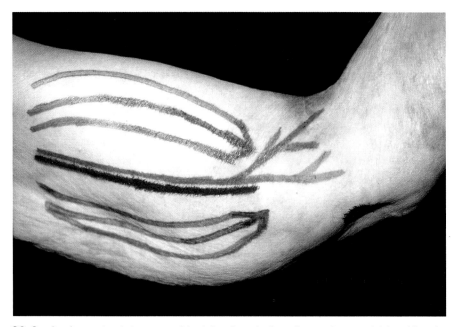

Figure 23-2. An important topographical landmark for dissection and identification of the MACN is the medial epicondyle of the humerus. In addition to this, the fascial plane separating the musculi biceps brachii and triceps brachii should be palpated and marked. The use of a proximal tourniquet helps to engorge the basilic vein, which allows it to be more easily identified. The entire upper extremity is prepared and draped with a stockinette. The donor site can be continuous with the head and neck ablative field.

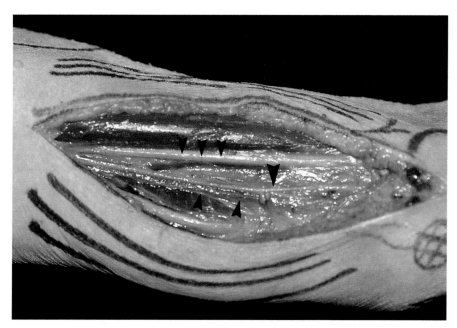

Figure 23-3. To expose the nerve completely, a longitudinal incision is made from the midarm to the midforearm, just medial to the midsagittal plane of the extremity. The dissection is begun superiorly through the subcutaneous tissue until the basilic vein (*two small arrows*) is identified. This vein pierces the brachial fascia and becomes more superficial as it descends in the arm. The nerve runs in close proximity to this vein, and after identification of the basilic vein is achieved, the MACN (*large arrow*) is easily identified and dissected. Care should be taken that this dissection is between the muscular fascia of the biceps and triceps muscles. It should be noted that the median nerve (*three small arrows*) lies just above the basilic vein and should be avoided. With the proximal nerve identified, the more distal branches can be traced until an adequate length of nerve is obtained. The anterior branch of the MACN divides into a consistent branching pattern in the area of the antecubital fossa and normally displays three to five large-caliber terminal branches. In patients with excessive subcutaneous tissue in the upper arm, the nerve and the basilic vein may be more difficult to identify. In these cases, it is important not to dissect deep to the muscular fascia as this will increase the risk of injury to the median nerve.

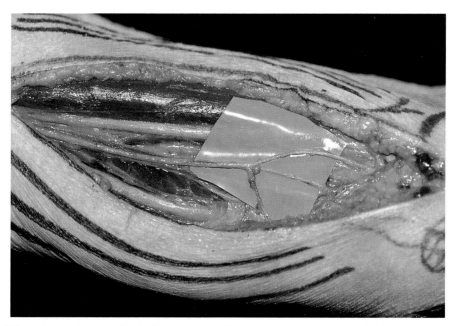

Figure 23-4. With the proximal dissection of the nerve complete, the division of the MACN is identified, and the distal branches are followed to obtain adequate length. The donor site is closed in two layers. As a rule, no drain is used, and the upper extremity is dressed with a light compressive dressing.

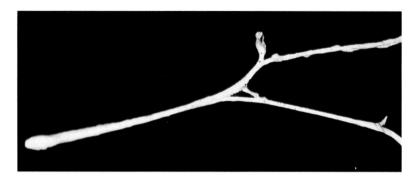

Figure 23-5. The caliber, length, and branching pattern of the MACN are consistent.

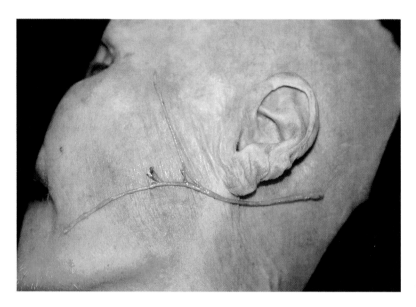

Figure 23-6. The nerve graft may be used to bridge facial nerve gaps that extend from within the temporal bone to distal sites on the face.

REFERENCES

1. Dellon AL, Mackinnon SE. Injury to the medial antebrachial cutaneous nerve during cubital tunnel surgery. J Hand Surg [Br] 1985;10b:33.
2. Izzo KL, Aravabhuni S, Jafri A, Sobel E, Demopoulos JT. Medial and lateral antebrachial cutaneous nerves: standardization of technique, reliability and age effect on healthy subjects. *Arch Phys Med Rehabil* 1985;66:592.
3. Kimura I, Ayyar DR. Sensory nerve conduction study in the medial antebrachial cutaneous nerve. *Tohoku J Exp Med* 1984;142:461.
4. Louie G, Mackinnon SE, Dellon AL, Patterson GA, Hunter DA. Medial antebrachial cutaneous–lateral femoral cutaneous neurotization in restoration of sensation to pressure-bearing areas in a paraplegic: a four year follow-up. *Ann Plast Surg* 1987;19:572.
5. Mackinnon SE, Dellon AL. *Surgery of the Peripheral Nerve.* New York: Thieme; 1988.
6. Mackinnon SE, Dellon AL, Patterson GA, Gruss JS. Medial antebrachial cutaneous–lateral femoral cutaneous neurotization to provide sensation to pressure-bearing areas in paraplegic patients. *Ann Plast Surg* 1985;14:541.
7. Masear VR, Meyer RD, Pichora DR. Surgical anatomy of the medial antebrachial cutaneous nerve. *J Hand Surg* 1989;14a:267.
8. Millesi H. Interfascicular nerve repair and secondary repair with nerve grafts. In: Jewett DL, McCarroll HR, eds. *Nerve Regeneration and Repair: Its Clinical and Experimental Basis.* St. Louis: CV Mosby; 1980:299.
9. Millesi H. Microsurgery of peripheral nerves. *Hand* 1973;5:157.
10. Millesi H. Nerve grafting. *Clin Plast Surg* 1984;11:105.
11. Millesi H. Technique of peripheral nerve repair. In: Tubiana R, ed. *The Hand.* vol. 3. Philadelphia: WB Saunders; 1988:557.
12. Nunley JA, Ugino MR, Goldner RD, Regan N, Urbaniak JR. Use of the anterior branch of the cutaneous nerve as a graft for the repair of defects of the digital nerve. *J Bone Joint Surg* [Am] 1989;71A:563.
13. Race CM, Saldana MJ. Anatomic course of the medial cutaneous nerves of the arm. *J Hand Surg* 1991;16a:48.
14. Sunderland S. *Nerves and Nerve Injuries.* 2nd ed. Edinburgh: Churchill Livingstone; 1978.
15. Woodworth RT. *Essentials of Human Anatomy.* 6th ed. Oxford, UK: Oxford University Press; 1978.

Sural Nerve Graft

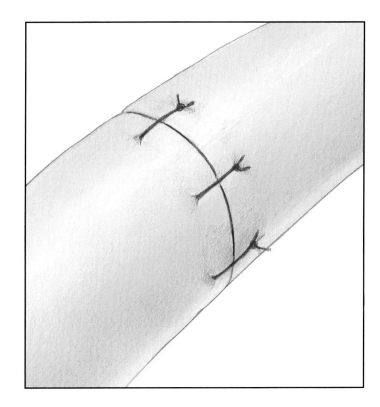

Mack L. Cheney, M.D.

The sural nerve is a commonly used donor nerve for the management of a variety of peripheral nerve repairs (1–5,9,12). It has a number of advantages that contribute to its utility, including the fact that it is a good diameter match for cranial nerve repair and that it has sufficient length (40 cm) for use in bridging extensive nerve gaps. In addition, the neurological deficit that results from the harvest of this cutaneous sensory nerve normally causes little morbidity. The nerve is relatively easy to harvest, making it possible for two surgical teams to work simultaneously at the donor and recipient sites, thereby expediting the surgical procedure.

FLAP DESIGN AND UTILIZATION

Two basic methods for harvesting the sural nerve have been described (6,11). Both the use of multiple transverse incisions and one longitudinal incision along the course of the nerve from the lateral malleolus to the popliteal fossa have been advocated. In addition, nerve and tendon strippers have been used to isolate and harvest the nerve from the lower leg. When using a nerve stripper, the sural nerve is identified through a small incision posterior to the lateral malleolus and is dissected proximally with the stripping instrument (7). Proximal division can be accomplished by placing gentle longitudinal traction on the graft and then utilizing the cutting edge of the instrument to sever the nerve. This technique is only appropriate when a simple nonbranching nerve graft is required because peripheral branches of the sural nerve cannot be preserved when using this instrument. A more direct approach to the nerve is achieved through a longitudinal incision starting behind the lateral malleolus and extending up the leg to a point where adequate nerve length is obtained. After sufficient length and an adequate branching pattern of the nerve have been identified, it is removed from its bed. Neuroma formation at the distal end of the transsected nerve is a potential complication after the harvest of the sural nerve. To prevent this, the distal end of the nerve should be placed within the body of the gastrocnemius muscle and stabilized with a suture (8).

The sural nerve is most commonly used in the head and neck to restore facial animation when there is a disruption of the facial nerve. Cross facial nerve grafts are often used in a two-stage procedure to achieve reanimation in long-standing cases of facial paralysis. The sural nerve is usually inset in a reversed orientation so that the distal end from the lower leg is sutured to the proximal branch of the nonparalyzed side of the face. The rationale for orienting the nerve in this fashion is that regenerating axons will not be lost through side branches as would occur if the nerve graft were placed in an antegrade fashion. By using a Tinel sign, the progress of nerve growth can be monitored. At the appropriate time, usually up to 1 year after the initial surgery, a free muscle flap is transferred to the face and reneurotized to the end of the cross facial sural nerve graft.

In addition to its usefulness as a conventional nonvascularized nerve graft, it may also be harvested as a vascularized graft (2–5). The vascular supply to the nerve may be based on a variety of sources, including an arterialized short saphenous vein, a cutaneous branch of the peroneal artery, or the muscular branch of the posterior tibial artery. A number of studies suggest that the use of vascularized nerve grafts when placed in poor recipient beds may lead to improved functional recovery after peripheral nerve repair (1,2,5,8).

NEUROVASCULAR ANATOMY

The sural nerve is formed by the union of the medial sural cutaneous nerve and a single communicating fascicle of the lateral sural cutaneous branch of the peroneal nerve (2,3). The dominant contributor, the medial sural cutaneous nerve, arises from the tibial nerve in the popliteal fossa between the superior heads of the gastrocnemius muscle. The nerve runs deep to the muscular fascia for a variable distance down the posterior calf and then pierces this fascia to lie in close association but deep to the short saphenous vein at the lateral malleolus. The nerve and vein run in a lateral compartment between the lateral malleolus and the tendon of the calcaneus. At this point, the nerve divides into several branches that pass around the malleolus distally and supply the skin of the posterior and lateral aspect of the ankle and the lateral surface of the foot (7). The nerve is devoid of major branches until it divides into two dependable branches on the lateral aspect of the foot. As the nerve courses proximally over the lateral head of the gastrocnemius muscle, it can be traced in a superficial plane over the muscular fascia if additional nerve graft length is required.

ANATOMIC VARIATIONS

Ortiguela et al. (10) described the course of the sural nerve from the distal thigh to the ankle in 20 lower limbs. The branches forming the sural nerve were identified and measured for length and caliber. In all limbs, both a medial sural cutaneous nerve and sural nerve were present. A lateral sural cutaneous nerve was identified in 19 of 20 limbs. In 16 of 20 limbs, a peroneal communicating branch from the lateral sural cutaneous nerve contributed to the sural nerve. In 80% of cases, the sural nerve was formed by a union of the medial sural cutaneous nerve and the peroneal communicating branch. In the other 20% of cases, the sural nerve originated from the medial sural cutaneous nerve only. In 94% of cases, the peroneal communicating branch

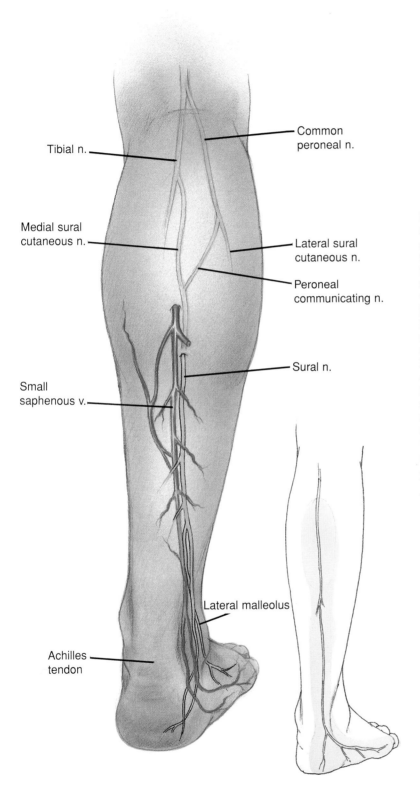

Tibial n.

Common peroneal n.

Medial sural cutaneous n.

Lateral sural cutaneous n.

Peroneal communicating n.

Sural n.

Small saphenous v.

Lateral malleolus

Achilles tendon

Figure 24-1. The sural nerve supplies sensation to the lateral surface of the lower leg and to the lateral and dorsal aspects of the foot. The sural nerve is most commonly formed by the union of two branches: the medial sural cutaneous nerve and a branch from the lateral sural cutaneous nerve, which is referred to as the peroneal communicating branch. The junction of the peroneal communicating branch with the medial sural cutaneous nerve is variable and may occur at any location in the calf. The medial sural cutaneous nerve is a branch of the tibial nerve and is the major contributor to the sural nerve in most cases. The medial sural cutaneous nerve and the proximal portion of the sural nerve run deep to the deep fascia of the calf between the two heads of the gastrocnemius muscle. In its distal course in the calf, it lies in a superficial plane over the muscular fascia. The point at which the sural nerve pierces the fascia is variable, but it is usually located in the midcalf. The sural nerve supplies sensory branches to the skin of the lower lateral calf, the lateral aspect of the calcaneus, and then the dorsal and lateral surfaces of the foot. It terminates as the lateral dorsal cutaneous nerve of the foot, which also supplies the lateral aspect of the little toe.

originated from the lateral sural cutaneous nerve. In addition, they also noted that the peroneal communicating branch was larger in caliber than the medial sural cutaneous nerve and, when present, was a useful source of nerve graft material.

POTENTIAL PITFALLS

Painful neuromas, although described in the literature, have been uncommon when the distal stump of the nerve is managed as described. The disadvantage of this nerve graft site is that the incision must be placed over the lower aspect of the leg. This makes it less desirable in female patients because the resulting scar tends to widen and is difficult to conceal.

PREOPERATIVE ASSESSMENT

Careful inspection of the cutaneous surface of the leg must be performed in the preoperative period prior to harvest of a sural nerve graft. Any evidence of ischemic changes in the skin should be noted prior to surgery. Patients who exhibit ischemic compromise of the leg are poor candidates for the harvesting of this nerve graft.

In addition, any evidence of previous lower extremity surgery that may have resulted in scarring or compromise of the general condition of the nerve should be noted and an alternative donor site selected.

POSTOPERATIVE WOUND CARE

The wound is not routinely drained but is wrapped with a gentle compressive dressing. Low-dose heparin administration may be indicated in patients who have an increased risk of deep venous thrombosis, and early ambulation is encouraged in all patients. In diabetic patients, early evidence of cellulitis is of particular importance and should be treated aggressively with intravenous antibiotic therapy.

Flap Harvesting Technique

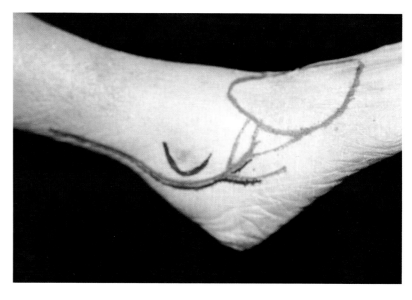

Figure 24-2. The key topographical landmark for locating the sural nerve is the lateral malleolus. The initial incision is planned posterior to this bony landmark in an attempt to identify the short saphenous vein as it courses behind the malleolus into the lateral aspect of the foot.

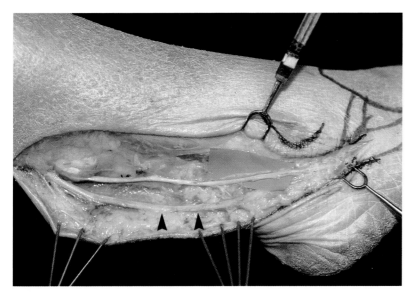

Figure 24-3. The dissection of the nerve is begun by identifying the short saphenous vein (*arrows*), which lies lateral to the nerve. The dissection is continued proximally over the lateral head of the gastrocnemius muscle to obtain an adequate length of the nerve graft. The distal dissection may be extended onto the lateral aspect of the foot where the nerve branches. This branching pattern of the nerve graft may be incorporated into the design of the repair, depending on the requirements of the nerve defect.

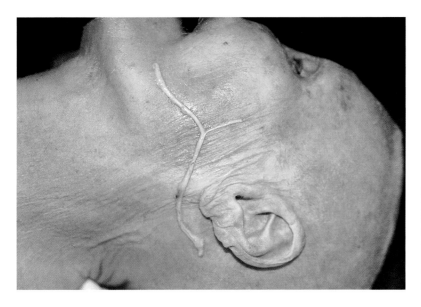

Figure 24-4. The sural nerve graft is useful in repairing long nerve gaps that extend from the temporal bone to the peripheral facial nerve. It should be noted that the sural nerve graft usually has only two primary nerve branches, limiting its use in situations in which a more complicated branching pattern must be reconstructed.

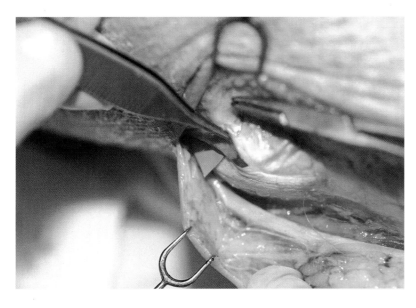

Figure 24-5. In an effort to prevent neuroma formation at the distal end of the sural nerve, the proximal sural nerve stump should be placed within the body of the gastrocnemius muscle. A slit is made in the muscular fascia, allowing placement and stabilization of the nerve stump within the body of the muscle. After a pocket has been made in the muscle, the distal end of the nerve is placed within the gastrocnemius muscle and stabilized with a permanent suture. The soft tissue of the donor site is closed in layers.

REFERENCES

1. Doi K, Kuwata N, Kawakami F, Tamaru K, Kawai S: The free vascularized sural nerve graft. *Microsurgery* 1984;5:175.
2. Doi K, Kuwata N, Sakai K, Tamaru K, Kawai S: A reliable technique of free vascularized sural nerve grafting and preliminary results of clinical applications. *J Hand Surg* 1987;12a:677.
3. Doi K, Tamaru K, Sakai K, Kuwata N, Kurafuji Y, Kawai S: A comparison of vascularized and conventional sural nerve grafts. *J Hand Surg* 1992;17a:670.
4. Gilbert A: Vascularized sural nerve graft. *Clin Plast Surg* 1984;11:73.
5. Gu YD, Wu MM, Zheng YL, Li HR, Xu YN: Arterialized venous free sural nerve grafting. *Ann Plast Surg* 1985;15:332.
6. Hankin FM, Jaeger SH, Beddings A: Autogenous sural nerve grafts: a harvesting technique. *Orthopedics* 1955;8:1160.
7. Hill HL, Vasconez LO, Jurkiewicz MJ: Method for obtaining a sural nerve graft. *Plast Reconstr Surg* 1986;1:177.
8. MacKinnon SE, Dellon AL: *Surgery of the Peripheral Nerve.* New York: Thieme; 1988.
9. May M: *The Facial Nerve.* New York: Thieme; 1986.
10. Ortiguela ME, Wood MB, Cahill DR: Anatomy of the sural nerve complex. *J Hand Surg* 1987;12a:1119.
11. Rindell K, Telaranta T: A new atraumatic and simple method of taking sural nerve grafts. *Ann Chir Gynecol* 1984;73:40.
12. Ruben LR: *The Paralyzed Face.* St. Louis: Mosby Year Book; 1991.

Subject Index

Subject Index